Diseases and Human Evolution

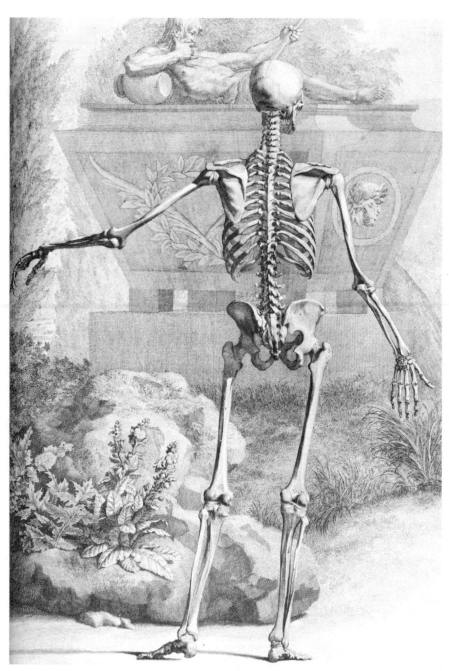

Bernard Siegfried Albinus, *Tabulae Sceleti et Musculorum Corporis Humani,* 1747, Plate 2

DISEASES
and HUMAN EVOLUTION

ETHNE BARNES

University of New Mexico Press
Albuquerque

© 2005 by the University of New Mexico Press
All rights reserved. Published 2005
First paperbound printing, 2006
Printed in the U.S.A.

11 10   2 3 4 5 6

Paperbound ISBN-13: 978-0-8263-3066-6
Paperbound ISBN-10: 0-8263-3066-5

LIBRARY OF CONGRESS CATALOGING-IN-PUBLICATION DATA

Barnes, Ethne.
Diseases and human evolution / Ethne Barnes.
p. cm.
Includes bibliographical references and index.

ISBN 0-8263-3065-7 (cloth : alk. paper)

1. Epidemiology.
2. Medical anthropology.
I. Title.
RA651.B365 2005
614.4—dc22

2005004169

Book design and type composition
by Kathleen Sparkes

Body text is Trump Mediaeval 9/14; 26P
Display type is Serlio and Frutiger Light

CONTENTS

PREFACE

We often ignore the invisible world around us, full of microbes and detritus; we go about our business unaware of our constant interaction with it. Most of the time no harm comes from this. But once in a while throughout our lifetimes, we all confront some invisible microbe or substance that challenges our immune systems to the point of causing disease. How we survive the onslaught depends on several factors—primarily, our genetic programming; the type of germ; and our health status, which includes nutrition, our age, and our own behavior.

For most of human history, geography determined what kind of microbes could attack humans. Geography restricted most microbes to specific regions of the world until humans began making the climb toward civilization with the development of agriculture and animal husbandry. Evolving commerce with its long-distance trade routes, crossing various geographic regions throughout the Old World, opened routes for many microbes to spread beyond their original areas. The pace for dispersing germs accelerated through time, particularly with European industrialization and colonization. Today we live in a global community, sharing many microbes that once remained limited to certain regions of the globe.

Human evolution can be viewed both as biological and cultural, with cultural evolution causing the most dramatic changes in human history over the past fifteen thousand years. As we have marched toward the modern world, we have affected the microbial world around us and created many of our own human diseases.

XII PREFACE

This book focuses on the changes in the patterns of human behavior through cultural evolution and how they have affected the development of human diseases. I have drawn on the work of many researchers in various scientific fields to put together a comprehensive picture of the history and major trends of human diseases. Complex details have been explained in the simplest terms for the benefit of the interested general reader and student. The purpose of this book is to provide basic knowledge to help readers understand how human behavior affects patterns of disease, so that they can better understand the diseases they themselves face.

I am grateful to my husband, Art Rohn, for his patience, editorial comments, and encouragement to research and write this book. Also, I thank Charles Williams III for supporting my research at ancient Corinth and for his constant encouragement with this project.

CHAPTER 1

INTRODUCTION

Recent interest in new diseases, such as HIV/AIDS and Ebola, and the resurgence of older diseases, such as tuberculosis, has raised important questions about the history of human infectious diseases. How did the various infectious diseases evolve? Where did they originate? What factors have hindered or facilitated diseases? How does a microorganism become a disease-causing agent (a pathogen)? Have infectious diseases changed through time? What can we do to prevent diseases from occurring and recurring?

In an attempt to answer these questions, many books and articles have been written over the years, some quite recently, from different viewpoints. Some writers have focused on the historical perspective of major diseases affecting civilization. Others have focused on the evolution of specific diseases from a medical approach. Some discuss the interaction between human behavior and the evolution of certain human diseases. This book brings together the various viewpoints in a multifaceted approach to the issues.

Human beings are unique in that we have evolved not only biologically, like all other creatures of this Earth, but also culturally. Changes in human behavior patterns with cultural evolution throughout the millennia have had the greatest impact on the evolution of human diseases. The study of human beings and their behavior through time, the province of anthropology, gives an objective perspective of how human behavior patterns and attitudes have influenced the evolution of human diseases.

The Meaning of Disease

The very word *disease* implies discomfort, or lack of "ease," within the body. Whenever the functioning of the body or any of its parts becomes impaired, disease occurs. Sometimes the impact of disease can be very minimal, while at other times it can be incapacitating and life-threatening. Most human diseases are caused by microorganisms from our environment, and human behavior patterns frequently influence how these microorganisms are spread.

Current perceptions of disease and its causes have roots in earlier belief systems; such perceptions also vary throughout the world. How people view their diseases depends upon how their culture interprets what constitutes a disease, and there are many different cultures with differing ideas about disease.

Modern Western medicine views the physical signs of disease as a biological process with a specific biological cause, while healers in other parts of the world may see the same physical signs of disease as the result of an imbalance within the body or with nature, a supernatural process, invasion by foreign substances, sorcery, or punishment for violation of rules governing human behavior (Murdock 1980). Not all human diseases are universally recognized as diseases. In areas where it is common to find the majority of the community afflicted with the same health problem for generations, people frequently accept the problem as part of their natural existence. This is common among peoples infested with parasites in underdeveloped countries, and among peoples suffering with goiters for lack of iodine in their soils, as in the highlands of Ecuador and Papua New Guinea.

The biological interpretation of disease in modern nations, developed by Western European civilization, rests on the premise of specific etiology (Dixon 1978). The European germ theory developed during the seventeenth century emphasizes specific causes for specific infectious diseases. Cure is obvious: just eliminate the causative agent by using medicines, surgery, radiation, or other intervention measures.

Modern public health measures employed to prevent disease follow the same premise of using tactics designed to attack specific germs that can invade water supplies, food sources, and living and working areas. Indeed, many infectious diseases that frequented our communities in the past have been greatly reduced or vanquished through public health measures and better standards of living. However, overzealous sanitizing of modern environments, water, and food sources can undermine natural human immune responses, leaving the seemingly protected population vulnerable to invading microbes able to sneak past the protective barriers.

The germ theory led to the antibiotic era that began in the early 1950s, dramatically reducing the threat of serious bacterial infections. Unfortunately, overuse and misuse of antibiotics in medical treatment and in animal feeds over the years has caused more harm than good, as the targeted microorganisms have figured out how to resist these drugs.

The "miracle" antibiotic drugs were never effective against viral infections; they could only be used against bacterial infections. The "miracle" drugs were oversold to the public to "prevent" secondary bacterial infections following viral infections, such as the common cold and influenza. This abuse contributed to the overuse of these drugs and their eventual ineffectiveness against life-threatening bacterial infections.

We are now experiencing a comeback from bacterial infections that once were considered defeated by antibiotics. This resurgence of bacterial infections results from their renewed vigor, gained from strains, often more deadly, that developed from antibody resistance.

Meanwhile, viral infections continue to rage unchecked among human populations, with new viruses silently making their way into our communities. Modern medicine is hard-pressed to cope effectively with viral infections. The common cold and influenza viruses continue to plague us, and the more deadly viruses, such as HIV, still challenge human control.

The massive efforts for the past decades to vaccinate whole populations of children against certain viral and bacterial infections, such as diphtheria, pertussis, tetanus, measles, chickenpox, and polio, have created new problems. Some of the targeted microbes are developing strains resistent to the vaccines, strains often more deadly than the originals.

The parasites that cause malaria have also revolted against the efforts of modern medicine by developing resistance to antimalarial drugs. Failed mosquito-control programs have added to this problem. Many of the health campaigns waged to control malaria-carrying mosquitoes have been disrupted by war and governmental neglect in many parts of the world where malaria is rampant, contributing to its resurgence.

Clearly, the theory of specific etiology, based on linear thinking as used in modern medicine, has failed to contain infectious diseases. Current public health measures may not be adequate to keep the new breeds of disease-causing microorganisms from spreading and creating new health hazards throughout the world. In addition, overpopulation of the world, with ever-increasing crowding of poor people in squalor within large cities, provides hotbeds for potential lethal epidemics.

Hippocrates, the father of modern medicine, was unaware of specific disease-causing microorganisms. He interpreted disease as an imbalance within the body and with nature. This early Greek physician, who flourished in the fifth century B.C. following his predecessors from earlier medical schools, recorded their medical knowledge for posterity. Man, as a part of nature, was susceptible to disease whenever disharmony prevailed, upsetting the balance of the essential qualities of the body. Hippocrates divided these essential qualities into four "humors," and it was the physician's job to direct treatment to restoring the balance between these humors (Sigerist 1945).

The Greeks were not the only ancient people to believe that disharmony within the body and with nature caused disease. The idea was common throughout ancient Asia. Medical writings spanning China's three-thousand-year written history focused on the cause of disease as disrupted harmony of the natural forces within the body, with treatment directed in ways to restore the natural equilibrium of these forces.

With the rise of Latin Christianity and the fall of the western Roman empire, religion began to play a key role in the concepts of disease throughout Western Europe. The medical knowledge accumulated from the ancient Greeks and passed on to the Romans became fragmented and mixed with local superstitions in this part of the world. During Western Europe's Dark Ages, disease was often linked to people's sins and the wrath of God. Meanwhile, physicians outside Western Europe, in the eastern Mediterranean region, retained the old beliefs of the early Greek physicians, following similar treatment regimes to restore the balance within the person's body (Sigerist 1945).

The Renaissance in Western Europe brought back some of the ancient Greek rational approaches to the treatment of disease as the new scientific era began to unfold the secrets of the human body and the microbial world. This laid the foundations for the development of modern medicine as we know it today. Robert Koch's discovery in 1876 of the bacteria causing anthrax led to the idea of specific etiology, or the germ theory, bringing modern science into the realm of medicine.

Today, modern Western medicine has become very technical and specialized, with an emphasis on treating body parts instead of the whole person. Somehow the thread of Hippocrates' teachings that treated the body as a whole by correcting imbalances of its constituent parts has been lost or overlooked. There is more emphasis on treating the diseased part and less emphasis on treating the person, and efforts are directed toward determining the causative agent of the disease in the affected body part and attacking it with high-tech agents.

Approaches to Understanding Disease

We can gain a better understanding of how human diseases evolved to what they are today by combining several different interpretive approaches. While anthropology provides insights into how human attitudes and behavior patterns influence the development of human diseases, we need to know more about other important factors that govern the evolution and spread of disease agents.

Medical science can tell us how a disease process takes place, how the immune system reacts to pathogens and other mishaps, and why some people are more susceptible to certain pathogens than other people are. The biological sciences provide understanding of the life cycle of microbes and parasites capable of causing disease, and of the mechanisms responsible for the spread of disease agents. The science of ecology deals with the interactions of living organisms and their environment, including human beings as well as microorganisms and other parasites that cause disease. All this information is necessary for the science of epidemiology to analyze disease patterns.

From all these approaches we learn what factors hinder or facilitate diseases, and we gain clues about how diseases evolved and about possible places of origin. To continue our search for more clues to the origin and evolution of human diseases, we need to combine these factors with an evolutionary perspective gained from historical evidence.

History provides many clues not only to diseases of the past, but also to human activities and attitudes responsible for the evolution and spread of diseases. Historical written records provide a major source of this information, but they are limited to a small portion of human history. Anthropological archaeology, besides adding to the historical information through reconstructions of past human behavior patterns and their impact on local environments, also provides important clues of human activities long before writing was invented.

Another branch of anthropology, known as paleopathology, the science of ancient disease, provides factual information from history. Paleopathologists can track through time the various diseases that leave recognizable signs on human skeletons and mummies excavated from archaeological sites. This information adds to our understanding of the evolution of human diseases and the interaction of disease with human cultural evolution.

Coming Together

As human beings have evolved to our present status within nature, so have the multitudes of microorganisms and parasites that have come into contact with us. Most of our microscopic associates create few, if any, serious threats to our bodies. Some have become important contributors to our health. Others act as microscopic predators on specific body tissues, creating disturbing situations leading to disease states that can be crippling or fatal, while some trigger over-reaction of host immune responses that can become disabling.

The vast majority of known diseases result from insults on the body created by the microorganisms we know as viruses and bacteria. Some diseases are caused by protozoa and rickettsiae. Some fungi (mycoses) also can invade the human body and cause disease. Microscopic and macroscopic worm infestations can also create disease.

The body's own response to intrusive environmental agents can create disease by overreaction to a foreign disturbance. Generally, it is the body's own immune-response mechanisms that determine the course of a disease process, regardless of underlying cause.

Sometimes disorder within the body's own physiology or structure can lead to a state of disease. Physiological disturbances can be caused by genetic upsets, nutritional imbalances, and environmental agents. Many times disease results from a combination of factors. Friendly microbes can become pathogens with changes in the host. Malnutrition often leads to lowered immune response to infection and poor tolerance of microbes and other parasites.

The human body is constantly adjusting and shifting responses to its internal and external environment in an attempt to maintain harmony within its integrated systems for a balanced state of health. Perhaps the ancient view of disease remains more accurate. Human beings, as a part of nature, constantly strive for harmony with the microbial environment around us and within us. Most of us are unaware that our bodies are engaged in this perpetual struggle to maintain our existence in a reasonably func-tional state. Dis-harmony creates dis-ease.

Germs, Genes, Geography, and Human Behavior

Many factors influence the development of human diseases. Human behavior has played the major role in the evolution and spread of diseases, and in return, some infectious diseases have had a major impact on the development of civilization. Human manipulation of the environment, beginning with early agriculture, has altered the way microbes and men have interacted for centuries. Every time we rearrange our environment, trouble begins. Our habits of daily living also affect how diseases develop. The spread of most agents of infectious diseases counts on poor hygiene habits and poor sanitation. Recent attempts to control the internal environment of our living, travel, and work spaces with closed air systems have also contributed to the maintenance and spread of many respiratory microbes.

Geography determines where diseases come from and influences what types of diseases will occur within each environment. In the past, most infectious microbes and parasites were confined to their place of origin within specific geographic regions. Human beings, sharing the same environment with these microbes for generations, adapted to them. However, changes in environment and human behavior fostered changes in local microbes. The movements of people have had the greatest impact, allowing several microbes to move out of their place of origin and adjust to new environments. Changes in local environments over the past five centuries, caused by overcrowded cities and more widespread population movements throughout the world, have greatly altered the ranges of many microbes. Today, massive population movements and rapid travel have blurred geographical boundaries that once separated different ecosystems and their resident microbes.

Human genetics adds another factor to disease. How an individual or an entire population responds to infection depends primarily on genetically inherited immune systems. Human populations adapt to the microorganisms in their immediate environment by the constant weeding out of individuals with inadequate immune responses. Microbe genetics likewise adapts to the immune responses of human populations. This constant balancing act creates a state of fluctuating equilibrium between human populations and microorganisms. Both human and microbe gene pools are polymorphic, containing a wide range of variability in their genes, equipped to adapt to changing circumstances.

CONCLUDING COMMENTS

We human beings are creatures of our environment, and we share our habitats with numerous other life forms, large and small. Changes we make in our environment affect the ways other life forms adapt to the same environment, and these changes alter the ways they interact with us. Today we human beings are on a rampage, rearranging our world to suit our peculiar desires. People are moving about the planet in ever larger numbers and traveling distances faster and farther than ever before. Our numbers are growing out of control and demanding more and more from fragile environmental resources. We blindly encroach upon areas we have avoided in the past, disturbing deadly microorganisms and unleashing them into our populations.

We continue to "stir the pot" of tiny life forms around us at an ever faster pace. We are mixing microbes from different regions that were formerly isolated from each other. Once-harmless microbes are gaining ground to select for disease-causing forms within their ranks, thanks to new environmental incentives.

Deadly viruses are being teased out of their slumbering isolation as wars, famine, and greed bring people into contact with them in greater numbers. Migrations and air travel bring people into contact with microbes that they have never encountered before.

Microbes also travel faster than ever before by hitching rides on air travelers from all over the world, finding new host and environmental challenges. Microbe evolution occurs much faster than human or animal evolution, and by stirring the pot of the microbial world, we are contributing to numerous evolutionary changes in many microorganisms.

An understanding of the history of human cultural evolution, combined with knowledge of disease drawn from a variety of disciplines, can teach us how we have arrived where we are today with our diseases and can help us to understand what to expect in the future. Perhaps we can begin to develop better ways of coping with diseases in the process of understanding how they have evolved. With this in mind, I have taken the liberty in this book to build on the knowledge gained from numerous works about diseases and human evolution by many researchers from a variety of scientific disciplines. In the following chapters, I attempt to pull together this bounty of information to trace the evolutionary history of the major diseases that have wreaked havoc on human populations in the past.

CHAPTER 2

THE WAR BETWEEN MICROBES AND MEN

The most successful human ancestor in evolutionary terms, *Homo erectus*, evolved around 1.5 million years ago, as far as we have been able to determine from the fossil record. This rugged-appearing hominid had heavy bony brow ridges, sloping forehead, large teeth, and no chin, but possessed the same basic body form we have today. *Homo erectus* was so well adapted biologically to his surroundings that he was able to survive for over one million years. Brain size gradually increased, while craniofacial and body features were eventually molded into those of the earliest *Homo sapiens*, the direct ancestors of modern human beings, about 400,000 years ago.

Homo erectus was an evolutionary success story, able to adapt to environmental changes and move into different environments throughout Asia, southern Europe, and Africa. *Homo erectus* knew how to make stone tools, and around 750,000 years ago (Stein and Rowe 1989), he learned how to make fire. The ability to make fire and keep warm during cold weather gave these early hominids the opportunity to move into the more temperate zones beyond the warmer regions of the Old World where they had evolved. These first technological advances by *Homo erectus*, the abilities to make useful tools and to control fire, set the stage for the dramatic evolutionary cultural events of later human beings—and for the evolution of human diseases.

Shifting back before human beings began their long climb up the evolutionary ladder, let us for a moment contemplate the environment of our planet when life began. Life made its first stirrings in the form of simple nucleic acids, the basic substance in all living cells, within the primordial sea. These simple nucleic acids eventually bonded together in a variety of configurations to create the first single-celled organisms.

The sequences of how the nucleic acids were bound together determined the form and function of cellular organisms and their progeny. Such genetic programming, carried within double strands of nucleic acid sequences known as *deoxyribonucleic acid (DNA)*, governs the development of all living organisms, with a few exceptions. Some viruses and viral particles manage to carry their genetic material within a single strand of nucleic acid, known as ribonucleic acid (RNA), instead of the standard two strands of DNA. The single RNA strand plays the role of genetic translator for DNA in the synthesis of protein building blocks in all other living organisms.

Once the building blocks of life were set in motion, evolution toward complex organisms began with specialization within the primordial cells. Packaging of the DNA into a nucleus and the development of specialized units, known as *organelles*, with specific functions within the cell made it possible for increasingly complex life forms to exist. The development of specialized tissues from collaborating cells led to different functioning organs within the integrated biological systems of higher life forms.

Not all life forms evolved to the same level of complexity. Many organisms remained microscopic in size and simple in form, able to adapt to the evolutionary changes taking place around them without making major biological shifts themselves. These microorganisms have become the most successful survivors since life began on Earth, having the ability to adjust to the myriad environmental changes throughout time and to survive under adverse ecological conditions today. Microbes have taken up residence all around us, and some have specialized in residing within and upon human beings. They inhabit our skin, hair, nasal and oral mucous membranes, eyes, gastrointestinal tract, and genito-urinary tract. All other life forms, both plant and animal, are similarly occupied by microbes. Some microbes have developed beneficial effects for their hosts, while others act as microscopic predators. Microorganisms have always been with us, adapting to our every evolutionary step (Dubos 1980).

Human beings have always lived in a virtual "soup" of microorganisms. The air we breathe, the food we eat, the water we drink, the ground we walk on, our pets, our homes, and our belongings are home to diverse forms of microscopic and near-microscopic life forms. Every day of our lives, without realizing it, we ingest, inhale, and come into contact with millions of microbes. The vast majority of the tiny organisms around us cause no harm as they share our environment. They are a necessary part of every ecosystem on Earth as contributing members of the life forces required to maintain order in our universe.

The microscopic world includes a variety of life forms that the human eye cannot perceive. There are strands of enclosed DNA and RNA, known as viruses; single-celled organisms known as bacteria and rickettsiae; single-celled animals known as protozoa; microscopic fungi; minute worms; and mites. Additionally, microscopic debris, pollen, scraps of matter, and chemical remnants are part of the microscopic world around us, and many people suffer from allergic responses to such foreign particles.

While much of the microbial "soup" that we live in is generally harmless—that is, does not cause disease or injury—several different kinds of microbes that have evolved along with us can cause bodily harm. These microscopic predators attack specific body tissues whenever the opportunity for invasion arises. Sometimes apparently harmless microbes known as *commensals*, living within or on us, can threaten the body when changes occur from disturbances in the body's metabolism. All microorganisms consist of populations of variants jockeying for dominance. When changes occur in their surroundings, dominance can be shifted to another, more adaptable variant that may be more harmful to the tissues. Sometimes the change promotes a variant that is less harmful to the body.

Our complex immune system has evolved to meet the numerous challenges of the diverse number of microbes within and around us to prevent harmful forms from destroying vital body tissues. Constant battles are waged between our defense system and invading microbes, with both sides locked into a struggle for control of territory and resources. This battle begins at birth (and sometimes before birth) and continues throughout life.

Our immune system cannot afford to ever let down its guard; instead, it must constantly check friendly microbes that can turn on us and become the enemy, as well as fighting off invading harmful ones, known as *pathogens.* The stresses of daily living or changes in our environment, nutrition, and behavior can alter the functioning of our immune systems, causing breakdowns in defense measures against harmful microbes and leaving us vulnerable to disease.

The Good, the Bad, and the Ugly

There are four major groups of microorganisms that cause problems for human beings. It is important to gain an understanding of how they operate as friends and foes, and how the human immune system reacts to them. A basic understanding of the interaction between microscopic agents of disease and the workings of the human immune system helps explain how infectious diseases have evolved in human populations.

Most parasitic microorganisms seek out only certain animal or plant species to be their host, and they target specific tissues within the body of the plant or animal that meet their special survival needs. Sometimes introduction into a new and different host environment triggers a change in the parasite's adaptive needs, allowing it to adjust to the new surroundings. Other times environmental changes in the host are incompatible with survival of the parasitic organism.

Bacteria

The food chain begins with bacteria, as they return vital nutrients to the Earth. Nitrogen-fixing bacteria recapture nitrogen from the air, returning it to the soil so that plants can exist, and in turn can sustain all other forms of life. Bacteria survive in all the different environments on Earth, existing primarily on dead and decaying matter in soil and water. They are the renewers of life, recycling old life for new.

Some bacteria can even attack nonliving materials such as oil (Ehrlich 1985; Postgate 1994). We could not survive without these microbes around to clean up after us and all other life forms with their constant recycling program. The numerous varieties and shapes of bacteria with different requirements have adapted to a wide range of environmental niches.

Bacteria, despite their single-celled form, are very complex biochemically, similar to the complexity of our own cells, but they can act independently in nature. They often live in colonies. Specialized enclosed areas within the cells of animals, known as *mitochondria*, may have evolved from bacteria entering into a symbiotic relationship with more advanced cells. Mitochondria have their own DNA, and they have considerable autonomy from the rest of the cell. They are primarily responsible for producing energy for the cell (Burnet and White 1972).

Some bacteria have adapted to harmless parasitic life on and within living tissues of plants and animals, feeding on the normal sheddings of dead tissue. Hundreds of different types of bacteria normally live in the human gastrointestinal tract, skin, mouth, and nasal passages, feeding on microscopic trash. Some bacteria are capable of infecting plants, insects, people, and animals to feed on metabolites of living tissue, changing their adaptive strategies according to the type of host (Wuethrich 1995).

Parasitic life is far less demanding in the procurement of food, and bacteria that have chosen this way of life have traded their ability to produce some of their own essential components needed for survival, for the same components ready-made by their host. Therefore, they cannot live away from their hosts for long, and many of them have reached a tacit agreement with their hosts to do no harm under normal conditions, while some have developed working relationships with their hosts. Human beings and animals carry in their digestive systems different types of bacteria that provide essential services to the host. The human gut depends on friendly bacteria to stimulate normal development of the mucosal lining of the intestines, to manufacture certain vitamins and amino acids, and to inhibit potentially harmful microbes from moving in and taking over (Dubos 1980).

Unfortunately, many bacteria can directly or indirectly harm the body's tissues and cause disease. Bacteria that have adapted to surviving on living tissues pose the greatest threat. Sometimes friendly bacteria living within the body's openings or on the skin surface can wreak havoc when one of their number steps out of line, or when the host environment changes and thereby causes changes in the bacterial population that can become threatening.

The bacterial cell is held together by a cytoplasmic membrane, and the majority of them can form a protective rigid cell wall or capsule that interfaces with the world outside them. The genetic material (DNA) is contained in chromosomes within a portion of the cell designated as the nuclear area. Many species of bacteria also have extrachromosomal material carrying small amounts of DNA (plasmids) outside the nuclear area, self-replicating independently of the nucleated chromosomes. Many of these independent chromosomes carry genetic resistance to antibodies and other substances, with the capability to synthesize toxins (poisons) and destructive enzymes. Some of the toxins are designed to kill competitor bacteria within the same species or related species (Mattman 1993).

Some of the extrachromosomal genes can produce threadlike strands (pili) with a hollow core that extend outside the cell. Such pili can transfer chromosomal material and its information to other bacteria (Slack and

Snyder 1978). Thus, resistance to antibiotics and chemical agents can be shared among bacteria, even crossing species.

The life cycle of bacteria is complex, as they pass through different stages of morphology according to shifts in the surrounding microenvironment (Mattman 1993). Bacteria can change forms, from the familiar, classical cell-wall-structured microorganisms that reproduce by dividing, to a variety of shapes without cell walls that elude most clinical tests. They can become threadlike, branching or wavy filaments that reproduce by budding, similar to fungi, or can become giant round cysts (L-bodies) that discharge large numbers of offspring. Sometimes large numbers of the same bacteria that have shed their cell walls will coalesce into flat sheets of growth called *syncytia*. Changing form helps bacteria adapt to alterations in their microenvironment. A human host taking antibiotics can stimulate bacteria to change form in order to evade chemical assault. Strong human immune responses can also trigger changes in bacteria trying to evade detection.

One type of bacteria, mycoplasma, manages to survive without ever forming a protective cell wall, but most other bacteria at some stage in their life cycle do form a cell wall for protection. Cell walls can be shed, and variable forms produced, to enable the bacterium to survive adverse conditions, growing and reproducing, able to revert to the parent form once conditions return to a more favorable state (Mattman 1993; Slack and Snyder 1978). These nontraditional forms are generally not identified by standard modern laboratory tests.

Bacteria have developed numerous ways to protect themselves from adverse conditions and to fight off intrusive biochemical agents in their microenvironment (Henis 1987). They have an evolutionary advantage over higher life forms because they can mutate quickly within a few generations— that is, in just a few days. Some bacteria can convert to a dormant spore form in nature when conditions become unfavorable, enabling them to survive for years under extreme conditions until their environment again becomes hospitable. The spores can resist chemical agents, high temperatures, sunlight, and cold.

Protozoa

The smallest animal life forms are the one-celled protozoa, some no larger than bacteria and others large enough to be seen with a magnifying glass.

Protozoa require moisture to survive. Over thirty thousand species live in water and moist soil, living singly or in colonies, and large numbers of them live on or within other animals and insects. Survival in nature can be tough for these minute creatures that require moisture to live. However, protozoa faced with a lack of moisture have developed the ability to form resistant dormant cysts during dry times (Bradbury 1987). Many parasitic forms utilize the cyst stage to transfer from one host to another.

Protozoa are encased in a thin elastic cell membrane, and the chromosomes containing the genetic DNA are confined within a membrane-bound nucleus, unlike bacterial chromosomes that are not bound within a nucleus. Other contents of the protozoan cell are packaged and bound by membrane into several specialized units known as *organelles*, each having a particular function (Gutteridge and Combs 1977). Most protozoa reproduce simply by dividing. Many of them move about by means of specialized cellular extensions.

Protozoa in nature feed principally on other microscopic animals, minute plant life, and bacteria, and are themselves food for small insects and animals in the food chain. They act as natural restraints on bacterial populations in nature and also contribute to soil fertility.

Certain protozoans have taken up residence in the gut of termites and the rumen of cattle, providing a necessary part of their digestion of food. Both termites and cattle depend on them to release enzymes that convert the cellulose of the plants they eat into digestible simple sugars, known as monosaccharides (Esch and Fernandez 1993). This mutual interdependency (symbiosis) between host and microbial protozoan evolved through time to benefit both parasites and hosts.

Several protozoa have adapted to parasitic life in a wide array of life forms, from earthworms and insects to animals and human beings. Many of these parasites undergo specific changes during their lifetimes as they come into contact with different microenvironments in their passage from one stage of development to another. Some also pass through a sexual stage, following a division into separate sexual forms known as gametocytes that combine to form an egg cell, the oocyst (Beck and Davies 1981). Many of them take up residence in the gut of their host and pass from one host to another through the feces of the infected host and feces-contaminated food or drink consumed by the new host. Some use an intermediate host, such as a blood-sucking insect acting as a vector, for one stage of development. The insect's bite can transmit the protozoa into the blood of an animal or human host where the parasite's life cycle continues in the blood or tissues of its new host. Sometimes more than one type of host is needed for the parasite to progress through different stages of development before the protozoa can mature into the adult form.

Several species of protozoa infect human and animal populations, especially in the moist tropical and subtropical regions of the world. Most of them cause relatively little harm, while others can cause terrible diseases in the digestive tract, blood, or tissues.

Viruses

All viruses are essentially strands of DNA or RNA, dependent on other life forms for their existence. They are found in all plant and animal life forms, including bacteria, protozoa, and fungi. Viruses can survive outside life forms, but they remain inactive and unable to replicate until they are reintroduced into an appropriate host. Viruses can be carried on wind currents in the air (Cooper and MacCallum 1984). They frequently attach themselves to organic and inorganic particles in water, especially in polluted waters (Bitton et al. 1987) where they thrive on bacteria. They can also cling to soil particles on land. Several viruses are carried about by insects.

Most viruses do no harm to the natural host life form, but many can become threatening under certain circumstances. Viruses gain entry into animal and human hosts through the skin, through the mucosal linings of the nose, mouth, throat, lungs, gut, urinary tract, bladder, and genitals, and the membrane covering the eyes (Cooper and MacCallum 1984). Some viruses can be passed from the infected host through the reproductive cells (gametes) to their offspring (Andrewes 1967). Most viruses are discharged from the infected host through body secretions and in droplets of moisture contained in the air breathed out from the host.

The viral nucleic acid (DNA or RNA) is protected by a protein coat known as the capsid, and some viruses also are surrounded by a fatty (lipid) envelope (Levine 1992). The protective coat is acquired by the new virus, known as a *virion*, as it leaves the host cell. Some viruses also carry other life-sustaining elements, such as complex proteins known as enzymes that promote certain biochemical reactions once the virus is activated (Cooper and MacCallum 1984). Each type of virus has its own distinct shape, size, chemical composition, and host requirements. Tiny RNA particles, referred to as viroids, virusoids or satellite viruses, which exist without a protective capsid, often depend on full-fledged viruses to gain entry into a host cell (Strauss and Strauss 2002). Otherwise they are not infectious.

Once a virus gains entry into its host, it attaches only to the target cells that can promote activation and reproduction, recognizing them by certain markers, known as *receptors*, on their surface. The virus enters the required target cell through one of the surface receptors and sheds its protective coating, freeing the viral nucleic acid to take over the cell for its own use in a step-by-step process. Activated viral nucleic acids begin to reproduce once they combine with the necessary amino acids of the host cell. Most viruses enter the cell's nucleus before activation. This may not occur immediately. Some viruses wait until circumstances within and around the cell change, triggering them into action. Some viruses prefer only one cell type, while other viruses use several cell types that originate from the same embryonic germ tissue. More than one type of virus can infect the same cell, and they can exchange genetic information to form a new type of virus. Many viruses release their offspring upon the death of the cell, while others release offspring from the living cell by extruding them through the cell membrane without destroying the cell (Levine 1992).

Some viruses may have evolved from the first primordial nucleic acids along with other primitive life forms, being able to make use of other beginning forms of life for survival. However, the similarity of viral nucleic acids to cellular genetic material in plants, animals, and microbes suggests that most viruses evolved from more complex life forms. This could have happened either as a gradual process of separation from primitive one-celled microorganisms, or as a result of runaway rogue nucleic acids from genetic material of more sophisticated organisms. In either case, they developed the ability to detach from their origins and evolve separately, by being able to take over the nucleic acids of the more complex cellular organisms for their own survival and reproduction (Andrewes 1967; Burnet and White 1972; Cockburn 1963; Levine 1992).

Regardless of how viruses evolved, they appear always to have been one of the determining factors for the evolution of life on our planet. Viruses that infect bacteria (phages) can carry genetic information from one bacterium to another. Viral genetic sequences from viral infections are known to have integrated into the genetic makeup of bacteria, plants, animals, and even human beings (Levine 1992; Mitchison 1993), where they may contribute directly to evolutionary change. Viruses are routinely pressured by host reactions to alter their genomes with host nucleic acids or leave parts of viral nucleic acids in the host genome (Lederberg 1993).

Evolution requires population balance between life forms. Infectious viruses act as part of nature's agents for population control within all life forms—bacteria, plants, animals, and human beings—weeding out susceptible individuals and promoting survival of the fittest (Cooper and MacCallum 1984).

Viruses adapt well to environmental changes, primarily because of the great diversity within their own ranks. Each virus type exists in several variant forms, and as certain strains can invade a host cell and become activated, other strains remain inactivated until the internal environment of the host becomes more favorable for them to become active. Viruses, particularly RNA viruses, can also mutate very quickly, and different strains existing in different animals that encounter one another within the same host can exchange genetic information between them to create a new strain, often to the detriment of the host (Blerkom 1991).

Rickettsiae

Rickettsiae resemble viruses in that they require a host cell to survive and reproduce. Morphologically and biochemically they resemble bacteria, they have some cellular structure, and they reproduce like bacteria. But this group has lost much of its independence and requires host cell biochemical actions for survival. They appear to have evolved from bacteria in blood-sucking insects—ticks, mites, and fleas. Rickettsiae primarily live in a symbiotic relationship with their insect hosts, and passage of their offspring to the next generation of insects often takes place through the reproductive cells, the gametes (Andrewes 1967; Levine 1992; Slack and Snyder 1978). The natural animal hosts of these blood-sucking insects have developed immunity and/or tolerance from long-term association with the rickettsiae introduced from the insects' blood meals.

Some rickettsiae can accidentally cause disease in susceptible animals and humans when natural hosts are not available, or when the accidental host intrudes into the natural cycling between blood-sucking insects and their natural hosts. Infected insects searching for blood meals transmit the organisms during blood feedings, either by infected feces deposited at the bite site, or by infected saliva.

The War Zone

Out of necessity for survival, all plants and animals have evolved basic, nonspecific methods for fighting off intruders into their tissues. Otherwise they could not exist as separate entities for long. The first lesson learned by all evolving life forms was how to distinguish one's own cellular material from foreign material. Any foreign material, especially proteins, had to be treated separately from one's own cellular makeup to keep out foreigners and prevent destruction of one's own cellular parts. Recognition of self was the first step toward developing a defense system against harmful intruders (Langman 1989).

By the time *Homo erectus* came on the scene, he brought with him from his prehuman ancestors a sophisticated defensive immune system developed from the simple evolutionary premise of distinguishing self from nonself. This system evolved to provide constant surveillance of the internal fluid portions of the body, probing the markers on cell surfaces to make sure they belonged to the individual and if not, alerting the body's defense mechanisms to destroy them. Evolutionary forces made sure that *Homo erectus* was well equipped to survive among the microorganisms of his time. These same forces continued to influence the development of a dynamic, complex defense system able to respond appropriately to a multitude of challenges from diverse foreign microbes encountered by *Homo erectus* on his wanderings throughout different environments. This has become our heritage: an extremely complex and adaptable immune system designed to protect us from the ever-changing microbial world around us.

The human immune system is equipped to react to virtually any microorganism with which it comes into contact. Just how the immune system reacts to foreign substances determines the disease process, and human immune systems are genetically diverse and variable in responses to microbial assault.

The complexity of the immune system is described here in very simplistic terms. There is much more to this intricate system that guards and protects our bodies from foreign invasion, much of which we still do not understand. This complexity alone could lead to chaos and damage the body's own tissues more than any pathogen could, if not for the checks and balances built into the system. Almost every immune response requires a dual code of signals before activation can occur. There is a constant feedback system between the chains of command and the effector cells, to ensure that the appropriate immune response is in action and that such action ceases when the battle is over (Langman 1989).

The physical barriers of the skin and mucous membranes lining the openings of the body constitute the first lines of the human defense system. Chemical barriers, such as the enzymes in tears that help flush out unwanted foreigners, also provide protection from invasion of microbic intruders.

Despite these defense barriers along the borders of the body's interior, some microorganisms have moved in and reside on the skin and mucous membranes of the eyes, nose, mouth, throat, gastrointestinal tract, and to a lesser extent the genito-urinary tract, living off the normal sheddings of skin and mucosa. They cause no harm and actually provide services by removing debris from these areas and in some instances by driving off hostile microorganisms. Some intestinal bacteria contribute important nutrients to our digestive system and help ward off other, harmful bacteria. Our bodies tolerate them primarily because they do not invade the body's interior and set off the internal surveillance system. However, if they happen to cause irritation of the skin or mucosa, the defense system reacts by sending inflammatory agents and special immune cells to the area to repulse the microbic irritant and repair damaged tissues.

Microbes that break through the physical and chemical barriers are immediately confronted by a network of special cells directly beneath the skin and mucosal barriers, where they act as guards or front-line soldiers. These cells belong to a group of multipurpose defensive cells, collectively known as *macrophages,* that are scattered throughout the body. Macrophages are responsible for cleaning up debris and removing foreign material from the body's tissues by ingesting them (phagocytosis). Encounter with a foreigner causes macrophage cells to present the foreign antigen to specialized lymphatic cells so they can take special actions against the invaders. The macrophages also secrete chemical messengers known as *cytokines* to sound the alarm. Release of the cytokines produces early, flulike symptoms of disease—aches, fever, headache, and malaise—as the immune system gears up for action. This is the beginning of a chain reaction of immune defensive measures with inflammation of affected tissues followed by repair and regeneration measures of damaged tissues. The entire immune response depends on the macrophages to sound the alarm and help the system identify the foreigner so that appropriate action can occur.

Some macrophages are fixed to certain areas of the body and named for their particular specialty area, while others move freely about the body through the circulatory system. Macrophage-type cells circulating in the blood are known as monocytes. Fixed macrophage type cells include von Kupffer cells in the liver, splenic macrophages residing in the spleen, microglial cells found in the central nervous system, alveolar macrophages scouring the airways of the lungs, Langerhans cells guarding skin tissue, and dendritic cells scattered around most organs and found within lymph nodes (Abbas et al. 1997).

The human immune system evolved to react to major microbial assaults with a very complex, two-pronged response system capable of detecting and destroying specific invaders. One part of this system was designed to detect free-roaming microbes within the circulatory and extra-cellular pathways of the body, while the other part evolved to detect microbes that have invaded cells of the body.

White blood cells known as *lymphocytes* act as the special forces within the immune system, while the macrophages and other phagocytic cells act as the front-line troops. Lymphocytes primarily roam the network of lymph vessels filtering the circulating blood system. The lymph vessels traverse one or more lymph nodes that house large numbers of various lymphocytes. The lymph nodes act as interrogation and holding centers for captured foreigners. Many of the invaders meet their end here. Full-scale invasion by foreign microbes triggers macrophages to transport their engulfed prisoners to the lymph nodes. Intelligence and command forces—specialized CD4 T cells—probe the captives to determine what course of action should be taken against the invasion. Orders are sent out to other special-force cells and all other cells participating in the battle.

CD4 T cells are among a group of lymphocytes that pass through the thymus gland where they are prepared for specialized actions. CD4 T cells are programmed to identify the foreign antigen presented by the macrophages and stimulate other T cells and B cells to take action. Certain CD8 T cells are programmed to call a halt to the immune reactions when the battle is over.

Lymphocytes coming directly from the bone marrow—B cells—are responsible for detecting and detaining microbes in the circulatory pathways under the authority of the CD4 T cells. The B cells are programmed to produce a group of proteins called immunoglobulins (natural antibodies) that bind with foreign antigens. This action allows macrophages and other phagocytic cells to more readily destroy the foreigners. Immunoglobulins are joined by circulating enzymes that help damage the foreigners, especially bacteria, so that they can be more easily destroyed by phagocytosis. Each B cell is programmed to produce only a certain type of immunoglobulin that reacts to a specific antigen. Once an immunoglobulin is activated by an antigen, the selected B cell mass produces the immunoglobulin specific for that particular antigen with all-out warfare against the foreign invader. One B cell can produce more than 10 million immunoglobulins in one hour, and they can make variations of the immunoglobulin (isotopes) that are capable of attacking the antigen in different ways (Nossal 1993).

The B cells must act quickly and effectively before the foreign invader has a chance to multiply and spread out of control. Time is of the essence, and it takes about five days for the appropriate immunoglobulin response to develop (Janeway 1993), while invading bacteria are reproducing every thirty to sixty minutes (Langman 1989). Once the attack is over, the B cells used in the battle retain the memory of the enemy, prepared to respond quickly if another invasion ever takes place. This is how we develop immunity toward certain pathogens.

Nature has equipped the B cell system with the ability to rearrange inherited genetic material within the immunoglobulins in countless ways (Janeway 1993; Nossal 1993). This allows the B cells to be prepared with millions of different kinds of immunoglobulin responses for any possible configuration of foreign material that may exist anywhere in the world. Evolutionary changes in pathogenic microbes can be met by this tremendous diversity of immunoglobulins. The outcome depends on how quickly and efficiently the appropriate immunoglobulin can be made, and how quickly and effectively the invading microbe can multiply and spread.

What happens if invader microbes manage to get inside tissue cells? With the first attack, immunoglobulins most often cannot be set in motion soon enough to stop cellular invasion. Once invaders penetrate the tissue cells, the B cells become ineffective because their immunoglobulins cannot cross the outer membrane of the cell. Foreigners gobbled up by and surviving in phagocytic cells cannot be reached by immunoglobulins. Hence the second arm of the immune system must take over.

Certain CD8 T killer cells respond to infected cells recognized by CD4 T cells when protein fragments (peptides) of the invader microbe are presented on the cell's surface by specific molecules designed for that purpose.

These special molecules come from areas within the cell known as the *major histocompatibility complex* (MHC). This system of identifying fragments of foreign material allows T cells to also identify microbes that change their outer surface markers to fool B cell immunoglobulins and slip into the cells. They have to shed their outer coats in the process of regenerating themselves, and loose particles of their genetic material (peptides) are picked up by the MHC molecules and transported to the cell surface for identification by the T cells. Even when invading microbes change their protein configuration with mutation, the T cells can often identify their foreign peptide fragments.

Each of the body's cells contains a network of microcanals (endoplasmic reticulum) connecting the nucleus to the cytoplasm of the cell. Certain regions within the chromosomes inside the nucleus generate the MHC molecules that travel through this network to do their job. Almost all types of cells that are not part of the immune system carry Class I MHC molecules, while phagocytic lymphocytes carry a different group of MHC molecules known as Class II molecules. There is a high degree of genetic diversity among the MHC genes, permitting a wide range of genetic responses to different foreign peptides. This variability ensures that some individuals within a population will survive to produce the next generation.

CD8 killer T cells stimulated by CD4 T cells are attracted to MHC I–bound foreign antigens on an infected cell. Once they confirm the identification, they attack the infected cell by punching holes in it and releasing chemicals to destroy the cell and attract phagocytic cells to clean up the debris. The killer CD8 T cells must work quickly, before the virus completes its replication cycle, or its finished progeny will be released to infect other cells when the cell is destroyed. This can set up a vicious cycle of CD8 T cells trying to contain the infection by destroying too many of the body's tissue cells (Paul 1993).

Class II MHC molecules are designed to take up foreign peptides shed from microbes regenerating inside enclosed pockets, known as *vesicles*, within phagocytic cells. While the bound foreign peptide displayed on the cell surface attracts CD4 T cells, the infected cell also sends out a signal from a surface molecule that is picked up by another protein on the T cell surface. This dual attraction mobilizes T cell responses and the release of cytokines by the CD4 T cell that stimulate the infected phagocytic cell to destroy the parasite living within its own vesicles (Paul 1993).

Immunity throughout the Life Cycle

The human immune system is most vulnerable in the first thirty-six months of life (Dubos 1980). The immune system in the newborn has not developed completely, and the newborn depends on about three months' supply of maternal immunoglobulins passed on before birth, plus maternal immunoglobulins passed to the infant during lactation. Mothers in poor health cannot provide sufficient protection for their infants, and this leaves them vulnerable to pathogens. Older infants being weaned from the breast become highly stressed with the sudden dietary and emotional changes, and this puts a strain on their immune systems. Most infants with compromised immunity will die from overwhelming gastrointestinal or respiratory infections under natural conditions.

By three years of age most children are immune to the microbes commonly found in their immediate environment. The immune system of children continues to adapt to its microbial surroundings. Some infections causing disease in adults often produce mild or no symptoms in children. By adolescence, children usually achieve immunity or tolerance to most of the microbes they grow up with.

The growth spurt of adolescence brings new physiological stress on the immune system, and unfamiliar roving microbes can trigger overzealous immune responses in the budding young adult. Normally quiescent commensal microbes can also become aggressive during this physiological upset and can provoke the immune system into action.

The immune system reaches its peak in development with adulthood. The thirties mark the high point of the strength of the immune defenses accumulated throughout the life of the individual. Loss of immune strength during the adult stage can happen with prolonged debilitation from injury, poor nutrition, irritating factors from the environment, or any physiological upset. Factors associated with the aging process can affect the immune system, and by the time a person reaches frail old age, his or her immune system is as vulnerable as that of the newborn. Respiratory diseases are as frequent amont the frail elderly as they are among infants.

Concluding Comments

Infection is not synonymous with disease. Most infections do not result in disease (Burnet and White 1972; Dubos 1980). Infection has to do with invasion by a potentially pathogenic microbe. The infection can be so mild that front-line phagocytic cells can easily contain it or a quick and effective immuno-globulin response is able to prevent full-scale invasion. Sometimes the invader successfully hides from the immune system, keeping a low profile so as not to attract attention. Sometimes a microorganism introduced into the human body finds the internal microenvironment incompatible for survival.

Weaknesses or breakdowns in our defense system, caused by genetic flaws, poor nutrition, or environmental or behavioral influences (or a com-bination of these factors), create the potential for disease. The very complex-ity of the immune system invites error in any one of the subdivisions within its ranks. Deficiencies within the immune system can leave the individual susceptible to certain diseases, while an efficient immune system provides resistance to disease. Variations in immune responses explain the variabil-ity in expressions of a specific disease, from infection without symptoms or mild symptoms, to transient serious illness, to chronic or persistent disease.

Health depends on the equilibrium between host and microorganisms, not on the eradication of microbes from the body. The primary aim of the immune system is to inhibit microbes from reproducing and colonizing within the body. The equilibrium between microbes and the host can fluctu-ate with changes within the host or the microbe (Dubos 1980). The human immune system is remarkable in that it can withstand numerous assaults by pathogens, foreign toxic materials, marginal or poor nutrition, injury, and general mayhem throughout the lifespan of the individual.

Hidden infections can reactivate months to years later to cause disease with changing circumstances within the host. Many microbes go stealth to evade immune responses. Often they do so when challenged by the immune system or medications, developing into chronic diseases. Several microbes identified by our immune system can change antigenic properties, perhaps more than once, and sneak past our defenses. Some diseases persist when host immunity is impaired.

Populations of specific microorganisms vary as much as do human pop-ulations and their immune systems. This variation (polymorphism) is neces-sary in all living organisms in order for evolutionary change to keep taking place to meet ever-changing environmental pressures. Usually within a microbe population a dominant form prevails in adapting to a specific micro-environment. Changes in the microenvironment can lead to changes in the dominant type of microbe. Sometimes changes in nutrition, medications such as antibiotics, or stress on the immune system from other sources can lead to biochemical changes within the body. Such changes can promote selection for more deadly varieties of friendly microbes, or less deadly strains of dangerous microbes. Mutations within a microbe population, particularly viruses, can lead to a strain more adept at getting around the immune system than previous types. The immune system's own variability, particularly within the B cell antibodies, constantly undergoes changes to meet the shifting challenges of microbes. Individuals within a human population may succumb to the onslaught of a disease, but some will have the right combination of genes and stamina to survive and contribute their genes to the next generation.

The balance of power between microbes and human beings shifts constantly, with each side jockeying for control, eventually leading to a state of fluctuating equilibrium. Individuals with poor immune responses will be weeded out, just as microbe variants that cannot adapt are weeded out. The selection process is repeated with every generation of microbes and people, and the battle goes on between them. Human evolution has been intimately entwined with microbe evolution, and changes in human behavior can upset the delicate balance.

CHAPTER 3

EARLY HUMANS AND THEIR DISEASES

Wanderlust

Part of the nature of human beings is the urge to wander, passed on in genes from our earliest ancestors. Many of us have the urge to just go somewhere else now and then. If we look closely at other natural urges, we will find that we also like to eat certain things at certain times of the year and avoid some foods most of the time. We also tend to want to be with certain people and avoid others. Our fascination with fire is as strong today as it was when our early ancestors learned how to master it. Pure clean water, usually taken for granted in modern society, has always been prized by humans. The need to feel safe and secure, especially as night falls, remains as important to us as it was to our ancestors. Our human nature requires comfort from other people in the form of nurturing and affection. We rely on each other for a range of creature comforts and for emotional support. We are not much different biologically and emotionally from our immediate human ancestors, archaic *Homo sapiens*, who evolved from *Homo erectus* nearly 400,000 years ago. We still share the same basic needs and urges from the distant past.

Early human beings wandered throughout their known world, following and hunting animals, and searching for clean drinking water, seasonal plant foods, shelter from the weather, protection from danger and the night, and contact with others. They most likely traveled and lived in small, closely related groups or bands within a specific territory familiar to the group for generations. Contact with other groups from adjacent territories would be necessary for social exchanges, especially for finding mates outside the group.

Environmental change in the habitat of early human beings most likely triggered the need to wander to another region for survival. Weather changes, such as long-term drought, excessive rains, or severe cold spells, or natural disasters, such as severe earthquakes or volcanic eruptions, could have signaled the need to leave and go somewhere else. Human groups also followed migrating animals, which they hunted for food from one environment to another.

Our early human ancestors, beginning with *Homo erectus*, managed to expand throughout the major continents of the Old World over several millennia. This led to long-term isolation of various groups of early wanderers and their genes from other groups of people. Eventual evolutionary changes among isolated groups of people adapting to various environments created the wide variability in human populations today. The divergence between gene pools brought with it changes in genetically driven immune systems adapting to different environmental microorganisms.

Evolutionary Hitchhikers

Homo erectus carried with him the internal and external parasites (ectoparasites) of his hominid ancestors, passing them on to *Homo sapiens*. Some of these microbes and minute creatures had become fixed into *commensal* (living together without harm) and *symbiotic* (living together with mutual benefit) relationships within a common ancestor shared by humans and apes long before they went separate ways around 7 million years ago. Similarities between some commensal and parasitic organisms of modern humans and apes support this idea of what we may call evolutionary hitchhikers (T-W-Fiennes 1967; Hare 1967).

The best example of this type of evolutionary link is the protozoa *Entamoeba coli* commonly found in the gut of humans. This microscopic creature helps clean up unwelcome intruders, feeding on bacteria and other microbes invading the large intestine (Beaver and Jung 1985). *Entamoeba coli* is a harmless protozoan that appears to have evolved along with humankind, living within our guts in harmony with our immune system. Similar *Entamoeba coli* also exist in Old World apes (T-W-Fiennes 1967), and this evidence supports the notion that it evolved from a protozoan found in a common ancestor of apes and humans.

Another small protozoan hitchhiker shared by both humans and apes, trichomonas (T-W-Fiennes 1967), probably also came from a common ancestor. Different species of this microbe live peacefully in the human intestinal tract, around the gum line in the mouth, and in the genito-urinary tract. Those living in the gut and genito-urinary tract can become irritable when their microenvironment is upset (Beck and Davies 1981), particularly in the vaginal canal of females.

Despite similarities, ape and human commensals and parasites generally do not mix well, and they frequently cause harm when they cross the species line. Evolutionary separation created different microenvironmental demands that required separate adjustments for the same types of internal and external parasites. Some parasites probably were not able to adjust to the changes evolving in humans or apes, or both, and new ones were added long after the split between humans and apes. Most human commensals and parasites were acquired once divergence from early apes began. As our human ancestors changed, so did the population of parasitic hitchhikers.

Biological divergence shaped significant differences between human and ape responses to similar potential parasites coming from shared environments. Most likely, selection was made within the ranks of the parasitic populations for the most suitable type of candidate with the best chance for survival within each specific type of host. Evolutionary selection of the most fit parasite also applied to other types of animal hosts when the prospective parasite had flexibility to adapt to a wide range of microenvironmental host changes.

The variability within immune responses of host populations also selected those individuals able to contain the invading parasite. Individuals unable to brake the invasion would sicken and perhaps die. Eventually an armed truce would result, and a state of fluctuating equilibrium would be reached among survivors. Some parasites became commensals as the hosts developed tolerance to them. However, populations of both hosts and parasites continue to carry the genetic material of the past, allowing the resurgence of individuals not previously selected.

Commensals under normal conditions generally remain harmless in their particular ecological niche in or on the host body. Upsets in their microecological zone can trigger a more virulent (infectious) variant of the commensal population to take over and harm the body's tissues. Human beings and animals debilitated from poor nutrition, injury, or other stresses on the body can become victims of their own commensals.

Commensals residing in the throat and mouth, especially Streptococci bacteria, can become virulent when their microenvironment changes. This can lead to acute or chronic infections of the nasal sinuses, inner ear, mastoids, and throat; dental abscesses; and periodontal disease. The earliest example of this was found in an archaic *Homo sapiens* skull known as the Rhodesian Skull from South Africa. This individual suffered from severe mastoid infection, dental abscesses, and caries (McKenzie and Brothwell 1967).

Intestinal commensals, especially *Escherichia coli* (*E. coli*) bacteria, can cause infection when the intestinal environment is altered or if they gain access to body tissues by accident (Hare 1967). Commensals living on the skin and in the nose, Staphylococci bacteria, can be harmful when they are inadvertently introduced to tissues below the skin by abrasion or wounds. Change can be brought about in the gut and mouth by poor nutrition and loss of nutrients required for tissue integrity and for proper functioning of the immune system. Infection by a pathogenic agent that alters the immune response and upsets the microenvironment can also trigger virulence in commensals.

Early human beings would have suffered the same consequences as modern people whenever the microenvironment of harmless commensals was changed and allowed a commensal to become a pathogen. Parasites that generally do little or no harm can become aggressive pathogens whenever the balance between them and their host is upset.

Herpes

The herpes virus group presents a good example of a long parasitic evolutionary history with both humans and apes. Herpes viruses also reside in a wide range of other mammals, birds, oysters, reptiles, fish, and amphibians (Cooper and MacCallum 1984; Honess and Watson 1977). This group of viruses evolved from a common primordial ancestor into a wide range of species to create parasitic relationships with specific hosts (natural hosts). Some of these viruses were attracted to the earliest human ancestors, who became their natural host. We find these viruses in human populations throughout the world today, even in isolated villages in underdeveloped countries (Black 1980).

Little was known about this group of viruses until the 1960s. Herpes viruses travel from one host to another through direct contact with the infected individual's saliva and other body fluids. Infection generally remains silent and does not cause any apparent disease. Occasionally after a long period of quiescence herpes viruses can be triggered into aggressive action and can cause disease. They appear not to act alone, and instead require some other agent of disease, genetic weakness, or physiological upset (or combination of such factors) to become *pathogenic* (disease-causing).

Herpes simplex virus is the best known of the human herpes viruses. Infection frequently remains with the host for life. Upsets within the internal environment of the host can affect the virus, creating conditions ripe for the development of herpes vesicles, small blisterlike sores. The vesicles tend to recur in the same site whenever conditions are right, generally where the skin meets mucous membrane. The most common site is around the lips of the mouth. *Herpes simplex* has produced a variant form that primarily infects the genitals of both men and women in a manner similar to the original *Herpes simplex*. This variant may have evolved much later, after the original virus had become well established in the human population.

Another herpes virus closely related to *Herpes simplex* has been identified in Asian monkeys, *Macaca mullatta*. This virus is known as B-virus, and it affects the monkeys the same way that *Herpes simplex* affects humans, but neither virus is tolerated by the other species. Monkey B-virus is deadly to humans (T-W-Fiennes 1967), indicating total evolutionary separation from the human virus. The virus can be transmitted to humans through bites from an infected monkey, carried in the monkey's saliva into the human bloodstream, where it rapidly overwhelms the unprepared immune system of the new human host. Macaque monkeys and humans must have acquired their herpes viruses separately but from within the same environment that contained the original ancestor of both types.

Epstein-Barr virus represents another type of herpes virus that is common in human beings. Infection generally remains silent, but it may cause disease when allowed to aggressively proliferate. Some individuals inherit immune systems poorly equipped to handle this infection. Mononucleosis is the most common manifestation of disease produced by this virus in temperate climates. This disease appears most frequently in late adolescence and early adulthood, at a time in the human lifespan when the body's immune system is the most aggressive and tends to overreact. The virus initially invades epithelial cells lining the throat, producing symptoms of fever, fatigue, sore throat, and swollen lymph glands. The virus moves on to invade lymphocytic B cells displaying similar surface receptors to those of the infected epithelial cells, which the virus uses to gain entry into targeted cells. Epstein-Barr virus integrates into about 10 percent of infected B cells, changing them to favor the presence of the virus. Here in these B cells the virus resides indefinitely, letting the infected cell reproduce it along with its own replication (Craighead 2000).

Epstein-Barr virus has been implicated in other diseases, when circumstances allow the virus to get out of control. For example, cancers of the B cells can develop, and cancerous tumors affecting the epithelial cells can lead to Burkitt's lymphoma in central African children and to adult nasopharyngeal carcinoma, frequently found in southeast China (Craighead 2000).

Human cytomegalovirus, another herpes virus, resides within epithelial cells of the salivary glands in the mouth and rarely causes disease. The virus is commonly transmitted by saliva or respiratory droplets between babies and young children, causing no harm. Adults can transmit the virus through seminal or vaginal secretions. Cytomegalovirus can cause a generalized infection when immune systems are compromised, and sometimes maternal infection can be passed to the unborn fetus (Craighead 2000).

Varicella-zoster virus is another herpes virus that many people have experienced during childhood with a great deal of discomfort. This virus causes chickenpox. The disease varies in severity depending on the host immune response. Some individuals retain the virus in peripheral (outlying) nerve endings following an outbreak of chickenpox, where the immune system keeps it quiet indefinitely. Upsets in the internal environment of the host following years of repression can trigger rapid new growth of the virus within the nerve endings where it has been hiding. Painful vesicles erupt along the course of the nerve, and this is known as herpes zoster or shingles. The virus can be transmitted from the lesions of shingles to individuals never before exposed to the virus.

Infections by herpes viruses among early human populations must have been common. The viruses can survive for years within human hosts. The hosts become carriers of the viruses, maintaining the infection within small, related groups for generations. The viruses reached a state of fluctuating equilibrium with human populations long ago. Susceptible individuals within each population continue to be born and develop disease produced by the viruses to the present day. The virus producing chickenpox could easily have survived quietly in adults for many years following childhood infection. Resurgence as *Herpes zoster* would have allowed the virus to infect the next generation of children. Since the human herpes viral infections are rarely fatal by themselves, they could easily be carried about within the small groups of early humans.

Roving Parasites and Opportunistic Microbes

Early human beings most likely remained within specific regions for many generations before gradually moving on. Humans as well as other animals interacting within their immediate home environment would also be interacting with the same groups of roving potential parasites. Many opportunistic microbes, particularly viruses, can adapt to more than one type of host. This explains similarities between the microbes found in different types of hosts within a specific environment.

Resident populations of humans and animals living within the same environment for centuries developed tolerance to most of the microbes in their habitat (T-W-Fiennes 1978a). However, the delicate balance between microbes and hosts would have been subject to fluctuations whenever changes occurred. A change could reflect any kind of shift affecting the host population, the microbe population, or the environment. Environmental and climatic changes can trigger genetic changes, and nutritional changes can lead to microenvironmental changes within the host that affect parasites. Behavior changes, particularly changes in daily living activities, can also affect microbe responses.

Hitchhiking parasites are everywhere, but few get accepted by potential hosts. Different environments around the world offer different sets of potential parasites. Each ecosystem is self-contained, with its own set of microbes, resident animals, insects, and human beings. Humans and animals moving into a new environment risk encountering new parasites unknown to their immune systems. Survival will depend on how well the intruder adjusts to the new parasites and how they adjust to the intruder. Successful adjustment will involve acquiring additional commensals and parasites found only in the new environment. This type of adaptation requires frequent exposure by the host over time to the potential parasite.

Confrontations with new parasites did not always end up in a standoff, with new resident microbes moving in under an arms truce. Early human beings wandering into new environments were exposed to numerous types of opportunistic microbes and minute creatures. Such parasites flourished in the soil upon which they walked, the air they breathed, the water they drank, the foods they ate, and in the animals and insects living in the area. The parasites were always looking for the opportunity to attack new hosts. Our ancient ancestors most likely learned to avoid those areas where sickness and death from unseen forces overwhelmed them and others of their kind.

Insect Carriers of Disease

Insects that carry disease, known as *vectors*, are found in every type of environment, from the cold Arctic to hot deserts. The rain forests of the tropical zones harbor the largest and most diverse types of vector-borne parasites dangerous to humans. Dense tropical forests may have been one of the areas avoided by our early ancestors.

Some insects, such as flies, carry diseases mechanically on their body parts to the host from sources of infection, such as contaminated soil, feces, open sores, and saliva of infected hosts. Viruses, bacteria, protozoa, and the eggs or larvae of infectious worms can be transported to new hosts through the secretions of insects. The transported infectious agents require access to the new host's body tissues through skin or mucosal abrasions and cuts, sometimes by ingestion, but primarily through the bite of insects.

Blood-sucking insects, especially mosquitoes, can transport infectious agents directly into the bloodstream of the host. More than two hundred viruses, known as arboviruses (Cooper and MacCallum 1984), and many microscopic protozoa and minute worms are transmitted by blood-sucking insects. Different environmental conditions favored the evolutionary relationship of specific parasites with their natural insect vector hosts and their natural animal hosts. Many creatures within the animal kingdom play natural host to insect-borne infections, including birds, rodents, bats, monkeys, and apes. Some vector-borne parasitic relationships with animals have spilled over into human populations. It is also possible that some of the arboviruses may have adapted to the earliest hominids and remained quiescent passengers throughout human evolution.

Most of the microscopic parasites carried by blood-sucking insects have adapted part of their life cycle to the microenvironment of the insect hosts without harming them. The insect becomes the intermediate host, while the eventual, targeted animal host becomes the definitive host. Generally the parasite requires a specific type of intermediate vector host or related vector hosts with specific microenvironmental conditions for certain stages of its development. The definitive animal host may vary, as long as the microenvironmental needs of the parasite are met. This relationship between insect and animal hosts allows the parasites to extend their range beyond their place of origin (Busvine 1980).

Human origins were tied to the warmer parts of the globe, where early groups of human beings living in or near the tropics would have been subjected to disease-carrying insects at some time in their lives. Early hunters would have been exposed to vector insects that pester large herds of game animals at certain times of the year. Parasites picked up from the hunted animals by the vectors could be transferred inadvertently to human hunters. Many of the parasites, living in equilibrium with their vector and animal hosts, would most likely have caused random havoc for the accidental human hosts.

Gathering plant foods from various food patches that harbored vector insect pests, particularly along water ways or densely forested areas where resting insect hordes could be stirred into action, would also have put people at risk of infection. Annoying insect pests would have been everywhere, just as they are today, but not all of them would have brought infection, and the nomadic habits of early humans would have limited the number of incidental infections from insect vectors.

The small numbers within early human groups and their nomadic ways made them less likely to become a prime source, or reservoir, for maintaining parasite infection from vectors. Most parasites carried by insect vectors require a constant supply of young hosts with immature immune systems, in order to maintain a reservoir of infection. As infected hosts mature, they generally become more resistant to the parasites within their environment. Small human groups with few offspring and relatively short lifespans, moving about, would have been a poor choice for most vector-borne parasites. Sporadic infection of early human beings, primarily intended for the natural animal hosts, was probably the rule.

Hitchhiking Insects

External parasites, known as ectoparasites, usually consisting of mites, fleas, and lice, commonly thrive on all species of living plants and animals. Many of them are so small that it is difficult to see them with the naked eye. Human beings have a long evolutionary history with microscopic mites that live in hair follicles and the sebaceous glands around the face without our knowledge.

Many tiny insects have evolved into a close parasitic relationship with a specific type of host plant or animal. Several of these ectoparasites have become species-specific, dependent on only one type of host for survival. The surface of the chosen host for these small creatures becomes their world.

One of the best known ectoparasites infesting humans is a tiny wing-less insect belonging to the louse family. This little six-legged creature has accompanied us throughout our existence. Both humans and apes share the same genus of lice, known as *Pediculus* (T-W-Fiennes 1967), most likely inherited from a common primordial ancestor. While only one type of *Pediculus* infests apes, three types infest humans: the head louse *P. humanus capitus*, upper body louse *P. humanus humanus*, and the pubic louse *Phthirius pubis*. The human head and upper body lice are actually the same, and they are quite similar to ape lice, while the pubic louse has evolved into a separate form.

Lice cement their eggs, called nits, to hairs on the head and body. Adults can live up to thirty days, and the female can produce five to ten eggs per day. The nymphs hatch from the eggs within four to fourteen days (depending on the temperature) and begin feeding along with the adults by piercing the skin surface of the host to suck for minute sources of blood (Esslinger 1985).

Generations of lice can survive on the host without having to move off to other feeding grounds. Fortunately for the lice, both apes and humans prefer close contact with others of their kind, allowing the lice easy access to new worlds. The host immune system has grown tolerant to these exter-nal parasites. However, bacteria living among lice populations can aggravate the tiny puncture wounds of the feeding lice, especially when there is an overpopulation of crowded lice. This results in an inflammatory reaction from the immune system that causes intense itching, signaling the host to take action and reduce the number of lice living in the infested area by scratching. Mutual grooming by both ancient humans and apes, with care-ful removal of these parasites, helped prevent overpopulation of these tiny creatures. Unfortunately, as we shall see later (see chapter 15), the human louse itself can be a victim of disease and can inadvertently transmit the infection to its host while feeding.

Human lice know no geographical boundaries. They are found from the Arctic Circle to the tropics, which indicates that they hitchhiked around the globe on our early ancestors while they spread out into different environments. The human pubic louse probably evolved when those lice inhabiting the hairs around the genitals were cut off for long periods of time from other lice populating the hairs of the upper body and head. Most likely this happened in temperate regions, when early human beings began to wear heavy clothing for protection against the cold. Such a change in human behavior led to long periods of separation of lice from the lower body and those on the upper body (Busvine 1980). Upper body lice are much more common among human populations inhabiting temperate to cold regions, and they prefer living among fibers of clothing when not feeding on their host. Pubic lice found the need to develop more robust claws on the posterior two pairs of their legs in order to cling more readily to pubic hair, rarely letting go during their life cycle, unlike the upper body lice.

Evidence for our long relationship with these tiny insects has been found on the heads of human bodies preserved by mummification. Ancient lice nits have been identified in mummy hair from ancient Egypt (Ruffer 1914) and from South America (Brothwell and Spearman 1963). Written documents dating back to early Egypt, India, and China mention head lice (Sandison 1967).

Ingestion of Parasites

Food sources and the manner of obtaining food can be linked to parasite acquisition. Drinking water sources contaminated with infectious excreta can also serve as a source of parasite infection. Microorganisms or offspring of larger parasites can contaminate animal or plant foods. Most animals adapt over time to the parasites associated with the food and drinking water sources from their immediate environment. Early human beings must have also adapted to the parasites in their local food and drinking water.

The first use of other animals as food by hominids most likely resulted from scavenging animal kills by other predators and finding defenseless, unprotected young animals. Hunting skills and hunting weapons developed as the taste for meat increased. Repeated close contact with other animals that were hunted for food also meant exposure to their parasites. Some of these foreign parasites were able to adjust to the hominid internal environment and eventually become accepted as part of the commensal population of human beings.

Divergence long ago in our evolutionary past from animal parasitic microbes to human parasitic microbes severed host reactions between animal and human hosts. Despite common origins and similarities, animal microbes can be deadly to unfamiliar human hosts. *Escherichia coli* bacteria, commensals within the guts of humans and bovines, differ significantly enough from one another that bovine *E. coli* introduced into the human digestive system can be extremely harmful. Recent reports of this happening with a popular fast food chain's hamburgers attest to this danger. Early human beings faced similar dangers, but their guts and immune systems were more likely adjusted to repeated exposure from butchering and consumption of raw and undercooked meat. The very young, sick, and old would have been most at risk.

The intestinal tracts of all animals provide fertile ground for parasitic life forms ranging from viruses to macroscopic worms. Human beings are no exception. However, new intestinal acquisitions are environmentally dependent. The type of parasites acquired depends on the type of parasites found in a specific environment.

Most parasitic protozoans, plus several types of parasitic worms (helminths), prefer tropical and subtropical regions. Passage from one host to another exposes their offspring to the environment. They need warmth and moisture to survive outside the original host until a new host can be found. Despite this need, some of the parasites that adapted to life in the guts of humans and other animals in warm, moist climates did manage to develop ways to survive host transfer in the more rigorous climates of the temperate zones after their hosts moved away from their places of origin.

Surprisingly, very few wormy parasitic newcomers adapted to the early human intestinal microenvironment and stayed on as resident hitchhikers. Nomadic human groups are far less likely to harbor intestinal parasites that require passage through the oral-fecal route and repeated exposure to infected feces (Polunin 1967). Not until humans became sedentary in their ways did intestinal roundworms (nematodes) and flukes (trematodes) become a nuisance.

The occasional intestinal parasitic worms acquired by early human beings were usually temporary residents, causing varying degrees of inflammatory reactions in the guts of their unintended hosts. Some of them probably provoked low levels of immune response, while most cases probably triggered severe diarrhea and intestinal cramping as the body tried to expel the irritating parasites. Dehydration and electrolyte imbalance would have been a severe consequence of such action, particularly in small children who cannot tolerate rapid fluid loss and tend to die quickly in such circumstances.

Trichinosis

Certain parasitic worms introduced into the digestive tract produce infective immature young, known as larvae, that can enter the host tissues through the intestinal wall. The larvae lie dormant in the body tissues, waiting for the infected animal to be killed and eaten by another animal. The gastric juices in the stomach of the feeding animal break down the protective capsules of the larvae and free them to enter the intestine of the new host. They penetrate the intestinal lining and develop into reproductive adult worms, able to produce new larvae that repeat the cycle of waiting in the host tissues for another hungry new host.

The larvae of the adult worms known as *Trichinella spiralis*, infecting the intestines of meat-eating hosts, can penetrate the intestinal wall and migrate through the host's circulatory system to muscle tissue. The larvae enter the muscle fibers, grow larger, and induce the muscle cell to develop a capsule around them where the larvae wait, sometimes for years, for the host to fall victim to another predator. Only meat-eating animals can be infected (Barriga 1981), but some cannibalistic rats maintain the infection in nature (Little 1985b).

Early human beings occasionally would have become accidental hosts by eating raw or undercooked meat of an animal infected with *Trichinella spiralis*. Omnivorous animals, such as wild pigs and bears, would be the most likely source of infection. Herbivores (plant-eaters) would not be infected. Infection with only a few of the infective parasites would most likely go unnoticed by the host.

Heavy infections would have occurred when massive numbers of larvae invaded the tissues at once to overwhelm the immune response. Serious disease can result when large numbers of the parasitic larvae pack into muscle tissues, damaging the muscles and interfering with normal muscle function, thereby crippling the host. The toxic effects of such a massive invasion alone can cause death (Little 1985b).

Tapeworms (Cestodes)

Many different types of tapeworms infect a wide range of animals. Most of them are host-specific, which indicates long evolutionary relationships between specific parasitic worms and their hosts. Some of the more opportunistic tapeworms can be accidentally accepted by an unnatural host if conditions are right. Tapeworms are probably the most ancient of intestinal parasitic worms, having lost most of their independent functions. Many of them have developed almost commensal relationships with their natural hosts. Infections in healthy animals generally go unnoticed or cause few symptoms.

Tapeworms are flat, segmented (proglottids) worms without a digestive tract. They absorb nutrients directly through the outer covering. The head, or scolex, attaches and anchors the worm to the intestinal wall. The mature segments contain reproductive organs, and the end segments contain mature eggs. Most tapeworm eggs are ingested by an intermediary host, frequently a herbivore, after passing out through feces of the original, definitive host. The digestive juices release the embryos from the egg into the intestine, where they penetrate the intestinal wall and migrate to the tissues, grow into larvae, and wait for the intermediate herbivore host to be eaten by the definitive host. The larvae develop into adult worms in the intestine of a new definitive host. Usually only one worm is allowed to flourish in a single host (Barriza 1981).

Early human beings were exposed to tapeworms primarily through the ingestion of raw or undercooked meat. Adult tapeworms of *Taenia saginata* and *Taenia solium* were introduced to the human intestine with the first hunters and gatherers. The tapeworms eventually adapted to life within the human intestine, as contact with the worms and their animal hosts increased during domestication of animals. *Taenia saginata* (beef tapeworm) uses herbivores for intermediate hosts. The human gut presented an ideal medium for the adult tapeworm, and human beings eventually became the only definitive host for this parasite once cattle were domesticated. This tapeworm can grow to enormous lengths, up to 50 feet, and can survive for twenty-five years (Beck and Davies 1981) in a healthy individual with little or no symptoms.

Taenia solium (pork tapeworm) primarily uses omnivorous swine as intermediate hosts for the passage of its immature young within cysts contained in muscle tissue. Human beings may also act as intermediate hosts, along with camels, dogs, monkeys, deer, sheep, and other animals, with carnivores the targeted definitive hosts. However, the human gut provided an ideal environment for the adult tapeworms, and humans soon became the preferred hosts once pigs were domesticated. These tapeworms are smaller than *Taenia saginata*, but they can grow up to 10 feet in length (Beck and Davies 1981).

The adult *Taenia solium* tapeworm produces few, if any, symptoms in the healthy host, but when the human host acts as the intermediate host for the encysted immature young, problems ensue. The eggs, ingested through feces-contaminated food or water, hatch in the small intestine, and the embryos migrate through the body, just as they would in the normal intermediate host. They are attracted to skeletal and heart muscle where they become encysted larvae (Little 1985a). The presence of small numbers of encysted larvae usually causes no symptoms. Large numbers of migrating larvae can cause serious illness and even death.

Noninfectious Disease and Dental Disease

The rigors of daily life would have left marks on the joints and muscles of the early hunters and foragers. Osteoarthritis with age, reflecting repetitive, forceful use of joints through activities associated with nomadic living, would be common. Trauma from accidents and confrontation with wild animals, other human beings, and natural disasters posed threats.

Teeth were rapidly worn flat from chewing coarse fibrous materials and abrasive foods eaten raw or undercooked (Molnar 1972; Smith 1984). The gums were easily irritated by dental use, which often left behind small bits of material trapped in the gum margins. This frequently resulted in periodontal disease, followed by early tooth loss and abscesses. Heavy use of the teeth offered some protection from dental caries by wearing down natural pits on the tooth surface before they could become impacted with caries-forming bacteria. Raw and undercooked foods also are not as caries-provoking as processed foods.

Early human nutritional needs were the same as those of modern humans. Moving about, scavenging and hunting for meat and foraging for seasonal plant foods, allowed human beings to meet their nutritional needs most of the time. Different ecosystems would offer different sets of food sources. Seasonal bouts of deficiencies in certain nutrients occurred when the plant sources could not be found. Competition with other animals or human groups for scarce food resources, seasonal weather upsets, and natural disasters would have strained early humans' ability to gain all of the nutrients and calories they needed to maintain health.

Disorders of human functioning, regardless of cause, would have hampered survival. Debilitating injuries, severe congenital defects, and flaws in immune functioning would have been lethal in a world that mandated only the fittest would survive.

Paleolithic Times

Homo sapiens arrived on the evolutionary scene around 400,000 years ago, bringing not only biological change but also cultural change. Culture replaced biology as *Homo sapiens'* most potent tool for evolutionary change. Archaic *Homo sapiens* began the steady climb toward modern humans during the Middle Pleistocene, when most of the world experienced much cooler conditions than today, and glaciers covered large portions of the northern regions of the world. Perhaps the advance of the Ice Age influenced behavior changes in our ancestors.

Climatic changes required adaptation. Archaeologists have found the remains of shelters constructed during this time. The shelters served as seasonal camps built near water sources, with food cooked over hearths. Stone tools increased in variety. Food procurement gradually became more organized and stable.

The best known example of one of these seasonal campsites is Terra Amata, discovered in the French city of Nice near the Mediterranean coast. This ancient site, dating to around 300,000 years ago, was situated within a small sandy cove with a freshwater spring nearby. It yielded evidence of repeated occupation by the same people returning each year in the late spring to exploit local food resources for a short while before moving on. They built temporary oval huts out of brush and stones. Hearths dominated the center of each hut, providing fire for cooking and warmth against the brisk, damp weather of that time. Traces of a wooden bowl were found, indicating the manufacture of containers to hold water and food. Pieces of red ocher discovered at the site may have been used for body paint. Butchered bones of many different types of animals (mostly young) include boar, wild ox, stag, elephant, and rhinoceros, along with shellfish and fish. Some animal bones had been fashioned into tools (De Lumley 1972).

The consumption of shellfish, particularly raw oysters, may have led to the introduction of infectious viral hepatitis into human populations. Numerous large coastal shell middens throughout the world, dating to the upper Paleolithic, show increased utilization of shellfish as a food source during this time. We know little about the antiquity of this disease, but many human populations around the world carry antibodies to various forms of infectious hepatitis. Usually exposure during childhood leads to few, if any, symptoms (Gust 1980).

Modern human beings began to appear somewhere around 100,000 years ago (Stringer 1992) during a time of gradual global warming. By this time human populations had advanced considerably in stone tool technology (Gowlett 1992) and survival techniques. Regional differences developed according to the adaptive requirements of different environments. The ability to adapt culturally as well as biologically to diverse environments became the key to human success. Eventually this success would allow human beings to tip the balance between them and nature, shaping the environment to meet their desires.

CONCLUDING COMMENTS

Beginning with *Homo erectus* at the onset of the Pleistocene around 1.5 million years ago and up until about 12,000 years ago, human beings depended on scavenging, hunting, and foraging for survival. Human groups remained small, and lived in balance with nature. Up until the appearance of modern *Homo sapiens*, the death rate appears to have been fairly equal to the survival rate of the young. Old age was rare, and few individuals reached their fifties because of the rigors of living in the wild. We can correlate this with the observation that captive wild primates and other wild animals generally survive much longer under controlled conditions than do their counterparts in nature.

Cultural changes, beginning with *Homo sapiens*, brought new technologies that improved the hunting and foraging way of life, slightly increasing the chances for more young and older individuals to survive. Nevertheless, the world remained populated by small, related groups exploiting their surroundings for food and shelter, until agriculture and animal husbandry were invented. The world population of hunters and foragers during the Paleolithic is estimated to have been between 5 million and 10 million (Coale 1974), compared to over 6 billion today.

Most of the infectious diseases that we know today did not affect early human beings (Black 1975; 1980). Their way of life and small numbers kept them safe from the crowd diseases that would develop later among large, dense human populations. Diseases incurred would have been occasional infections acquired from animals (zoonoses) and from opportunistic infectious agents present in the environment. Human beings living within a particular ecosystem for several generations would have developed immune resistance or tolerance to the potential pathogens they encountered on a regular basis. Individuals with poor immune responses would have been weeded out. Seasonal nutritional deficiencies would have posed more of a threat than would infectious diseases.

For most of human existence, nomadic hunting and foraging for food in small groups was a way of life. We still react with the same instincts and survive with the same basic immune system in our modern world. However, by altering our natural environment to meet our particular desires, modern human beings have created new stresses unknown to our ancient ancestors.

THE SEEDS OF CHANGE

Prologue

The final retreat of the massive ice sheets of the pleistocene took place between thirty-two thousand and ten thousand years ago, accompanied by fluctuating changes in the global environment. The subarctic tundra regions contained many of the last big game animals, such as mammoths, mastodons, and woolly rhinoceros. Massive herds of hoofed animals, such as wild bovines, wild horses, reindeer, and other deer, roamed the steppes of Central Asia, Europe, and North America. Pleistocene peoples living in present-day France and Spain revealed the creative side of human nature with rich artistic expressions in cave paintings. Stone tools became more refined and diverse, with many of them intended for use in working ivory, bone, antler, and wood (Smith 1972). Human migrations expanded into New Guinea and Australia, followed later by migrations to the New World and to South Pacific islands.

Our ancestors refined and broadened their technology and skills of food procurement to better exploit a broader range of food resources found throughout the world's various ecosystems. Food items included just about everything edible that was available to them: numerous small and large forest animals, as well as the large animals from the grasslands, along with fowl, mollusks, grubs, nuts, tubers, fruits, legumes, bulbs, greens, and seeds. Even then, notions of what was considered food, and practices of how and when it was procured, varied among different peoples. Grinding stones were now used to pulverize acorns, nuts, and seeds (Henry 1989). Fishhooks, nets, and harpoons, along with skin boats, were used to reap bountiful supplies of fish, shellfish, and marine animals along the edges of the seas, rivers, and lakes (Piggott 1965).

Global temperatures and moisture patterns shifted dramatically by the end of the Ice Age, thirteen thousand to ten thousand years ago. Many of the big game animals disappeared as the tundras shrank. The temperate zones and bordering ecological zones grew warmer with increased moisture, allowing woodlands to expand into former steppe regions. The climatic shifts altered the distribution of the plants and animals in many ecological zones. Plant and animal diversity increased with the expansion of ecotones, the transitional zones between different environments (Butzer 1964; Henry 1989), and human populations were quick to take advantage of these diverse offerings.

Depending on environmental conditions, food sources and food procurement techniques varied. Some peoples relied more heavily on marine resources than on other sources of food, while others relied more on hunting. Hunting groups that depended on large herds of herbivores eventually learned to control small herds for their own use, guiding them to selected grazing and watering areas. This way, fresh meat and hides were always readily available on the hoof, with no need to go looking for them. This type of animal control, along with selective breeding and culling, eventually led to taming and domestication of sheep, goats, cattle, reindeer (Herre 1969), and possibly other deer (Dennel 1992).

Marine exploitation, herding, hunting, and food foraging were so successful that several different human populations around the globe continued to pursue this way of life up into modern times. Pastoral peoples and maritime cultures of old continue in some parts of the world today, but many of them have modified their ancestral technologies with modern equipment. Political pressures forced most of them to change their way of life by the end of the twentieth century.

Only a few remnant populations of hunters and foragers survived until the mid-twentieth century in scattered parts of the world. They provided a living history of our ancient past, and also taught us how readily humans can learn new ways, as modern tools and hunting weapons reached them. New ideas travel fast and are adapted quickly if they readily fit into the scheme of things. People tend to pick and choose what they wish to incorporate into their way of life, and so it was for ancient populations on the verge of revolutionizing food procurement methods through farming. Many peoples adopted the ideas associated with cultivation, while others chose not to incorporate farming into their way of life.

The Best of Times

The end of the Ice age brought a period of optimal climatic conditions and abundance, allowing human groups to thrive and increase somewhat in numbers. This modest increase came about as infant survival rates and adult longevity were promoted by the bounty and diversity of plant and animal food resources, and by changing technology.

Seasonal camps along the fringes of expanding woodlands in the uplands of the eastern Mediterranean region of western Asia began to take on a different character as people adapted to the changing ecotones associated with the woodlands. They built their shelters near permanent water, and exploited the plentiful food resources available to them in varying adjacent ecological zones (Butzer 1964; Henry 1989). The diversity of plant growing seasons with elevation changes, and the different types of animals living in nearby ecological niches provided a steady source of food for much of the year. Excess amounts of plant foods could be preserved and stored for use when growing seasons ended, making it more desirable for people to stay in one place.

Wild sheep, goats, pigs, cattle, gazelle, and deer became the major meat animals in the eastern Mediterranean region of southwest Asia (Butzer 1964). Wild barley and wheat grew in dense stands along the fringes of the upland woodlands, and the people living there were quick to take advantage of this bountiful supply of food. The cereal grasses increasingly became valuable portions of their diet. Stands of cereal grasses at different elevations ripened at different times, making it easier for people to amass large stores of these food resources (Henry 1989). Harlan (1967) estimated that a family could collect over a ton of wild wheat grains in a three-week period. The wild cereal grains most likely were cooked as gruel, roasted, or ground into flour to make a doughy paste for baking on stone slabs.

Ancient peoples, such as members of the Natufian Culture, thrived in the region adjacent to the eastern Mediterranean Sea, known as the Levant, from 12,500 to 10,500 years ago. The Natufian population exemplifies the success of human existence following the end of the Ice age. Gazelle provided their main meat supply, supplemented by smaller animals, fish, and wild fowl. Wild cereal grains became the major staple food, supplemented with nuts (pistachios and almonds), lentils, and other plant foods. Their numbers increased, and they eventually built permanent settlements with stone-walled dwellings housing several families and storage pits (Henry 1989; Miller 1992).

Plentiful and varied food supplies, along with improved climatic conditions, allowed human groups to experience optimum health conditions. Scattered, small, permanent and semipermanent settlements appeared near readily available freshwater springs and clear streams. People managed to live in relative comfort in harmony with nature.

Slight shifts in climate in the Levant region around eleven thousand years ago decreased precipitation amounts. This shrank the Mediterranean woodlands and permanent water sources. Declining food resources for the growing human populations living there forced most of the Natufians to eventually abandon their homes and return to nomadic hunting and foraging. Some of them took matters into their own hands by carefully tending and cultivating the cereal grains that had become their most important food resource (Henry 1989). Constant selection of certain cereal variants led to domestic forms that were easier to manage and that brought greater yields.

Changing Times

The earliest archaeological evidence for plant cultivation comes from the eastern Mediterranean region of west Asia around eleven thousand years ago, with domesticated barley, and einkorn and emmer wheat, followed by legumes, such as the lentil and pea (Miller 1992). Sheep domestication also occurred at this time in the uplands of what is now Iraq, followed by the domestication of goats, pigs, and cattle (Butzer 1964; Herre 1969). Early forms of agriculture were mixed with herding, hunting, foraging, and fishing. This new adaptation has been labeled the Neolithic (New Stone Age). Eventually agriculture became the dominant way of life for humans wherever plant cultivation took over.

Plant cultivation and animal husbandry gradually spread throughout the Mediterranean region, into Europe, north Africa, the Caucasus, Central Asia, and into the Indian subcontinent (Zohary and Hopf 1993). Wheat and barley became the staple crops of Europe and west Asia. New plants in different ecological zones were added to the growing list of domesticated plants. Rye and oats became popular in the colder regions of Europe. Grapes and olives found a place in the Mediterranean diet (Sauer 1993). Pearl millet and sorghum, along with other local grains, were domesticated in north Africa (Harlan 1992). The wild ass (donkey) came from northeast Africa (Herre 1969), and Zebu cattle were domesticated in India (Butzer 1964) as wheat, barley, sorghum, and millet spread into the northwestern part of the Indian subcontinent from the west (Sauer 1993).

Signs of agriculture appeared in the woodlands of northern China around nine thousand years ago, or possibly earlier. Climatic conditions there resembled those in the eastern Mediterranean woodlands (Chang 1986). Local types of millet were domesticated, along with Chinese cabbage, soybean, buckwheat, adzuki bean, peach, and persimmon.

The earliest evidence for domesticated rice comes from south China around seven thousand years ago (Crawford 1992). The wild ancestors of domesticated rice ranged over a broad, tropical to subtropical belt from south China to Southeast Asia and into the Indian subcontinent, along with the swamp water buffalo (Zohary and Hopf 1993). This animal was easily domesticated and became a fixture for wet rice cultivation as rice farming expanded throughout the region (Clutton-Brock 1981). Domesticated rice gradually became the major staple food throughout Southeast Asia, and spread north into northern China, Korea, and Japan, and west into India.

Agriculture in Southeast Asia developed independently with nonseed tropical plants, such as banana, yams, taro, sugarcane, breadfruit, and sago. Certain types of jungle fowl (chickens), ducks, geese, and Asian pigs also became domesticated here (Butzer 1964), and they spread throughout Asia.

New World agriculture evolved independently of the Old World. Over one hundred fifty plant species were domesticated in the Americas. Some of the first cultigens developed in Mesoamerica included maize (Indian corn), beans, squash, amaranth, and chiles, dating back to 6500 B.C. (Patterson 1973). The potato, quinoa, peanuts, sweet potato, tomato, and manioc appeared among numerous cultigens domesticated in the Andean region of South America. Signs of the oldest domesticated plants going back ten thousand years come from two cave sites in the Andean region, Guitarrero Cave with beans and chile peppers, and Tres Ventanas Cave with tubers (Moseley 1992). The only animals that could be domesticated in the New World were dogs and turkeys in Mesoamerica, and the guinea pig, muscovy duck, llama, and alpaca in the Andes of South America.

New World agriculture had far less impact on the evolution of human diseases than did Old World agriculture. The primary reason for this was the inclusion of a large number of domesticated animals with farming in the Old World, and earlier development of civilizations with trade routes traversing a wide range of separate geographic regions. Close contact and daily living with domesticated animals became a major source of new human diseases gained from animal microbes. Extensive trade contacts and the massing of large numbers of people in ancient cities provided exchange routes for and mixing of numerous microbes from different regions.

The development of agriculture changed the way human beings interacted with their environment and with each other. Plant cultivation required careful management of the local terrain to promote the growth and expansion of selected crops. The incorporation of domestic stock into farming in some areas of the Old World altered the arrangement of local environments. Changes forced on the local ecology also meant changes in the world of parasites. Disease patterns among sedentary farming peoples began to take on a different character than disease patterns among nomadic peoples.

Farming involved varying approaches, depending on the environment. Slash-and-burn gardens with semipermanent settlements characterized tropical and subtropical forest zones. Multiple planting areas could take advantage of the variations in growing seasons at different elevations in both temperate and subtropical areas. Farming of river bottom land required more planning around periodic flooding. Wherever cultivation went, it altered the landscape, and the balance between humans and nature began to tilt.

Agriculture spread out from the various regions of origin mentioned above, and became the dominant form of human subsistence between 7000 B.C. and 3000 B.C. throughout the world. Many peoples not willing to settle down were gradually pushed into less desirable regions, such as deserts, rugged mountains, and tropical forests. Many coastal cultures eschewed agriculture to continue fishing and shell fishing along with gathering. Nomadic herders dominated the steppe grasslands and highlands that were less suited for agriculture.

The invention of the ox-driven plow in the eastern Mediterranean revolutionized agriculture. Cultivation expanded into areas not previously farmed. Alluvial river valleys attracted large-scale farming with the ox and plow. Farming villages became the common habitat for humans. Market towns developed to handle exchanges of excess foods and goods as trade intensified. The new way of life required changes in social organizations to cope with the increasing interactions between larger numbers of people. The development of metal technology improved tools and weapons. Trading networks and commerce developed between different regions. Ever increasing numbers of people banded together in urban settlements. Eventually another way of life evolved—civilization, with large populations living in cities. The microbial pot was stirred with increasing vigor, allowing more and more new human diseases to develop.

Changes in Disease Patterns

Changes in human behavior toward the environment altered disease patterns. The new disease patterns varied according to geographic region, but the common theme involved human manipulation of the local environment (T-W-Fiennes 1978). As we trace the origins of agriculture around the world, especially from the eastern Mediterranean region of west Asia, to north Africa, the Indian subcontinent, Southeast Asia, and East Asia, we find the focal regions for the evolution of human diseases that continue to plague humanity today.

Nature's rule, following any kind of environmental shakeup, whether manmade or natural, provides for the return to some form of environmental state of fluctuating equilibrium among all living things within that particular environment. This means that, in both microbe and host populations, the majority will reach a point where they become tolerant of each other. Equilibrium remains in a fluctuating state because of the variation in every population of living things in nature. Minor variants less adaptable to one state of equilibrium may achieve major status with changes in the environment.

The first major manmade environmental changes began with agriculture, stirring up the delicate balance between human beings and microbes. Each key area for the development of agriculture became the focus for the development of diseases peculiar to that region. Gradual genetic adjustments by both humans and microbes over time in any given environment eventually establish a new order of fluctuating equilibrium between them. However, any disruption of that balance results in disorder, followed by disease and death. Climatic changes; nutritional changes; famine; war; overpopulation with pressure on natural resources; further alterations of the environment, such as deforestation and irrigation; and introduction of new microbes, new animals, new plants, or new human migrants would tip the balance in favor of the microbes. In time, if there are no further insults, the delicate fluctuating balance resets itself among the survivors.

Early farmers used simple tools for cultivation, which reshaped their environment with minor disturbances of the local ecosystem. We can see this today wherever primitive agriculture is still practiced. Minor disturbances created few changes in the environment and caused relatively few adjustments between microbes and man. However, major changes came with increasing use of greater portions of the local environment for cultivation, compounded in many areas of the Old World by animal husbandry and advancing technology in farming.

Cultivated fields, food storage areas, and refuse areas in both permanent and semipermanent settlements, regardless of geographic location, attracted insects, rodents, and other small creatures. Protection of stored foods from animal and insect pests has always been a problem, and humans have devised numerous ways to insulate stored foods from them with varying degrees of success. Flies soon settled into a domestic mode among human habitats, as did various beetles, mites, mosquitoes, spiders, mice, rats, birds, reptiles, snails, and microbes.

Farmsteads and villages acted as magnets, drawing in small creatures from the surrounding environment. Reed mats, thatched roofs, and refuse areas became particularly alluring places to take up residence. Wild rodents and birds, the most notorious carriers of infectious viruses (Cooper and MacCallum 1984), were drawn to human settlements. Places where human and domestic animal excreta accumulated also became breeding grounds for parasites. Long-term relationships between humans and their small, unwanted, acclimated companions generally resulted in a new order of fluctuating environmental equilibrium, as long as pest population growth was kept in check.

Rodent-borne Diseases

Problems arose with rodents whenever rodent population growth exploded or new rodent species arrived on the scene. Perhaps that explains why cats, domesticated in northeast Africa, began to earn a place in human settlements around five thousand years ago (Beadle 1977).

The first rodent to take advantage of established human domiciles was the house mouse, *Mus musculus*. This small, furry creature, descended from wild ancestors in Central Asia, quickly adapted to the changes brought by agriculture. Moving into human houses, hiding by day and feeding by night, this little mammal could survive very well from food droppings and stored food goods, particularly grains (Hanney 1975). Life became much easier under the protective shelter that humans provided, insulated from harmful predators and surrounded by readily available food. Damage to human food supplies by burgeoning populations of rodents can be devastating, and early farmers must have had various ways to control them.

Expanding trade networks developing across Central Asia allowed the house mouse to spread outside its homeland. Safe passage was easy for the mouse, hidden away in caravan baggage and able to survive for long periods without water, as long as food was available. House mice moved to homes in the eastern Mediterranean, Europe, north Africa, and the Indian subcontinent, and eventually all over the rest of the world. Highly adaptable, the house mouse can even survive temperatures as cold as 14°F and can live off frozen foods (Hanney 1975).

Rats also moved into the domestic circle around human habitats. The most acclimated rat, the black rat (*Rattus rattus*), became a member of the household much later in time, as we shall see in chapter 14. The concentration of food resources in cultivated fields, barnyards, and storage areas brought wild rodents into unusual contact with humans. Displacement of wild rodents from their natural habitat by human intervention also forced them into greater contact with people, as they struggled to survive the upsets in their environments.

Occasionally wild rodent populations explode beyond the carrying capacity of their natural food resources. Shifts in seasonal moisture patterns can prolong growing seasons of natural food sources for the rodents and allow them to rapidly increase in numbers. When the seasonal moisture returns to its former pattern or decreases, the natural food supply shrinks and can no longer sustain the increased rodent population. This can lead to spillover of excessive numbers of hungry rodents, which would normally avoid people, into human habitations in search of food.

Several wild rodent populations serve as reservoirs for microbes that can be potentially dangerous to humans. Generally, rodent-borne microbes are species-specific, preferring to inhabit a certain species or subspecies of rodent host. The infected natural hosts are not affected by the microbes, making it possible for the microbial population to be sustained. Occasionally infection from the natural rodent host can be transferred to another type of rodent, including those rodents that have become acclimated to human settlements. Humans in turn can become accidental hosts to the infection by their close association with infected rodents living with them.

Microbes carried by both wild and acclimated rodents can be transmitted to humans by bites from their fleas or other blood-sucking insect vectors, such as sandflies, and sometimes directly by breathing in dust laden with their infectious urine and saliva. The types of microbe that produce diseases that rodents can transmit depend on the geographic location and local environmental conditions.

Many of the new rodent-borne viral diseases being discovered today, such as Lassa fever and Hanta viral infections, are most likely old diseases that are just now gaining recognition by the scientific community. These viral diseases, and many others, could not possibly be detected before the development of high-technology equipment capable of identifying them. Sporadic episodes of mysterious diseases linked to rodents that appear today probably also occurred among Neolithic populations.

Insect-borne Diseases

Blood-sucking insects, including flies, gnats, midges, mites, lice, mosquitoes, and ticks, cannot only can be annoying, but also can transmit dangerous microbes from wild animals and birds to human communities wherever opportunistic, vector-borne microbes exist in the local environment. These insects can become infected with a variety of arboviruses, bacteria, rickettsiae, protozoa, fungi, and some tiny nematodes (roundworms) known as microfilaria (Clements 1992: Gillett 1971).

All blood-sucking insects require a stable animal host reservoir for their blood meals. Interactions between a particular blood-sucking insect, its host, and a microbe developed whenever the opportunity for such interactions existed within a given environment. The initial infection might have occurred in the insect at any stage of its development, or in the animal host. Long-term interactive exchanges of the infective microbe between animal host and insect vector frequently led to microbial dependency on both for development and procreation (Esslinger 1985).

When farmers cleared fresh land for agriculture, they often caused upsets in the interaction between blood-sucking insects and their natural animal hosts. Agricultural changes altered breeding sites for blood-sucking insects by making them less favorable or more favorable. Deforestation, water management projects, and the crowding out of natural animal hosts, combined with increasing density of sedentary human populations, forced blood-sucking insects to substitute humans and their domesticated animals for their natural hosts.

Some insects, naturally catholic in taste, readily adjusted to human hosts as they became a dependable blood source by living in large numbers in the same place. Other insects, despite the opportunity to dine on human blood, retained their preference for a specific or similar animal host, shifting to humans only when animal hosts were not available. Insects biting both humans and infected animals transfer infection to humans. Domesticated animals in early farming communities often served as substitute animal hosts to become accidental links between infectious agents and humans (Andrewes 1967).

Most individuals growing up in areas where certain insect-borne diseases are endemic eventually reach a level of tolerance or resistance to the diseases as they mature into adults. Those individuals unable to do so perish in infancy or early childhood, or suffer chronic ill health or early death as adults. Tropical regions have the highest number and variety of vector-borne diseases, followed by semitropical regions. Colder climates have fewer varieties of vector insects and much less insect-borne disease. Arctic mosquitoes that breed in ice melt pools, although annoying when they swarm during the summer months, do not appear to carry disease-causing microbes (Andrewes 1967).

Mosquitoes have been the major universal insect carrier of many different disease-causing microbes. Several thousand species of mosquitoes occur throughout the world, in every environment except where the ground is frozen throughout the year. The majority of mosquito species prefer the warm, moist tropic and subtropic regions of the world (Clements 1992). Thus, most of the mosquito-borne microbes are found in these regions. Agricultural changes in the tropical-subtropical belt extending from the eastern Mediterranean, north Africa, and the Middle East, through the Indian subcontinent, to Southeast Asia, and into eastern Asia, created new opportunities for bloodthirsty mosquitoes and their infective microbes, particularly the protozoa causing malaria (see chapter 5).

Most of the mosquito-borne microbes dangerous to humans are transmitted by two subfamilies consisting of Anophelines and Culicines. The

Anophelines carry the malaria-producing plasmodium protozoa, while the Culicines are best known for transmitting arboviruses. Many of these viruses have been accidentally introduced into human populations from time to time, spilling over into human communities from their natural cycles between mosquito vector and natural animal host. This happens mostly when human beings intrude into their territory. The reservoir for many of these viruses can be found in wild birds and rodents that may nest around human habitats. The resulting viral infections include inflammation of the brain (encephalitis), inflammation of the membranes covering the brain and spinal cord (meningitis), bouts of joint pains and fever, and severe hemorrhagic fevers that are deadly. Both Anophelines and Culicines can transmit the tiny offspring of microfilarial worms to humans in tropical regions (Gillett 1971; Orihel 1985). These minute worms take up residence in various tissues of the body, depending on the species, and move about through the lymph and blood system (see chapter 7).

Adult male and female mosquitoes feed on nectar and juices from flowering plants. Adult females take blood meals when they are ready to reproduce. They require blood protein for the development of the eggs (Clements 1992; Muirhead-Thomson 1951). Females lay their eggs in or near water, which is required for the survival and development of the hatching larvae. The females are fussy about the sites where they will lay their eggs, and each type of mosquito chooses the site with concern for the proper requirements for the development of the offspring. Most mosquitoes prefer standing water in pooled areas, while some prefer the banks of moving water. Many species prefer clear water, while others like brackish water. Some lay their eggs in moist imprints in grassy surfaces or muddy soil that eventually becomes inundated with rainwater. Grassy marshes provide excellent breeding grounds for many mosquitoes. Some species have adapted to salt marshes and tidal pools. Some mosquitoes have even adapted to human habitats, breeding in manmade containers that hold water, in irrigation ditches, rice paddies, human and animal footprints, and impounded water. No matter what water source is used, the offspring of all species require protection from wind and wave action. The tiny larvae also need food, in the form of plankton, decaying vegetative matter, or animal and human excreta, depending on tastes. Water temperature and light also affect the choice of egg-laying sites. Some mosquito larvae require full sunlight, but most prefer partial or complete shade. Temperature tolerance varies as well, from warm to cold, but not the extremes of each (Horsfall 1962).

Some mosquitoes can travel long distances on the wind, up to several hundred miles, in search of suitable blood meals. Most prefer to stay close to the ground in the immediate area where blood meals are easily accessible. Neolithic farming communities expanded many mosquito habitats by increasing breeding grounds with irrigation and impounded waters, plus a plentiful supply of blood meals. Some mosquitoes in tropical and subtropical regions readily took up residence with humans and became acclimated to them. Most mosquitoes avoid the high heat of the day, becoming active only at night or when the light is subdued at dusk and dawn. The cooler indoor temperatures with subdued or absent light provided by simple village structures were just as good as their natural daytime resting places in nature. Other mosquitoes preferred to maintain their natural resting places in vegetation around or near the houses and enter after dark to feed on sleeping residents. Their resting places are often greatly enhanced by the village residents as they plant favored bushes and sow crops nearby (Gillett 1971; Horsfall 1962).

Togetherness in a Crowded Village

Increasing numbers of people living together promotes the exchange among them of several infectious diseases, depending on hygiene habits and sanitation methods. Simple cleanliness in many cases acted as a barrier to the spread of diseases. (The following chapters will focus on the evolution of several diseases that began with village life and agriculture in various parts of the world.)

Within the paleopathological record, we find evidence of changes in disease patterns on ancient human skeletal remains associated with the establishment of settled agricultural communities. Signs of anemia appear in far greater numbers within settled populations than in hunting and foraging groups (Stuart-Macadam 1992). Anemia is often an indicator of bacterial infection, as the host pulls iron out of the blood circulation to keep it away from the pathogens. Many bacterial parasites depend on the host's iron supply for survival, and by inducing anemia the host augments the immune system's defense against the microbes (Kent and Dunn 1996; Weinberg 1992).

Most children growing up and surviving in the new order of interaction between infectious agents and human beings would eventually have developed tolerance or resistance to the microbes they came into contact with on a daily basis. Individuals unable to develop appropriate immune responses were generally weeded out at an early age, although some individuals with inadequate immune responses managed to survive with chronic or recurring disease that shortened their lives.

As more and more people crowded together in close living quarters, they were more likely to maintain certain contagious infections within the group. Although most adults and older children grow tolerant or resistant to local diseases, the frequent appearance of newborns assured fresh hosts with little resistance in the settlement for local pathogens.

The growing dependence on specific cultivated foods also brought the threat of nutritional imbalances when food sources were in short supply. Poor nutrition leads to poor immune responses to infection, as well as to nutritional disorders.

Diseases transmitted by mouth from fecal contamination would have found favor in ancient crowded villages and cities where sanitation was poor. Open sources of drinking water could easily become contaminated with animal and human excreta, either directly or indirectly from rainwater runoff. Infants and small children, in particular, would have been very vulnerable to microbes traveling this route. Flies breeding in accumulating waste products would also have contributed to oral-fecal infections. Many of our ancestors, always in search of clean drinking water, may have been aware of the problems associated with fecal contamination and may have taken measures to prevent it. Nomadic peoples, always on the move, escaped most of the oral-fecal route of accumulating contamination.

Intestinal Roundworms (Nematodes)

Ever larger human groups settling into permanent villages increased people's chances of becoming infected with intestinal roundworms. Infective worm larvae in feces passed out by the host contaminate commonly used soil, handled objects, and plant foods. Contaminated fingers transfer the infective larvae to the mouth.

Most intestinal roundworms require a certain amount of time outside the host for development of the infective larval stages. They prefer shaded, warm, and moist areas, where eggs and larvae can survive for weeks, months, or even years. The eggs cannot cannot be infective until the larvae complete their development outside the host. This takes anywhere from a few hours to several weeks, depending on the type of roundworm and appropriate conditions (Little 1985a).

Human beings in tropical and subtropical regions usually prefer to defecate in shaded areas that remain warm and moist, creating ideal breeding grounds for infectious larvae. Direct sunlight kills the larvae, as do freezing and high heat. Rainwater runoff from defecation areas can spread the infected larvae to other places around human habitations and increase the risk of infection. Toddlers carrying the worms and defecating indiscriminately within the settlement greatly increase the infection rate. Human feces sometimes used to fertilize cultivated plants also expose people to infective larvae when they tend their fields and gardens. Some worm eggs can even be carried on dust particles and breathed into the lungs.

The more frequent contact people have with infected fecal material, the greater the chances of maintaining the worm population within the group. Sedentary living became the ideal situation for intestinal roundworms, and young children became prime targets because of their habit of placing soiled fingers in their mouths. Most individuals growing up with intestinal roundworms tend to develop tolerance or resistance to the worms as they reach maturity. Heavy infestations with disease manifestations generally are limited to the very young, especially when immunity has been compromised by poor nutrition, particularly protein deficiency, or by other diseases (Beck and Davies 1981).

About eleven major groups of nematodes can invade humans, most of them accidentally. The most common intestinal roundworms that have plagued humans since Neolithic times are the large Ascaris roundworms, hookworms, and the small whipworms and pinworms.

Ascaris lumbricoides is the largest roundworm infecting human beings. These roundworms most likely adapted to humans when pigs were domesticated (Beck and Davies 1981). Pigs carry a similar roundworm, *Ascaris suum*, that can infect humans. The human roundworm can also infect pigs (Little 1985a). Close association between humans and pigs for centuries allowed the Ascaris roundworm to adapt to humans. This would have been an easy transition for the worm because of the similarities between human and pig physiology.

Ascaris lumbricoides spread with its human carriers throughout the world, except where it is too cold and dry for the larvae to develop outside the host. The warmer and moister regions of the world allow the worms to thrive in greater numbers. Female Ascaris worms can produce up to twenty thousand eggs per day. Adult worms survive for a year or more in the host intestine. Females reach lengths of 8–12 inches, while the males are shorter (Little 1985a). Once the infective larvae are ingested by the host, they hatch out of the eggs in the small intestine, penetrate the intestinal wall, and migrate to the lungs. After doubling in size, they move up the bronchial tubes in the lungs to the back of the throat where they are swallowed, finally returning to the small intestine. Here they develop into adult worms. Small numbers of migrating larvae with the initial infection usually produce few symptoms. The immune system becomes increasingly alarmed with subsequent infections or with massive numbers of migrating larvae, resulting in pneumonitis, fever, and a cough that produces phlegm containing worm larvae. This will clear up as the larvae move out of the lungs. Large numbers of adult worms in the small intestine can cause gastrointestinal upsets and abdominal bloating and pain (Beck and Davies 1981).

Ascaris worms do not tolerate high fevers suffered by the host, and they can be adversely affected by other physiological upsets. When the host has a high fever, the worms seem to panic and try to escape from the small intestine in both directions. Large numbers trying to escape through the intestinal route can produce blockage of the bowel, while those worms moving in the other direction can block the bile and pancreatic ducts or penetrate the liver. Worms that do manage to reach the upper end of the alimentary canal will escape through the nose or get coughed out through the mouth (Little 1985a).

Ascaris infestation is frequently associated with a smaller type of intestinal roundworm known as the whipworm, *Trichuris trichiura*, particularly in tropical and subtropical regions. The tiny larvae are ingested, hatch in the small intestine, and penetrate the tiny intestinal projections known as villi, where they continue to develop for three to ten days. They move back into the intestine and end up in the cecum, the upper portion of the large intestine, where they grow into adult worms. Large populations of these worms can crowd into the colon and rectum. They attach to the lining of the intestinal wall, where they can survive for several years (Beck and Davies 1981).

Small children become the major hosts of whipworms. Little children with heavy infestations display abdominal pain, diarrhea, weight loss, and anemia. Older children and adults usually incur only light infestations with little or no symptoms. Pigs and dogs also carry these worms (Little 1985a), suggesting that one of them may have been the original host.

Pinworms, *Enterobius vermicularis*, another small, threadlike intestinal worm, commonly occurs throughout the world. These tiny worms are most prevalent in temperate regions. They also live in the cecum and colon of the large intestine. The female moves to the rectum when ready to produce eggs, and crawls out of the anus while the host sleeps to deposit her eggs on the skin around the rectal opening. The larvae require only a few hours outside the host to develop and become infective. The sticky eggs clump together, adhere to clothing, objects, dust particles, and fingers, and hence can easily be transmitted to other hosts. Intense irritation and itching in response to the eggs encourages the individual to scratch and transfer the eggs under the fingernails (Little 1985a). Symptoms are generally mild unless there is a heavy infestation, and then symptoms develop similar to those of whipworms. The worms most likely originated in Europe, and there is no known animal reservoir.

Hookworms

Two major types of hookworms profited from human manipulation of the environment. The hookworm known as *Ancycostoma duodenal* originated within the eastern Mediterranean region, Middle East, and Nile Valley in north Africa. Ancycostoma spread along with the domesticated animals into the tropical regions of Africa and Southeast Asia, and eventually into the South Pacific. Another hookworm, *Necator americanus*, thought by some researchers to have originated in the New World, was actually brought to the Western Hemisphere with slaves from west Africa. Necator prefers the tropics but can adapt to warm temperate regions (Little 1985a).

Many animals, such as dogs and pigs, can swallow hookworm eggs after they have passed from the infected host. The eggs can pass through them without harm (Beck and Davies 1981). This aids the spread of these worms. The larvae can only hatch and develop outside the host, feeding on bacteria and organic debris in the soil, until they transform into an infective, nonfeeding form with a sharp, pointed tail. They can move around in the soil to avoid drying rays of the sun, and to gain a vantage point for contact with the skin of a warm-blooded host. However, they must be careful not to use up their energy reserves. Soil type, moisture, and temperature affect the larvae. They cannot survive in clay soils, dry soils, or freezing temperatures. Most larvae do not survive long enough to infect a host. Infection is favored with ideal environmental conditions: high rainfall, shaded loose soil, and warm temperatures (Chandler 1945).

The larvae penetrate the host's skin, causing inflammation and itching at the site of entry. They move deeper into the skin tissues to gain entry into tiny blood vessels where they can move through the circulatory system to the lungs. There they grow and develop for about a week before moving up the bronchial tree to be swallowed and end up in the small intestine. Here they attach to the intestinal wall with cutting plates in their mouth parts, where they feed on the host's blood and tissue fluids. Ancycostoma can also enter the host through the oral-fecal route, and breast-fed infants can be infected from their mother's milk (Little 1985a).

Small numbers of migratory larvae gaining entry into the body produce few, if any, symptoms. Large numbers of larvae can provoke severe immune reactions with fever, nausea, headache, shortness of breath, and a dry cough as they break into the bronchial tree. Development of the worms into adult form in the small intestine frequently causes abdominal discomfort. The major problem with hookworms results from blood loss as they bite into the intestinal wall. Large numbers of adult worms can cause serious loss of blood, over 100 ml per day, leading to severe anemia. Even small numbers of worms can produce anemia with continuous removal of iron-containing red blood cells. The iron would normally be recycled for new red blood cells. Diets low in iron and protein also contribute to the problem. Severe hookworm anemia can bring on heart failure, and can cause poor growth and development in the young (Beck and Davies 1981).

Noninfectious Disease and Dental Disease

The Neolithic brought changes in human behavior patterns. Farming and village life led to alterations in daily living activities that brought about changing patterns of repetitive functional stress on joints and muscles. Patterns of osteoarthritis changed to reflect the new work requirements.

Trauma from accidents now included accidents resulting from the hazards associated with agriculture and the developing new types of work. Human conflict also appears to have increased throughout the Neolithic as populations increased and competed for resources. New and improved weapons developed over time, and warfare became more common as civilization evolved.

Dental wear patterns changed from flat wear to a more angular wear on teeth with dietary changes and dental use. Chewing tough, fibrous material and abrasive foods gave way to chewing fewer fibers and softer processed foods (Molner 1972; Smith 1984). Teeth did not wear down as quickly, leaving natural surface pits exposed to caries-causing bacteria. Cooking pulverized grains and other plant foods broke down carbohydrate bonds, releasing simpler forms that readily mix with saliva for easier digestion. Unfortunately, this mixture tends to leave a sticky film on teeth, an ideal medium for the growth of oral bacteria that form dental caries. The greater the reliance on cultivated foods, the greater the frequency of caries. Increase in oral bacteria also led to increase of periodontal disease and dental abscesses, with early tooth loss.

Nutritional needs were best met in the ecotones with abundant and diverse food resources. Early agriculture, combined with hunting, gathering, and fishing, provided optimum nutrition. Surplus foods could be stored and used to guard against hunger when food sources diminished during seasonal weather fluctuations.

Dietary changes brought on by more intensive agriculture created new problems with nutrition as people became more dependent on food crops. Caloric needs could be met, but nutritional needs were often neglected. More food did not always mean good nutrition. Overdependence on processed grain crops with few supplementary foods, especially protein foods, created nutritional deficiencies (Cohen and Armelagos 1984). Poor nutrition hampered immune systems and led to more disease.

Individuals suffering from debilitating injuries, congenital defects, and chronic illnesses that were not life threatening had a better chance for survival in a Neolithic village than in earlier groups that were frequently on the move. Their survival depended more on cultural acceptance than on the manner of subsistence.

CONCLUDING COMMENTS

For more than a million years our ancestors survived by hunting and foraging in small nomadic groups. Most diseases occurred at random, and acquired parasites were few. By the end of the Ice Age, between thirteen thousand and ten thousand years ago, human adaptation to environmental changes in many parts of the world dramatically altered human interaction with the environment and the patterns of human disease. The seeds of agriculture and the domestication of animals revolutionized human existence.

Humans began to settle down in one place to manipulate and alter their local environment with cultivation and the keeping of stock animals. Progressive forms of agriculture and stock raising, in many instances, breached the threshold of environmental tolerance of human interaction. This led to a reordering of the environment and the interactions between human beings and all other living organisms, both plant and animal, within the disturbed ecosystems. Many microbes and other parasites reacted to the new order by developing affinities to the human upstarts. Repeated exposure to infectious agents within the settled environment challenged human immune systems on a continuous basis, increasing the chances of infection, particularly chronic states of infection.

Eventually, as the new orders settled, the relationships between infectious agents and human population reached a level of fluctuating equilibrium within the disturbed ecosystems. Most individuals developed tolerance or resistance to local infections, while a lesser number, born with immune systems unable to fight off the infections, remained vulnerable, thereby helping to maintain the infection within each generation of the population. But the new order of fluctuating equilibrium between humans and microbes was to be breached again and again by new pressures from human and natural events throughout the course of history, drastically upsetting this delicate balance.

Neolithic cultural changes were not accepted uniformly. Many human populations preferred not to cross the environmental threshold with farming and domestication of animals, but remained a part of nature, surviving by hunting, foraging, and fishing, and living in small nomadic or seminomadic family groups. Those groups of people that clung to earlier ways of life continued to maintain the old disease patterns, as long as they remained separated from Neolithic peoples.

Increasing emphasis on agricultural crops as the main food sources for Neolithic peoples, along with alterations of the local environment, brought about dietary changes that were not always beneficial. Plentiful food supplies may have helped to increase numbers of people, but the quality and length of life may have been lessened because of repressed immunity resulting from poor nutrition interacting with disease. Growing dependence on specific food crops also meant greater vulnerability to famine brought on by climatic changes, such as long-term drought, and social upsets such as war.

Early Neolithic populations primarily increased in density while causing little change in the global population. Once agriculture became established throughout the world and agriculturalists adjusted to their newly
created environmental orders and new disease patterns, the global population began to gradually increase. This became possible with moderate
increases in infant survival rates (Pennington 1996) wherever basic nutritional needs were met. The global population as a whole began to expand to
an estimated 200 million to 400 million by A.D. 1, setting the stage for later
population explosions (Coale 1974).

The Neolithic development wrought many changes between humans
and the microbial world. Most of the diseases that haunt us today go back
to the development of centers for early agriculture and civilization, extending in a broad belt from the eastern Mediterranean to north Africa, the
Middle East, the Indian subcontinent, Southeast Asia, and East Asia.

Disease patterns changed, and continued to change with every progressive step toward the world as we know it today. Patterns of disease varied
according to the different geographic regions, wherever agriculture and civilization developed. Increasing population densities strained and polluted
environmental resources, leading to further insults and shakeups of local
ecosystems. Far-reaching trading networks, crossing different geographic
regions, led to trade in disease-carrying agents between different regions of
the world. The microbial pot was being stirred with increasing vigor, and disease patterns changed with each new human venture.

CHAPTER 5

MOSQUITOES, MALARIA, AND GENE WARS

Shifting Paradigms

Neolithic farmers planted the seeds of change that altered the way human beings interact with their environment. The delicate balance between all life forms within numerous ecosystems became increasingly subject to human intervention. Cultivation of the land disturbed the natural order of plant, insect, and animal interaction. Growing human populations demanding more cultivated foods created greater environmental disturbances. Wherever agriculture became a prominent way of life, it changed the environment. Forests were cleared, water management systems altered dry lands and alluvial river valleys, and controlled grazing of domestic stock contributed to changes in vegetation.

Mosquito populations have survived evolutionary changes for more than 25 million years, adapting easily to shifts in their menu of available blood sources, from giant reptiles to mammals and birds. Large Pleistocene mammals played a major role in the survival of many types of mosquitoes. With the demise of the Ice Age mammals, mosquitoes that depended on their blood for survival shifted to any available large, warm-blooded animal within their range (Edman 1991). The larger and more numerous the animals, the better the mosquitoes' chance of survival.

Blood meals are important for the development of the fertilized eggs within the female, but the developing young that hatch from these eggs also have special needs. The specific water and food requirements of young larvae limit the range of the parent mosquitoes, and this limitation frequently influenced the selection of host animal types. Environmental upsets that altered the selection of their natural animal hosts forced the majority of mosquitoes to adapt to other animal sources of blood again and again.

Small groups of nomadic hunters and foragers were not the most desirable hosts for mosquitoes that depended on a steady source of mammal blood. Human blood contains less of the amino acid isoleucine than does the blood of other animals. This amino acid is necessary for protein synthesis in egg production within the female mosquito. Smaller amounts of isoleucine lead to smaller numbers of eggs (Edman 1991). Steady supplies of human blood would have to be available on a regular basis to make up for fewer eggs produced with each blood meal, and even then, most mosquitoes would still prefer animal blood if it were available.

Neolithic farmers taking up permanent residence within mosquito territory presented a different paradigm for mosquito interaction dependent on large animals. The shift from their natural animal hosts to human beings depended on the appetites of the indigenous mosquitoes, the presence or absence of natural hosts, the introduction of domestic animals, climatic conditions, and changing breeding and resting areas. Some mosquitoes adapted to the growing, densely packed human habitation sites that crowded out their natural animal hosts. They were primarily attracted to the domestic animals locked up in man-made structures, particularly cattle and pigs, and second to humans in houses. Natural daytime resting places in dense vegetation, caves, hollow trees, and overhanging stream banks were frequently replaced with dark regions of houses and animal shelters, particularly structures made of mud and thatch.

Warm houses and stables allowed some temperate zone mosquitoes to remain active throughout the winter months in parts of Europe. Deforestation, land cultivation, and water management systems wiped out many customary places to breed, but they also created new breeding sites for mosquitoes. Life for the newly acclimated mosquitoes was good, with plenty of places to breed and rest, and bountiful supplies of blood meals for the females, all within easy range.

This new paradigm brought human beings into repeated contact with tiny protozoan parasites known as plasmodia, carried by Anopheles mosquitoes. These parasites depend on the internal environment of the female mosquitoes for reproduction, and they use animal hosts to incubate their offspring.

Only certain types of Anopheles mosquitoes and their animal hosts will tolerate the parasites. Some of the plasmodia have adapted to humans along with
their mosquito carriers. Human infection with plasmodia produces malaria.

The evolutionary relationships between the definitive mosquito host,
the intermediate animal host, and the plasmodium parasite are ancient.
When humans became part of the cycle is debatable (Carter and Mendis
2002). Small groups of Paleolithic hunters and foragers in the tropical and
subtropical zones most likely suffered infection by some of the malaria parasites. The infection was probably short-lived, sporadic, and infrequent in
small groups of nomadic peoples frequently on the move. Most of the infected individuals probably had few symptoms. Hunting and foraging groups
surviving today where malaria is endemic do not have the severe malaria
characteristic of their sedentary agriculturalist neighbors. Traditional
nomadic peoples rarely maintain any of the genetic hemoglobin disturbances
associated with generations of sedentary peoples living in malaria endemic
areas (de Zuleta 1980; Livingstone 1986).

The animal hosts for the Anopheles mosquito act as the reservoir for
the plasmodium parasites. When animal hosts are few and far between, the
mosquito cannot obtain enough infectious plasmodial forms to maintain the
parasite population within its ranks. The parasite cannot be transferred
between infected mosquitoes, and if the infected female mosquito cannot
inject the parasite into an animal host, it dies with her. If the animal host population does not contain the infective forms of plasmodium, biting mosquitoes will not become infected, and the disease cycle will be broken. This cycle
would have been difficult to sustain in small nomadic groups of ancient
hunters and foragers (Grmek 1989).

The Neolithic agricultural revolution brought humans into greater and
more constant contact with Anopheles mosquitoes and also with their plasmodium parasites, particularly the more deadly forms. Malaria became a
major, established Neolithic disease. The plasmodium parasites thrived in
densely populated human settlements as the repetitive cycle of infection
between humans, mosquitoes, and plasmodium flourished (Livingstone 1986).

The Vectors of Malaria

Nearly five hundred species of Anopheles mosquitoes exist throughout the
world, but only a small percentage of them willingly bite humans (Busvine

1980). Not all Anopheles mosquitoes biting humans can sustain the plasmodia. Also, variation in susceptibility to the plasmodia exists within the same species, and each species has several variants. Not only do the mosquitoes have to be able to accept the parasites, they must survive long enough for them to reproduce and transmit their infectious offspring (Beck and Davies 1981; Horsfall 1972).

Infective mosquitoes need to live close to human dwellings in large numbers for the cycle of malaria to be maintained in the human population. The mosquitoes must be able to ingest a large number of infective forms of the parasite, and they must be willing to bite humans repeatedly. The cycle requires sufficient numbers of human and animal hosts to maintain the presence of the parasites. Climate and environment also have to be favorable for long-term mosquito survival and breeding (Beck and Davies 1981; Horsfall 1972).

Regardless of the limitations on the transmission and maintenance of malaria, Anopheles species capable of sustaining malaria parasites exist in almost every part of the world. Infected African slaves brought malaria to the New World. The parasites gained access to local Anopheles mosquitoes as they dined on the blood of the slaves. Thus, local Anopheles capable of accepting the plasmodia spread the disease in various parts of the Americas. Similarly, infected individuals from malaria-infested regions introduced malaria to Europe, parts of Central Asia, the Near East, and the Pacific Islands, and this danger still exists today. The introduction of the malarial plasmodia into new Anopheles species created new strains of the parasites, some with greater or less vigor, depending on the new mosquito environment (Bates 1949).

The most important mosquito vectors relevant to the rise and spread of malaria come from the regions of the Old World where agriculture and animal husbandry took over, pushing out and replacing their natural wild animal hosts. Various Anopheles species and strains adapted to different geographic regions, differing in their choice of breeding places and blood feeding habits. Most Anopheles mosquitoes prefer cattle and other domestic animal blood over human blood, and will bite humans only as a second choice. All of them hide from the sun during the day, like vampires, seeking dark, shaded places to rest. Some females prefer to lay their eggs in clear pools of water, others prefer brackish water pools. Sunlight also plays a role in the selection of a breeding place. Soil disturbance caused by humans greatly enhances mosquito breeding places by creating places for water to puddle (Horsfall 1972).

The most notorious and prolific carriers of the deadliest form of malaria, caused by falciparum parasites, belong to the *Anopheles gambiae* group of tropical central Africa. Gambiae females lay their eggs in rain pools or wherever water is trapped and receiving direct sunlight, shunning shaded areas. Gambiae eggs are tough, able to withstand drying out of water pools during the dry season, and able to survive the ravages of wet season floods by clinging to grass stems (Horsfall 1972).

Infected gambiae mosquitoes traveled down the Nile River into Egypt, and from there some variants, carried by ships, spread the falciparum parasites to warm, moist subtropical agricultural regions of the eastern Mediterranean. Some infected gambiae were accidentally transported by ship to Brazil in 1930. The invaders were soon eradicated, however, following an outbreak of malaria in 1938 (Burnet and White 1972).

The clearing of land by farmers for cultivation and the trampling of soil by stock animals created ideal breeding places for these mosquitoes. Hoofprints, wallows, cultivation furrows, roadside ditches, borrow pits, and wheel tracks, along with deforestation, provided ample rain pools for the eggs. Gambiae mosquitoes quickly adapted to human settlements and developed a preference for the blood of humans as well as domestic livestock. Gambiae females enter houses or sleeping sheds at night to feed, but they normally spend the daylight hours resting along stream banks, in termite mounds, or in other sheltered, dark and cool places (Horsfall 1971; Russell et al. 1943).

Anopheles funestus is another common tropical African mosquito vector for falciparum parasites, found in the same regions as the tropical gambiae. Funestus mosquito eggs are more susceptible to drying than gambiae eggs, and the larvae prefer clear water with partial shade. These mosquitoes also readily bite humans, entering houses to feed at night. The females remain there to rest until they leave to lay their eggs. Smoking fires will drive them out to their natural resting places in dense stands of grass, hollow trees, and along stream banks. Funestus will also feed on domestic cattle and goats (Horsfall 1971; Russell et al. 1943).

The rise of agriculture and animal husbandry in the Indian subcontinent created new havens for *Anopheles stephensi* mosquitoes and their malaria-producing plasmodium parasites, known as vivax. These mosquitoes adapted easily to human settlements, attracted primarily by domestic cattle. Some variants developed a preference for human blood, while others only turn to humans as a second choice. They enter cattle sheds and houses to feed, and the larvae thrive wherever water is contained in any kind of cavity or manmade container. They will breed in wells, cisterns, flowerpots, roof gutters, and masonry reservoirs (Horsfall 1972).

A. *Stephensi* is found in the Indus Valley, where the great Harappan civilization developed from early farming villages, from around 2700 B.C. to 1700 B.C. (Fagan 1996). Malaria carried by this mosquito may have played a role in the demise of this early civilization (de Zuleta 1980).

The early shipping trade from India to the Middle East spread *A. Stephensi* mosquitoes and their malaria-producing vivax parasites westward to oases around the Persian Gulf, the irrigated river valleys of Mesopotamia, and eastward into Burma (de Zuleta 1980) and Thailand.

The spread of malaria throughout Europe was facilitated by a group of mosquitoes known as the *Maculipennis* complex, primarily consisting of three major types with several variants: *M. atroparvus*, *M. labranchiae*, and *M. sacharovi*. They followed the agricultural revolution, as land was cleared for cultivation. Because they were naturally attracted to any large animal within range, they turned to humans and their domestic animals as the blood sources of choice. Preferring to attack under cover, they sought out manmade shelters (de Zuleta 1980).

All three types within the *Maculipennis* complex prefer to breed in coastal marshes. Some atroparvus variants will also breed in sunlit freshwater pools, and in Spain they adapted to breeding in rice fields when rice cultivation was introduced by the Arabs. Some sacharovi mosquitoes can breed in sunlit brackish inland marshes, and some labranchiae mosquitoes will breed in surface water covered by algae, such as springs, cisterns, pools, or ponds. Adults of all three types can survive for a certain period of time during the winter months in an inactive state, surviving on fat reserves stored in the fall. Many of them remain active in the warmth of human or domestic animal shelters during the cold months (Horsfall 1972). The incubation period of the plasmodium parasites injected into human hosts during the winter months is prolonged, and thus symptoms of malaria do not develop until summer arrives (Burnet and White 1972).

Labranchiae moved into the Mediterranean region from north Africa, thriving along the Mediterranean and Dalmatian coasts, especially Italy, southern Greece, and Asia Minor. They also moved up along the shores of the steppe zone around the Black and Caspian Seas, and the upper Arabian Peninsula. Sacharovi arrived from West Asia to range along the coasts of northeastern and central Italy, Sardinia, and the Balkans. Sacharovi mosquitoes also entered central Russia, the trans-Caucasus, the Middle East, and eventually western China (Horsfall 1972; Russell et al. 1943). Atroparvus appears to be indigenous to Spain, spreading up the coast of Western Europe, and it may have been introduced to the coastal areas of Italy by ships (de Zuleta 1980).

Vectors responsible for malaria in the temperate regions of Europe and Central Asia belong to the *Anopheles clavinger* mosquitoes. Primarily a woodland species, they can withstand the long winters and cool summers of temperate regions. When the females become active, they will bite any large animal that enters their territory. The cold-adapted larvae can remain dormant beneath iced-over breeding pools throughout the winter (Horsfall 1972; Russell et al. 1943).

Some clavinger variants also exist in the woodlands of Asia Minor, the Levant, and parts of north Africa. The larvae require acidic water, preferring small ponds rich in vegetation, marshes, and shallow rock pools. The females will lay their eggs in cisterns and wells, especially in the Levant region where they are the major malaria carrier. Other variants along the east coast of the Black Sea near the Caucasus Mountains spend the summer in mountain streams and the rest of the year along the coast. Some readily enter houses within their territory, while others prefer stables of domestic animals. They will travel long distances to feed and breed (Horsfall 1972; Russell et al. 1943).

Several different Anopheles mosquitoes in Asia can transmit malaria parasites. One common group of malaria vectors in Asia, the *Anopheles minimus* complex, ranges over most of tropical and subtropical Asia, from India to China. The females prefer to lay their eggs in margins of clear, flowing water sources with partial shade, and the larvae cling to overhanging plant roots or filaments of green algae. The grassy edges of irrigation ditches and rice fields provide ideal breeding places, and the females are attracted to humans and domestic animals. Agriculture enabled these mosquitoes to become acclimated to humans, increase in numbers, and spread throughout Asia. They prefer to rest during the day under beds in bamboo and mud huts, clinging to wall hangings, and in wood piles. Many variants prefer human blood, while some will bite humans and domestic animals equally. Originally they would bite any large animal within range (Horsfall 1972; Russell et al. 1943).

Another successful Asian mosquito vector of malaria parasites is *Anopheles sundaicus*. These mosquitoes, found along the coasts of India and Southeast Asia, prefer brackish waters with floating mats of algae. Their numbers increase during the dry season when tidal pools become brackish with the lack of rain. Larvae can also survive in saline pools formed by domestic animal urine, and in rice fields. They easily adapted to human settlements, entering houses and cow sheds to feed indiscriminately on human beings, cattle, or water buffalo. Some variants bite humans only when there is no other choice (Horsfall 1972; Russell et al. 1943).

Evolution of Malaria

The distribution of malaria and the mosquito vectors of malaria parasites in the Old World followed the origins and spread of agriculture and animal husbandry. Malaria spread with ever increasing human contacts over a tropical-subtropical belt extending from the Mediterranean region, sub-Saharan Africa, Mesopotamia, the Indian subcontinent, and Southeast Asia, with incursions into the neighboring temperate zones at various times throughout human history. The extensive spread of malaria was possible because the plasmodia carried by humans could infect the many varieties of blood-sucking Anopheles mosquitoes indigenous to each region. Expanding trade routes, the slave trade, migrations, invasions, and manmade environmental disturbances facilitated the spread of malaria and several mosquito vectors of malaria throughout the world (de Zuleta 1980).

Malaria actually consists of four different diseases with similar symptoms, caused by four different types of plasmodia: *Plasmodium malariae*, *Plasmodium vivax*, *Plasmodium ovale*, and *Plasmodium falciparum*. Other plasmodia infect reptiles, birds, and other mammals (Busvine 1980), but not humans. Some of the plasmodia infecting monkeys and apes appear similar to those infecting humans, and this strongly suggests that the human types evolved from the primate types. The reverse phenomenon occurs also, where primates contract the plasmodia from humans in endemic malarial areas. This seems to be the case with chimpanzees in west and central Africa with *P. vivax* and *P. malariae* (T-W-Fiennes 1967).

Vivax causes most of the human malaria infections in the world. South and Southeast Asia appear to be the place of origin for *P. vivax*, where it has an identical counterpart, *P. cynomolgi*, affecting macaque monkeys.

These monkeys once ranged from Southeast Asia throughout the Indian subcontinent, the Middle East, and the Mediterranean basin, adapting to temperate climates as well as tropical and subtropical climates. With the agricultural revolution and increasing human populations pushing the monkeys out of their natural habitats, vivax could have switched from the monkey host to the human host (Livingstone 1984) with a mosquito vector willing to bite both monkeys and humans. *Plasmodium malariae* may have originated alongside *P. vivax* from another monkey plasmodium known as *P. knowlesi.*

Plasmodium ovale and *Plasmodium falciparum* most likely evolved in tropical Africa. Ovale infects monkeys as well as humans in west Africa. Chimpanzees in west and central Africa carry a plasmodium, *P. reichenowi*, similar to the human falciparum plasmodium. However, reichenowi infecting chimpanzees is carried by different Anopheles mosquitoes than those transmitting falciparum to humans (T-W-Fiennes 1967). Some of the chimpanzee plasmodia may have been transferred and adapted to humans as they crowded out the chimpanzees from their natural range in west Africa when agriculture was introduced to this region. Gambiae and funestus mosquitoes could then have picked it up from the infected human hosts.

Most likely, all of the plasmodia types evolved from free-living opportunistic protozoa in the tropics long before modern humans appeared, perhaps adapting to primate animal gut environments after being ingested. With invasion of the bloodstream and adaptation to red blood cells for incubation, the plasmodia would have been available for blood-sucking mosquitoes (Busvine 1980). Apparently the internal fluid environment of the female Anopheles mosquito triggered reproduction within the mosquito. Eventually, the cycle between mosquito and animal host developed, replacing a cycle between animal gut and moist external environment.

The four different plasmodia that cause malaria vary in ability to cause disease. Malariae parasites produce the mildest form of malaria, suggesting *Plasmodium malariae* as the oldest of the human plasmodia (Chandler 1945), followed by ovale and vivax. Ovale appears to have evolved in response to natural resistance to vivax within certain west African populations, generally producing a fairly mild form of malaria. Vivax is the most adaptable of the malaria parasites, since it can survive in several different vectors and temperature zones. *Plasmodium vivax* produces the most common form of chronic malaria. Falciparum has high virulence and causes deadly malaria, suggesting that this parasite had a more recent introduction into human populations than the other plasmodia. The other three plasmodia types may have been more virulent when first introduced to humans, but then reached a maintenance level of equilibrium with their human hosts.

The Lives of the Plasmodia Parasites of Malaria

All four types of plasmodia responsible for malaria have similar life cycles and produce similar disease symptoms. The life cycle includes a nonsexual reproductive phase in the human host, alternating with a sexual reproductive phase in the female mosquito. Time for completion of this cycle varies with each species, varying from eight to thirty-five days, and fluctuates with environmental temperature changes (Yaeger 1985).

Once the offspring of the parasites are injected into the host, a long process begins in which the young plasmodia reproduce and transform themselves through a series of multiple divisions. Some of them eventually develop into immature sexually reproductive male and female cells known as gameteocytes. The gametocytes circulate in the peripheral bloodstream, waiting to be sucked up by the female mosquito. Only these forms of the parasite can survive and develop into reproductive parasites in the mosquito. All other immature forms included in the mosquito's blood meal are digested and destroyed in the mosquito's gut.

The male and female gametocytes escape digestion and mature within the mosquito gut into complete male and female reproductive cells known as gametes. The mature male and female gametes unite and produce a fertilized egg, the zygote. The zygote elongates into an ookinete, able to move about on its own. This mobile egg penetrates the mosquito's stomach wall. Once outside the mosquito's stomach, it forms a round sac-like structure, called an oocyst, in the outer membrane of the stomach wall. The oocyst then expands rapidly with numerous developing immature offspring, known as sporozoites. The overextended oocyst ruptures and releases them, and the fledgling sporozoites migrate to the mosquito's salivary glands. The bite of the mosquito releases the sporozoites along with the mosquito's saliva into the victim's bloodstream (Beck and Davies 1981; Yaeger 1985).

Within a half-hour following the bite of the mosquito, the sporozoites travel through the bloodstream to invade the cells of the liver. For some unexplained reason, the liver cells suffer little pathology from the invading parasites. The liver cells provide the nourishment for the sporozoites to develop into schizonts that divide and multiply, producing thousands of the next immature phase of the parasite, known as merozoites.

The liver cells release the merozoites by the seventh or eighth day. Once released, merozoites trigger reaction from the B cells of the host's immune system to manufacture specific immunoglobins (antibodies), IgM and IgG, against them. The immunoglobins mark them for destruction by phagocytic macrophages located in the spleen, liver, and bone marrow before they enter the red blood cells. Infected red blood cells are also targeted for destruction (Jones 1975a).

Merozoites that can escape the reactions of the immune system invade the red blood cells to complete the next phase of their development. Some of the vivax and ovale merozoites also enter other liver cells for another round of division within the liver. Vivax and ovale parasites can easily maintain a constant supply of their progeny in the liver cells of the host for long periods of time, creating recurrences of malaria. Falciparum and malariae lack the ability to maintain a store of their progeny in the liver cells, so malaria does not recur, unless merozoites can be maintained in the blood tissues (Beck and Davies 1981; Yaeger 1985).

The final and most devastating assault on the human body by the plasmodia parasites takes place in the red blood cells. The disk-shaped red blood cells are responsible for transporting life-giving oxygen from the lungs throughout the body tissues and taking away the gas waste product of cellular respiration, carbon dioxide, to the lungs to be expelled. This takes place within the hemoglobin in the red blood cells.

Utilizing the oxygen carried within the hemoglobin molecule and subsisting on the globin proteins, the merozoites divide and transform into another immature form, known as trophozoites, that in turn divide and transform into schizonts. Each schizont, thriving on the oxygen and broken-down proteins within the hemoglobin, produces new merozoites, varying in shape and number according to plasmodium species. With the final destruction of the red blood cell, these merozoites are released into the bloodstream and gain entry into other red blood cells to repeat the cycle. The classic overt signs of malaria—chills, fever, and sweating—occur during this phase of release of the merozoites from the red blood cells. As the number of merozoites increases, the number of viable, circulating red blood cells decreases, producing anemia in the host. Following a number of these red blood cell cycles, some trophozoites transform into immature sexual gametocytes (Beck and Davies 1981; Yaeger 1985).

How long the gametocytes, the only infective agents of the parasite, can remain viable in the human host's bloodstream depends on the species of plasmodia. The gametocytes of vivax can persist in the blood for one to three years, while gametocytes of malariae can persist indefinitely, and gametocytes of falciparum generally last no more than one year (Benenson 1970). This assures the spread of malaria by way of human carriers traveling to other regions where susceptible Anopheles mosquitoes can become infected. However, maintenance of the infection in the new region depends on several factors: the numbers of mosquitoes and their blood feeding habits, the number of human hosts, climate, and environmental conditions.

Vivax Family

Plasmodium vivax is the most common and widespread of the infectious plasmodia, responsible for about 80 percent of all malaria, and the only plasmodium species represented in the cooler temperate zones. Within eight days of infection, each invading sporozoite finding its way into the liver can produce more than ten thousand merozoites. The merozoites released from the liver into the circulating bloodstream are slow to invade the red blood cells. This allows the host immune system's phagocytic macrophages time to destroy most of them, limiting the number invading red blood cells. The macrophages can eventually destroy all of the merozoites coming from the liver as the disease progresses (Yaeger 1985).

Vivax merozoites only invade young red blood cells. They complete the asexual reproductive cycle within the infected red blood cell within thirty-six hours after invasion. The red blood cell swells as twelve to twenty-four new merozoites develop. They are released into the bloodstream by the damaged cell by the forty-eighth hour, to repeat the cycle in uninfected red blood cells. The infectious sexual gametocytes appear in the host's bloodstream after one or more red blood cell cycles. Temperate zone vivax strains can undergo a prolonged incubation period in the liver cells for up to ten months while the mosquito vectors lie inactive throughout cold weather. Sporozoites can also remain dormant in liver cells for several years (Beck and Davies 1981; Yaeger 1985).

All stages of development can overlap within the host in the beginning of the infection. Eventually, the red blood cell cycles synchronize to occur at the same time, every forty-eight hours (Beck and Davies 1981).

Malariae Family

The malariae plasmodium coexists with vivax in tropical areas, but it is quite rare and spotty in distribution. The incubation period in liver cells takes about thirteen days, with about two thousand merozoites produced by each sporozoite, far fewer than those produced by vivax. Smaller numbers of merozoites produced results in fewer parasites entering the blood, and the long time it takes for them to enter red blood cells allows macrophages to destroy most of them (Yaeger 1985).

Unlike vivax, *Plasmodium malariae* invades only older red blood cells, and it takes seventy-two hours for six to twelve merozoites to develop and be released from the infected red blood cell. The red blood cell cycle synchronizes from the beginning. The parasite, the smallest of the four plasmodia infecting humans, uses less hemoglobin in the red blood cell. This leaves the infected red blood cell near normal size. There are fewer infectious gametocytes produced as well, but they can remain at very low levels in the host bloodstream for many years (Beck and Davies 1981; Yaeger 1985).

Ovale Family

Plasmodium ovale primarily occurs in tropical forests of west Africa among human populations resistant to vivax. Small enclaves of ovale plasmodia also exist in Papua New Guinea and the Philippines (Livingstone 1984). The parasite closely resembles *Plasmodium vivax* in certain aspects of the red blood cell cycle, but in other ways it more clearly mirrors *Plasmodium malariae*. Ovale can have a prolonged latent incubation period, anywhere from one to four years, before the sporozoites become activated in the liver cells to produce red blood cell infection. Each sporozoite can produce up to fifteen thousand merozoites (Jones 1975a). Nonsexual reproduction by division progresses slowly in the liver cells. Once released from the liver cells, the merozoites prefer to invade only young red blood cells, sometimes two merozoites to a cell, where each schizont produces eight to nine merozoites within a forty-eight-hour cycle. Like vivax sporozoites, dormant ovale sporozoites can be maintained in liver cells for many years (Beck and Davies 1981; de Zuleta 1980; Yaeger 1985).

Falciparum Family

Plasmodium falciparum, the most deadly of the human malaria parasites, has spread throughout the tropical and subtropical parts of the world, with many different variants adapting to different regions. The incubation period for sporozoites in the liver cells is only six days, and each sporozoite produces about forty thousand merozoites. Once the merozoites leave the liver cells, they cannot reinfect those cells, and none remains behind to cause recurrence. Without further infection from mosquito vectors, the disease generally lasts no longer than ten months. Upon release from the liver, the merozoites rapidly invade the red blood cells with little loss of merozoites to phagocytosis by macrophages. The merozoites have no preference for young or older red blood cells, and will invade any red blood cell that is available (Beck and Davies 1981: Yaeger 1985).

Unlike infected red blood cells from the other plasmodia that continue to circulate throughout the bloodstream at all times, falciparum-infected red blood cells stick to the lining of small blood vessels within the capillary beds of the internal organs. The falciparum infection alters the surface of the parasitized red blood cell so that it can adhere to the small blood vessel walls. This protects the parasite by keeping the infected red blood cell away from the phagocytic macrophages anchored in the spleen and liver. Clumps of these infected red blood cells can block the flow of capillary blood to the brain, lungs, and kidneys, causing serious damage to these organs.

Release of the new merozoites, usually from eight to twenty-four of them, from infected red blood cells occurs within thirty-six to forty-eight hours after invasion. They quickly invade other nearby red blood cells, and it is common to find more than one, frequently several, merozoites invading the same red blood cell. Rapidly increasing numbers of merozoites can lead to dangerously low levels of functioning red blood cells, and this can cause severe anemia and collapse of tiny blood vessels. The release of infectious gametocytes from infected red blood cells occurs relatively late in the course of the disease, and they circulate throughout the body to surface areas where the mosquitoes can pick them up (Beck and Davies 1981; Yaeger 1985).

The Disease Complex

Severe anemia is caused by the massive destruction of infected red blood cells. Normally aging red blood cells, with an average lifespan of 100–120 days, are recycled through the spleen and liver along with damaged red blood cells. Localized macrophages digest and break down the old and damaged cells, releasing hemoglobin components for reuse (Williams et al. 1989). The presence of high concentrations of red blood cells destroyed by the parasites causes the macrophages to proliferate, enlarging the spleen and causing congestion of the liver.

Normal red blood cell recycling involves disassembling of the globin proteins with amino acids directed to the general pool of amino acids for reuse. The heme iron recycles into newly formed red blood cells forming in the red bone marrow as the old ones die. High losses of functioning red blood cells cause the bone marrow cells to enlarge with increased production in an attempt to replace those rapidly being destroyed. Excess heme iron recycled from hemoglobin not used directly in the synthesis of the new red blood cells gets stored in the liver. The liver converts excess iron to bilirubin to be excreted through the bile (Williams et al. 1989). The breakdown of too many red blood cells at one time increases the amount of excess heme iron building up in the liver, which in turn creates too much bilirubin. Excess bilirubin circulates in the bloodstream, producing a jaundiced yellow color of the skin and eyes that is frequently seen with chronic malaria.

The symptoms of malaria, outside of a feeling of general discomfort and low-grade fever, usually do not appear until after one or more red blood cell cycles of the parasite have been completed. When a large number of red blood cells rupture, simultaneously releasing the merozoites, the immune system swings into high gear and the classic symptoms appear: shaking chills, high fever, and profuse sweating that may last for several hours. The high fever causes headache, accompanied by backache, muscle ache, abdominal discomfort, and nausea. The entire episode can last eight to ten or more hours, followed by a feeling of relief coupled with exhaustion. This respite lasts only a short while before the cycle repeats itself with the release of another new brood of parasites into the bloodstream. The first attack may last a week, a month, or longer, with recurrences. The attack can be deadly for the very young and for those individuals with compromised immune systems (Beck and Davies 1981; Benenson 1970).

The different forms that the plasmodia take creates confusion for the immune system; different species and even different strains of the same species challenge the immune system with a wide array of antigenic properties. The major assault on malaria parasites by the immune system begins with the release of the first merozoites into the bloodstream from the liver. The stimulated phagocytic lymphocytes and macrophages increase production up to two hundred times their normal rate in an effort to eliminate the parasites from the blood. They are also stimulated to engulf parasitized red blood cells and other foreign material. They may even attack normal, uninfected red blood cells in their zeal to destroy the invader (Barriga 1981).

Immunoglobins that mark the merozoites for destruction cannot identify other forms of the parasite. B cells must produce different immunoglobins to recognize each form. Immunoglobins designed for a specific strain of plasmodium may not recognize another strain of the same type. Eventually, without reinfection, the healthy immune system will acquire resistance or tolerance to whatever parasitic variants and their different forms exist within the host, and malaria symptoms will disappear.

The parasitic form within the liver and the infectious gametocytes for some reason appear not to provoke the immune system, allowing these forms to survive for varying periods without causing any symptoms of malaria. Some immune systems become overzealous in response to falciparum malaria. They create new immunoglobins against the immunoglobin-antigen complex formed by their own immunoglobins as they combine with the antigens of the parasite to promote their destruction by phagocytosis. Chaos ensues, and the disease takes over, particularly in very young children (Barriga 1981).

Benign Tertian Malaria/Vivax Malaria

Malaria caused by *Plasmodium vivax* begins with mixed stages of development and release, with feelings of general discomfort and low-grade fever, until one synchronized brood dominates to begin the forty-eight-hour cycle of chills, high fever, and sweating. The initial cyclic series diminishes in intensity for about the first two weeks, depending on strain and host immunity, followed by a symptom-free period that lasts about two weeks. Another, less intense attack follows with a series of short-term recurrences of newly released merozoites from red blood cells that continues for about two months. Finally, a prolonged period of inactivity (latency) occurs as the red blood cell-produced merozoites die out (Beck and Davies 1981; Yaeger 1985).

Relapses frequently take place after six to nine months, and continue over a period of two to three years, as new merozoites are released from the liver. Relapses can be triggered by a physiological upset, such as pregnancy, alcoholism, or another infection. Usually the malarial infection dies out after relapse in the absence of reinfection (Beck and Davies 1981).

Quartan Malaria/Malariae Malaria

Plasmodium malarie produces symptoms similar to vivax malaria, but follows a seventy-two-hour cycle, sometimes with more severe attacks. Short-term recurrences of newly released merozoites from red blood cells can occur after several weeks, months, or years, in the absence of reinfection. This results from persistence of merozoites in red blood cells at low levels (Yaeger 1985).

This particular plasmodium can invoke a peculiar immune response that seriously damages the kidneys, a condition known as quartan malarial nephropathy. This disorder appears to result from the reaction of the immune system, in individuals with high counts of circulating antimalarial immunoglobins to a specific malariae strain. Reinfection with this strain produces an immune reaction that binds the immunoglobin-antigen complex to the membranous covering of the glomeruli, the lobulated collections of capillary blood vessels in the kidneys. This blocks blood flow through the kidneys and eventually causes kidney failure (Beck and Davies 1981; Yaeger 1985).

Ovale Benign Tertian Malaria/Ovale Malaria

Plasmodium ovale causes symptoms similar to those of vivax malaria, with a similar forty-eight-hour cycle. Ovale plasmodia produce a mild, short-term disease. Fever is less intense than in the other malarias, with a slower build-up of merozoites in the bloodstream. Relapses caused by the release of merozoites from liver cells occur less frequently with ovale malaria than with vivax malaria, and usually persist no longer than one year (Beck and Davies 1981; Yaeger 1985).

Malignant Tertian Malaria/ Falciparum Malaria

Plasmodium falciparum causes the most dangerous type of malaria, with many complications that can be life-threatening. Early symptoms may mimic the flu or a cold. The first cyclic attack may be hardly detectable or with sudden chills less pronounced than in vivax malaria. The temperature rises quickly, is sustained for many hours, then dips, rises again, and eventually peaks, followed by a short sweating period. The cycles can vary from thirty-six to forty-eight hours, and one cycle of released merozoites may extend into the next, with little or no break between the cycles. The initial attack is frequently followed by recurrences during the first month, with periods of rest between attacks gradually increasing after three to five months. The disease generally does not last longer than one year, and there are no relapses (Beck and Davies 1981).

Many of the complications from falciparum malaria result from blocked capillary blood flow to major organs. Thus, the effects of falciparum infection can vary according to host immunity, numbers of parasites, and organs involved with impeded blood flow.

The massive numbers and aggressiveness of released merozoites in their attack on the red blood cells can lead to severe anemia as the number of healthy circulating red blood cells dramatically declines. Excessive numbers of merozoites combined with the reaction of the immune system also produce extremely high temperatures, headache, delirium, cyanosis (bluish discoloration of the skin), and hemorrhage within internal organs from back-up pressure in blocked capillaries. Coma and death can follow within a few hours. Collapse of the entire circulatory system can occur with massive invasion of the network of small blood vessels surrounding the organs in the abdomen. The victim becomes markedly cold with clammy skin, and dies (Beck and Davies 1981).

Cerebral malaria develops when the small blood vessels of the brain are blocked. Cerebral malaria occurs primarily in young children with an overzealous immune response to the merozoites through a build-up of immunoglobin-antigen complexes in the tiny blood vessels. Children suffering from malnutrition rarely develop cerebral malaria since their immune systems cannot produce enough immunoglobins to form the complexes (Barriga 1981). Symptoms of cerebral malaria may appear suddenly or gradually, with behavior changes or seizures, followed by coma and death (Beck and Davies 1981).

When blockage affects the liver, the victim can suffer extreme nausea, severe and constant vomiting, gastric distress, pronounced jaundice, and hemorrhaging into the stomach. This is known as the bilious form of malaria. Blockage in the intestinal capillary beds, known as the choleric form of malaria, produces profuse diarrhea and severe dehydration (Beck and Davies 1981).

Individuals suffering from repeated infection with the same strain of falciparum, and those treated inadequately with quinine, can have such massive destruction of the red blood cells that hemoglobin from these cells builds up in the blood and exceeds the liver's ability to break it down. The excess hemoglobin shows up in the urine as the kidneys try to eliminate it.

This is known as black water fever since the urine turns dark red (hemoglo-
binuria) from the fractured hemoglobin. Black water fever begins suddenly
with a severe chill and extreme exhaustion, followed by a rapid rise in temperature, and pain over the kidneys. Nausea, vomiting, and a rapid, feeble
pulse ensue. Renal failure and death occur in about 50 percent of affected
individuals (Beck and Davies 1981; Yaeger 1985).

Variants of falciparum parasites in pregnant women can adhere to
small blood vessel walls of the placenta and infect the red blood cells nourishing the fetus. This can lead to premature delivery, anemia, and death for
both infant and mother. Surviving mothers can eventually develop immunity to these variants in succeeding pregnancies (Fried and Duffy 1996).

Mixed Plasmodial Infections

Individuals can be infected with more than one plasmodium species, and the
different species are antagonistic toward one another. Vivax and falciparum
plasmodia frequently occur together in most endemic areas (Burnet and
White 1972). The dominating plasmodium will display the major symptoms.
Falciparum dominates over vivax, while vivax dominates over ovale and
malariae. Once the dominant species has run its course, the suppressed
species can then take over and cause malarial relapse (Yeager 1985).

Endemic versus Epidemic Malaria

Endemic malaria occurs wherever a large human population maintains some
degree of constant infection of one or more of the malarial parasites with
reexposure throughout life. Young children, individuals with compromised
immune systems, and women pregnant for the first time are typically most
affected by the disease, and often suffer a high death rate.

Children who survive the ravages of repeated attacks of malaria gradually develop some immunity or tolerance to the malarial parasites with age.
Adults can withstand repeated infection by the same plasmodium parasite
if their immunity becomes well established. However, acquired immunity
to one type or strain of plasmodium parasite does not provide protection
from a newly introduced one.

Most endemic malarial areas coincide with poor agricultural regions.
Generally low mortality (death) but high morbidity (disease) from chronic
malaria exists among adults where malnutrition interferes with proper

immunity. Chronic malaria with fatigue verging on exhaustion and mental disturbances prevails with poor nutrition and reinfection.

Malaria can be maintained within an endemic area as long as people receive a sufficient number of mosquito bites each night to keep the plasmodia within the human population (Livingstone 1986). Tipping the balance between numbers of biting mosquitoes and numbers of human hosts can lead to a gradual reduction and demise of the malarial parasites. Long-lasting climatic changes, such as cold or dry spells affecting mosquito numbers; environmental or manmade changes affecting mosquito breeding places; and cultural practices, such as use of net barriers or insecticides, affecting transmission to humans, can shift the paradigm.

Epidemic malaria occurs on a seasonal basis with a rapid rise in the mosquito population when the environment is more conducive to breeding. Loss of immunity, and poor nutrition from crop failures, can also lead to seasonal outbreaks. Epidemic malaria can occur when introduced to a human population for the first time, either by a human carrier or by an infected mosquito vector, or when a new strain of a plasmodium is introduced. There tends to be greater mortality and morbidity among all age groups with epidemic malaria.

Surviving the New Order through Genetics

Malaria's greatest threat is to the very young with immature immune systems unable to handle initial and repeated infections. Newborns can gain some protection from a healthy maternal immune response to malaria, but the greatest protection from malaria parasites for the newborn comes from the continuation of fetal hemoglobin circulating in the baby's blood for the first few weeks of life. Fetal hemoglobin, designed for oxygen uptake from the mother's circulatory system before birth, gradually becomes replaced with mature hemoglobin after birth. Fetal hemoglobin takes up and gives off oxygen at lower oxygen tensions than does mature hemoglobin. Malaria parasites cannot survive in fetal hemoglobin; they require the higher oxygen tension of mature hemoglobin to survive and complete their red blood cell cycle. But these protections are short-lived as fetal hemoglobin is replaced by mature hemoglobin and the mother's protective antibodies fade, leaving the baby to cope with its own developing immune system.

Throughout all of the regions where malaria became endemic during the Neolithic agricultural revolution, genetic responses evolved (Livingstone

1986) to combat malaria. Genetic responses developed primarily to protect the very young from the ravages of malaria and increase their chances for survival. Hemoglobin mutations developed to mimic the properties of fetal hemoglobin that retard malaria parasite development and allow the young victim to survive to adulthood.

Over four hundred hemoglobin variants (Pauling 1994) have evolved in response to malaria, with different populations exhibiting different genetic responses. The very complexity of the hemoglobin molecule invites variations to occur. Many of the hemoglobin variants are scattered and confined to small population groups, but some have widespread distributions. Hemoglobin variants, as well as malaria, spread to different regions of the world with population movements, migrations, and the slave trade. Some populations acquired more than one hemoglobin variant as a result of mixing among different populations (Livingstone 1986).

Wherever malaria did not exist, no specific genetic hemoglobin variants associated with the disease developed. Native Americans, in particular, have no hemoglobin variants responsive to malaria (Black 1980). Hemoglobin variants are maintained only by endemic malaria selection, and Livingstone (1986) estimates that it only took twenty to thirty generations (about five hundred years) for a hemoglobin variant to reach a stable frequency level within a gene pool affected by endemic malaria.

Normal hemoglobin consists of two pairs of unlike proteins, known as globin chains, each holding an iron-containing heme group. Each globin chain is produced by a separate gene that can produce many such variations. One pair of globin genes are clustered on chromosome 16 and code for the alpha globin chain and its embryonic precursor, as well as a zeta globin chain. The other pair of globin genes cluster on chromosome 11 and code for embryonic precursors to fetal (gamma), beta, and delta globin chains. This makes it possible for several variants to occur with only slight alterations in the combinations of amino acids that make up the globin chains (Steinberg and Embury 1994).

Most adult hemoglobin contains two alpha and two beta chains. Some adult hemoglobin substitutes two delta chains for the beta chains. Hemoglobin forming in the embryo gives way to fetal gamma and alpha hemoglobin within the first few months of pregnancy. Fetal gamma hemoglobin persists for up to six weeks after birth, before giving way to beta or delta globin chains (Steinberg and Embury 1994; Williams et al. 1989).

Most mutations in globin genes occur with substitution of one amino acid for another. Some mutations cause reduced or absent hemoglobin molecules, and/or allow persistence of fetal hemoglobin. Combinations of these mutations can occur in the same individual (Adams 1986). Varying degrees of protection from malaria parasites can be obtained with a variety of hemoglobin changes, as long as the normal activities of the nonparasitized red blood cells can be carried out.

Some abnormal hemoglobins can be potentially dangerous in themselves. The major problem with these variants occurs when an individual inherits the same dangerous abnormal variant globin chain (haplotype) from both parents. This is known as being homozygous for the abnormal hemoglobin. The double dose of the same genetic variant can be fatal in the most severe hemoglobin abnormalities. The individual who inherits the dangerous abnormal variant from only one parent, and who is thus heterozygous for the abnormal hemoglobin, can be protected by the normal globin chain inherited from the other parent, while gaining some measure of resistance to malaria from the abnormal globin. Individuals homozygous for a severe abnormal hemoglobin variant may die out, but the majority of heterozygous individuals will survive to produce the next generation of the affected population.

Wherever endemic malaria persisted for several generations, abnormal hemoglobin variants attained a high frequency. Following Mendelian genetics, when each parent carries a gene for a severe abnormal hemoglobin variant, 25 percent percent of their offspring will receive the trait from each parent and succumb to the disorder caused by the variant. Twenty-five percent will not receive the trait, and they will be vulnerable to malaria. Fifty percent will receive only one gene for the trait and will gain some protection from the disease (Pauling 1994).

Sickle Cell

Sickle cell variant hemoglobin, known as hemoglobin S, results from a genetic substitution on the beta globin chain. One amino acid, glutamic acid, is replaced by another, valine. This substitution appears to be specific in response to falciparum plasmodia. Infected red blood cells with one abnormal beta hemoglobin tend to alter the cell's normal shape, a process known as sickling, when oxygen is released, inhibiting the parasite's growth in the red blood cell with lower oxygen tension. The infected cell's lifespan is also shortened by the defect so that the parasite cannot complete its development. Sickling also tends to pry loose infected red blood cells sticking to the walls of the capillaries, which are swept along in the blood flow through the spleen and liver where the phagocytic macrophages can destroy them. Infants born with this variant tend to have high levels of protective fetal hemoglobin for a longer period of time (Eaton 1994; Nagel 1994).

While the heterozygote for hemoglobin S gains protection from falciparum malaria, the homozygote loses. Red blood cells with two of the same variant beta hemoglobins are more fragile than normal red blood cells, and the abnormal beta globins readily interact with each other when oxygen leaves the cell. This process alters the normal shape of the red blood cell so that it loses its flexibility. Normal disk-shaped red blood cells are flexible so that they can squeeze through the tiny blood vessels of the capillaries. The rigid, misshapen sickle cell has difficulty squeezing through the tiny capillaries. High numbers of them can pile up and block tiny blood vessels, causing tissue damage. The lifespan of sickle cells is considerably shorter than that of normal red blood cells, even without parasite invasion, leading to chronic anemia (Steinberg and Embury 1994).

Babies born homozygous for sickle cell anemia will generally show no signs of the disease during the first months of life, because of high levels of unaffected fetal hemoglobin. Sickled hemoglobin usually appears during the second year, followed by episodes of illness and anemia. As the anemia progresses, the infant experiences colic-like symptoms and feeding difficulties. About half of the babies born with this disorder will die from it during this time. As the surviving infants grow older, they suffer painful bouts in joints and other areas, associated with masses of sickle cells piling up and blocking capillary blood flow to the affected areas. These episodes, referred to as sickle cell crises, can be precipitated by infections causing high fevers, commonly *Streptococcus* pneumonia (Powers 1994), as well as malaria parasites.

The young child in sickle cell crisis becomes irritable and unwilling to move as joints and bones suffer from lack of oxygen. The affected tissues become inflamed and swollen, and if blood flow does not return, the affected tissues can die. The hands and feet are affected the most in very young children. As they grow older, ribs and the long bones of arms and legs more often become affected. Sickle cell crisis often allows other infectious processes to invade affected tissues, particularly the *Salmonella* bacteria. Repeated crises can lead to severe anemia with heart failure or stroke. If the child can survive the first years of life, the crises generally decrease during the remainder of childhood, but increase dramatically during late adolescence (Powers 1994). Homozygotes rarely survive beyond this age (Grmek 1989).

Malaria infection with sickle cell disease in the homozygote is often fatal, particularly in a situation of poverty and poor nutrition. New red blood cells cannot be produced fast enough to replace the short-lived sickle cells and infected cells. The body becomes starved for oxygen and dies (Glader 1994; Ohene-Fempong and Nkrumah 1994).

The uneven distribution of sickle cell genes reflects the origin and spread of *falciparum plasmodium*. Falciparum appears to have entered African human populations as agriculture intensified (Su, Mu, and Joy 2003). The highest frequencies for sickle cell exist in the low-lying wet regions of west Africa, followed by central and eastern Africa. Rural ethnic groups whose members do not marry outside their own ranks maintain the highest frequencies of the abnormal hemoglobins (Ohene-Frempong and Nkrumah 1994).

Embury and Steinberg (1994) defined five different mutations in beta globin haplotypes capable of producing the sickle cell trait. This means that sickle cell developed independently in at least five different focal populations, all of which were exposed to the same malaria parasite for several generations. Three main foci of origin of the sickle cell trait in Africa are central west Africa (Benin haplotype), central tropical Africa (Bantu haplotype), and the Atlantic west African region (Senegal haplotype). Another haplotype has been identified in the Eton peoples in Cameroon. Eastern Saudi Arabia and parts of India are the focal point of origin of another haplotype that resembles the Senegal haplotype. More haplotypes may be discovered with future research.

Gene pool exchanges through contact with other populations spread many of the sickle cell genes to other parts of the world. The Benin haplotype spread to north Africa primarily by way of the slave trade, and was then introduced to western Saudi Arabia and scattered areas throughout the Mediterranean in low frequencies (Nagal 1994). Conquest of the south and east coasts of the island of Sicily by north Africans brought the sickle cell gene to the local population (Tentori and Marinocci 1986).

The Arab-Indian haplotype, first identified in eastern Saudi Arabia, has been found in fifty different tribal groups in central and south India. This suggests a central focus of distribution that may have stretched along the Indus River. The ancient Harappa civilization in the Indus Valley could have been the focal distribution point for this haplotype (Nagal 1994). The resemblance to the Senegal haplotype and the evolutionary response of sickle cell to *Plasmodium falciparum* strongly suggests that the Arab-Indian haplotype has African roots. Trade routes from north Africa, the Arabian Peninsula, and the Indus Valley may have been responsible for the spread of falciparum and the development of a genetic variant similar to the African Senegal haplotype of sickle cell in the Indus Valley.

Hemoglobin Variants C and E

Other amino acid substitutes on the beta globin chain produce milder symptoms than hemoglobin S. These hemoglobin variants are known simply as hemoglobin C and E (Barriga 1981). High frequencies of hemoglobin C exist in many populations in central west Africa where hemoglobin S genes are in low frequencies (Livingstone 1986).

The hemoglobin E variant became one of the most common hemoglobin variants in the world (Kinney and Ware 1994), with widespread high frequencies in several Southeast Asian populations. Obviously *Plasmodium falciparum*, once introduced into these populations, promoted genetic hemoglobin changes similar to the African responses. Population movements spread the mutant genes from at least two different focal areas, with haplotypes known as the Cambodian and Thai haplotypes. These haplotypes overlap at the junction of Cambodia, Thailand, and Laos, and the highest frequencies of both can be found among three different tribal groups at Assam in India near the border with Burma (Winichagoon et al. 1990). Some of the hemoglobin E haplotypes, along with falciparum, followed trade routes along the Himalayas from the east into Bhutan, Nepal, and Tajikistan. The Veddas in Sri Lanka also responded to falciparum with a hemoglobin E variant (Livingstone 1986).

Hemoglobin E variants did not develop in all populations of Southeast Asia. Some populations developed a different response to the malaria parasites—ovalocytosis, large amounts of abnormal elliptical-shaped red blood cells. This genetic response occurred independently in different regions at different times. Indonesian and New Guinea native peoples have high frequencies of this disorder (Livingstone 1986).

Duffy Negative Blood Group

While all human populations can be divided into the four major ABO blood groups and Rh factor, there are other lesser known blood groupings that also react differently to various antigens. The Duffy negative blood group happens to have a total negative effect on vivax parasites. This does not appear to be a specific genetic response to malaria (Livingstone 1984), unlike the abnormal hemoglobins. Vivax plasmodia just cannot penetrate Duffy negative red blood cells to cause infection (Desowitz 1981).

The highest frequencies of this blood group occur among African pygmies, throughout populations in west Africa, and in most of east Africa. The Duffy blood group is rarely found outside of Africa, except, strangely, for some individuals in Iceland and Bhutan. Obviously, more than one mutation event created this blood group, and we do not know what triggered its origins. Other blood groups may have similar resistance to malaria parasites, as well as to other parasites (Livingstone 1984).

Vivax malaria does not exist wherever the Duffy negative blood group dominates in African populations. With vivax absent, *Plasmodium ovale* takes over. Ovale parasites can penetrate Duffy negative red blood cells and produce malaria, and so can falciparum parasites (Beaver and Jung 1985). Ovale plasmodia primarily exert their influence in west Africa, and wherever Duffy negative resistance to vivax occurs (Livingstone 1984). Perhaps a variant of vivax mutated to produce ovale when resistance by this blood group thwarted its survival when it was introduced to Duffy negative populations.

G6PD Enzyme Defect

Most people carry an enzyme known as glucose-6-phosphate dehydrogenase (G6PD) in their red blood cells. This enzyme helps protect the red blood cell from oxidation, the taking away of its oxygen molecule by certain chemical substances, known as oxidants. Oxidation fragments the red blood cell. Normally G6PD protects the red blood cell from being robbed of its oxygen, by increasing glucose metabolism in the cell. This binds up the oxygen molecules so that the oxidants cannot steal them.

Two main types of the G6PD enzyme, A and B, are both found on the female X chromosome. The male, receiving both Y and X chromosomes, gets only one of the two types of G6PD enzyme, and if the enzyme is missing, he inherits a deficiency of G6PD. Females receive two X chromosomes, one from each parent. One X chromosome with normal G6PD enzyme will protect a woman from complete deficiency if one is missing. When both X chromosomes are missing G6PD, she also inherits a deficiency of G6PD.

By helping the red blood cell hold on to its oxygen, this enzyme maintains a favorable oxygen tension desired by falciparum parasites (Beck and Davies 1981; Greene 1993). Without the enzyme, the red blood cell is vulnerable to oxygen thieves, and the loss of oxygen from the red blood cell hinders the survival of the falciparum parasite. Several populations throughout the malaria belt have developed numerous variations of G6PD deficiency in response to the disease (Livingstone 1984). Most of these variants do not cause any problems unless the red blood cells become overwhelmed by oxidants, stealing oxygen and reducing the amount of oxygen carried in the bloodstream. Some variants have very little G6PD activity, making them very sensitive to oxidant stress. Antimalarial drugs act as oxidants, along with several other synthetic drugs. When individuals with certain types of G6PD deficiency take these drugs, severe anemia and blood loss through the kidneys can occur (Greene 1993).

Five major classes (Greene 1993) and over a hundred genetic variants of G6PD deficiency display variable responses to oxidant stress (Young 1975). The most common variants occur with the B type of G6PD, while type A variants are primarily found among black Africans. West Africans have a variant highly susceptible to the oxidizing effects of antimalarial drugs. Another variant in China, called the Canton variant, also reacts to certain oxidizing drugs.

Another major G6PD variant found in the Mediterranean basin can cause severe reactions with exposure to broad beans known as fava beans (*Vicia faba*). Fava beans contain natural oxidants damaging to G6PD-defective red blood cells. The frequency for this G6PD variant reached high levels within endemic malaria areas of the Mediterranean region in response to falciparum parasites. While the G6PD deficiency provides some protection against the parasites, the deficiency also leaves the red blood cells vulnerable to the oxidants in fava beans.

Not everyone with this variant reacts the same way with fava beans, indicating that some other inherited factor prevents severe oxidizing reactions. Also, boiling the beans renders the chemical agent responsible for the reaction harmless. Without the inherited modifying factor or the removal of the oxidizing element, severe acute hemolytic (red blood cell–damaging) anemia results as massive numbers of the red blood cells fragment and self-destruct. Some people have such a sensitivity to the beans that just inhaling the pollen can trigger a reaction (Grmek 1989).This particular variant of G6PD deficiency predominates in Greece, southern Italy, Sicily, Sardinia, Anatolia, Corsica, and the Mediterranean coast of north Africa. Kurdish Jews have the highest frequency (50 percent of males), followed by Sardinians

(Young 1975). Ironically, fava beans have been a staple food in these areas for many centuries. Pythagoras warned the populace of the dangers of eating fava beans in the sixth century B.C. (Grmek 1989).

Thalassemia Syndromes

Thalassemia consists of a group of hereditary hemoglobin abnormalities responding to malaria parasites primarily by reduction or deletion of either pair of alpha or beta globin chains. Sometimes the delta globin chain substituting for the beta globin chain can be affected in the same manner as beta globin (Grmek 1989).

Close to a hundred different point mutations affect the beta globin genes (Kazazian et al. 1990), with each variant specific to a certain population. Gene deletions primarily produce alpha variants (Antonarakis et al. 1986). Both alpha and beta variants result in deformed red blood cells with increased rigidity, which makes them susceptible to fragmentation by oxidation. Red blood cells with deformed beta globin fragment twice as easily as red blood cells with deformed alpha globin (Shinar 1990). The deformed and short-lived red blood cells make it difficult for malaria parasites to survive, thereby providing protection against the disease. Individuals inheriting defective globin genes from both parents risk serious anemia from too many defective red blood cells.

Some individuals inheriting a single defective alpha gene from one parent derive some protection from malaria parasites. They also become silent heterozygote carriers of alpha thalassemia, a serious anemia disease in itself when too much of the alpha globin is missing.

Heterozygotes may be missing one of the two haplotypes in one of the globin chains making up the pair of alpha globin chains, or they may be missing either a whole alpha globin chain or a haplotype from each alpha globin chain, resulting in mild anemia or none at all. Sometimes only one haplotype exists with the other three haplotypes absent, resulting in HbH disease with mild to moderately severe hemolytic anemia. Total absence of alpha globin is fatal, and the unborn baby with this disorder (Bart's hydrops fetalis) generally dies from severe hemolytic anemia before birth (Adams 1986).

Alpha thalassemia occurs throughout Southeast Asia (Livingstone 1986), with extremely high frequencies in India (Nagal 1994). Missing one alpha chain appears more often than the other forms, providing protection against malaria parasites. Alpha thalassemia also appears in some areas of

Africa, most often missing a haplotype from each alpha globin chain (Embury and Steinberg 1994).

Beta thalassemias can be found in the Mediterranean basin, Africa, India, China, and Southeast Asia. Many variants exist throughout the regions, and it is not unusual for an individual to have two different variants. Combinations of one of the thalassemia variants with one of the sickle cell variants provide additional protection against malaria (Ohene-Frempong and Nkrumah 1994).

Expressions of beta thalassemia include silent carrier, intermediate forms, and severe forms. Intermediate forms often result from genetic modifying factors interacting with the beta globin defect, causing mild to moderate chronic anemia. Some intermediate forms can regress or become inactive as the individual grows older. Homozygotes inheriting two copies of the same variant can have mild to severe anemia, depending on the site of mutation (Kazazian et al. 1990). Homozygotes with severe defective beta globin (Cooley's anemia) suffer from severe hemolytic anemia, delayed growth and sexual development, bone deformities, and fragile bones. Death usually occurs in childhood or early adolescence (Grmek 1989).

The Mediterranean beta variants originated with the ancient Greeks, who spread them throughout the Mediterranean wherever they established their colonies. This included parts of Italy, Sicily, Corsica, Cyprus, Crete, Sardinia, portions of north Africa, and Anatolia. Alexander the Great's army carried the beta variants to the Caspian Sea region, the Middle East, Central Asia, and the Indian subcontinent (Grmek 1989).

Isolated inbreeding populations carry the highest frequencies of the beta variant defects (Caffey 1957). The secluded descendants of ancient Thracian tribes, the Pomaks of Thrace in Greece, carry high frequencies of one particular variant, hemoglobin O Arab. This same variant also exists within a population on the northern side of Mount Rhodopi in Bulgaria (Loukopoulos 1986).

Persistent Fetal Hemoglobin Hemoglobinopathy (PFHH)

The short period of protection of the newborn against malaria provided by fetal hemoglobin can be genetically extended. Mutation within the gamma-globin complex, frequently by substituting for missing or reduced beta or delta globin chains, extends the life of fetal hemoglobin. This mutation generally occurs in association with the mutated abnormal sickle cell and thalassemia hemoglobins (Loukopoulos 1986; Kinney and Ware 1994).

Mixed Hemoglobin Abnormalities

With the mixing of different populations came the mixing of different hemo-globin abnormalities. Many combinations involve the sickle cell hemoglobin heterozygote, ranging from persistent fetal hemoglobin hemoglobinopathy (PFHH) to thalassemia variants. Combinations of hemoglobin C and E are uncommon (Kinney and Ware 1994), but beta thalassemia combined with hemoglobin E does occur in Southeast Asia, leading to severe hemolytic ane-mia (Winichagoon et al. 1990). Combinations of hemoglobin C and beta tha-lassemia cause only mild anemia. Combinations of hemoglobin S and alpha thalassemia also produce mild anemia (Loukopoulos 1986), and combined hemoglobins S and C may produce latent anemia in middle age.

Concluding Comments

Malaria became a significant human disease when agriculture and animal husbandry became a way of life during the Old World Neolithic. Mosquitoes carrying malaria parasites easily adapted to human beings and their domes-ticated animals. Human disturbance of land and forests also expanded the breeding grounds of the mosquito vectors. As more and more people crowded into communities, malaria parasites thrived, and movements of people and trade goods spread the disease and genetic responses to it throughout the Old World. Thus human behavior exacerbated the malaria problem, waxing and waning with changes in population densities, farming methods, trading prac-tices, and the damaging effects of war (Jones 1909).

Most likely *Plasmodium vivax* was the first malaria parasite estab-lished within growing population centers, and vivax continues to be the dom-inant cause of malaria today. *Plasmodium malariae* played only a minor role in the spread of malaria, keeping a low profile alongside the dominant vivax species. Vivax had the advantage of being able to adapt to the temperate zones favored by many early civilizations.

Most likely both *Plasmodium vivax* and *Plasmodium malariae* origi-nated in South or Southeast Asia and spread eastward and westward with increasing human trade and migrations. Vivax may have been more virulent when it first arose in human populations, causing more serious disease than it does today. Once it became established as a major disease in ancient pop-ulations, it may have evolved into a less virulent form as human populations adjusted to it.

Human skeletal remains of rice farmers with evidence of thalassemia, from the four-thousand-year-old site of Khok Phanom Di on the coast of central Thailand (Tayles 1996), verify the existence of malaria in Neolithic Southeast Asia. Writings from the Brahmin priest Susruta in India mentioned the symptoms of malaria associated with mosquitoes during the sixth century B.C. in ancient India (Gillett 1971), supporting the paleopathological evidence of a long association with the disease.

The more deadly falciparum malaria spread from tropical Africa throughout the Mediterranean basin, and eastward into areas of West and Southeast Asia. Early dynastic records suggest falciparum malaria was present in the Nile Valley (de Zuleta 1980), coming down the Nile River from its central African origins with infected *A. gambiae* mosquitoes and infected humans. Tests on Egyptian and Nubian mummy tissues verify that *Plasmodium falciparum* reached ancient north Africa (Miller et al. 1994).

Strong evidence of genetic responses to malaria in the form of thalassemia have been documented in six-thousand-year-old skeletal remains from the Levant (Hershkovitz and Edelson 1991), western Anatolia, and northern Greece (Angel 1966), proving a long association with malaria in the eastern Mediterranean. Hippocrates' writings from the fourth century B.C. describe the symptoms of both vivax and falciparum malaria compiled from earlier works (de Zuleta 1973). High frequencies of thalassemia (Grmek 1989) developed in various regions of Greece, and ancient Greek colonists spread their mutant genes and malaria to other parts of the Mediterranean basin.

Expansion of the later Roman Empire spread malaria to parts of Western Europe, and kept malaria on the move throughout its holdings. Malaria remained a serious problem in the Mediterranean region up until the early part of the twentieth century when modern eradication programs were carried out to eliminate the disease (Carter and Mendis 2002; Jones 1909).

The problems of malaria varied from region to region, depending on local human behavior and manipulations of the local environment. Some of the ancient populations resorted to draining swamps to destroy the mosquito's breeding grounds, with great success. Ancient Etruscan farmlands in Italy managed to be virtually free of malaria until taken over during the late second century B.C. by Roman landlords who destroyed the old system and allowed marshy areas to develop, increasing the incidence of malaria (Trentori and Marinucci 1986).

Vivax malaria spread as far north as the Arctic Circle in Russia, and was carried to the Americas by the slave trade, where it reached as far north as southern Canada. Vivax malaria disappeared from Western Europe by 1921 with improved housing, separation of livestock from houses, and changes in agricultural practices (Horsfall 1972; Russel et al. 1943). It disappeared from North America and Russia by the 1950s. Falciparum malaria spread throughout the tropical and subtropical zones around the world, and continues to be a worldwide problem, despite the World Health Organization's global eradication programs that began in 1956. Extensive use of DDT during the mid-twentieth century had some success, but no lasting effect, as eradication programs faded during years of political turmoil in many underdeveloped countries.

Malaria has been on the rise in many parts of the world, primarily from lack of effective eradication programs aimed at breaking the cycle between mosquito, environment, and humans. Southeast Asia has experienced the greatest increase in malaria (Beck and Davies 1981), and infection with *Plasmodium falciparum* has become more difficult to treat now that the parasites have become resistant to antimalarial drugs (Beaver and Jung 1985). Over 500 million cases of malaria appear each year around the world, causing approximately 2 million deaths, mostly of young children (Tishkoff et al. 2001). Increasing populations, accompanied by poverty and poor nutrition, and poor land management in malaria-infested areas, coupled with decreasing control of the disease, have created a serious world health problem today.

CHAPTER 6

INVITATION TO A MINUTE WORM

The Schistosomes

Background Check

Hundreds of millions of years ago certain tiny, free-living, hermaphroditic flatworms living in water adapted to parasitic life inside water snails. They evolved and diversified along with their snail hosts. The snails came to act as protective incubators for their tiny offspring, allowing the immature worms to divide and multiply within the snail, free from predators. The growing flatworms helped themselves to the readily available food supplies from the snail's glycogen (sugar) stores. As the young worms reached adolescence, they returned to the water to grow into mature adults and reproduce the next batch of parasitic young. Meanwhile, their free-living cousins continued to develop and mature in the open water.

Along the evolutionary pathway, some of the tiny, parasitic flatworms eventually found that the internal environment of other creatures could serve the needs of the maturing adults and the reproduction of eggs much better than the open water. The gut and circulatory system of fish, and eventually amphibians and reptiles, offered alternative fluid pathways for adult survival. These enclosed environments offered protection and "creature comfort" with ample food sources readily available in the gut or blood of the host, and the snail continued to act as incubator for the growing young. The new hosts to the adult flatworms also helped spread the worms to other areas where the eggs, upon leaving the host, could find new snail populations willing to accept them.

Eventually some of these parasitic flatworms, known as trematodes or flukes, managed to adapt to the blood circulation of evolving warm-blooded birds and mammals. This greatly enhanced their mobility, and infected migratory birds helped spread the parasites over thousands of miles, wherever a susceptible snail population would accept them. These particular trematodes prefer to inhabit the veins within the circulatory system of warm-blooded animals, while trematodes infecting cold-blooded animals reside in the arteries. These tiny blood flukes, known as schistosomes, thrive on the oxygen and nutrients of red blood cells (Basch 1991).

A wide variety of schistosomes occur around the world, wherever there are appropriate snails, animal hosts, and water sources for them to complete their life cycle. Most of the snail hosts prefer quiet waters with aquatic vegetation, and a warm, but not overly hot, climate. Many of them have adjusted to alternating wet and dry seasons. Animals accustomed to eliminating in or near the same water source they drink from ensure the continuing passage of parasites between snail hosts and animal hosts.

The schistosomes are fussy about what kind of snail they will use to incubate their offspring. Their evolutionary ties to the snail remain strong. Each schistosome species usually depends on one species of snail to incubate the young, and different variants of schistosomes, separated geographically, favor the specific variant of snail species of that region. The growing adolescent flukes are less fussy about the animal host. Some schistosomes attracted to large mammals will take whatever large animal comes their way, whether four- or two-legged.

Unlike their hermaphroditic adult cousins infecting cold-blooded animals, adult flukes infecting warm-blooded animals have evolved into sexually reproducing pairs. Male and female flukes bring together and mix different genes to produce greater genetic diversity among their kind. This genetic diversity provides a pool of genetic variability for quicker adaptation to changing environments, increasing the odds that one of their variants will survive change.

The Onerous Guest

There are several species of schistosomes, each consisting of a complex of related flukes with similar habits. The different species vary in size and habits, but basically they follow the same cycle of life. The tiny schistosomes resemble roundworms more than flatworms. The adult male, approximately 5–11 mm long (less than one-half inch) and about 1 mm in diameter, is smaller than the female. Both male and female adults have an oral sucker opening into the alimentary tract on the head end, and below it a ventral sucker used for attachment to blood vessel walls. The male's ventral sucker grows larger and more powerful than the female's. The sucker attachment keeps the fluke from being carried away with the blood current.

The fluke ingests red blood cells through its oral sucker opening for dismemberment and absorption. Nutrients, particularly glucose, can also be absorbed through the outer body surface, the tegument. Female schistosome consumption of red blood cells has been recorded as high as 330,000 per hour, while males consume up to 39,000 per hour (Erasmus 1987).

The most unusual feature of the male is the gynaecophoric canal, a large groove or slit-like pouch in its belly, designed to hold the adult female in a constant copulating embrace. The mature female, thinner and longer than the male with smaller suckers, can reach a length of just under 20 mm (three-quarters of an inch). She deposits her eggs within the small branches of the host's veins, known as venules, which empty into the tiny capillaries draining adjacent organs. Depending on the species, the female can produce anywhere from twenty to two thousand or more eggs each day (Jourdane and Theron 1987). Most adult flukes can survive for three to twelve years, while some species have been known to survive for over thirty years (Von Lichtenberg 1987).

The eggs generally form an oval shape with a spiked expansion of the outer shell at one end. The embryo forms within a thin membrane adhering to the thicker outer shell. The outer, permeable shell allows fusion of nutrients into the egg, and the growing embryo can release substances out of the egg. The secretions from the embryo help the egg penetrate the tissues of the host. Once the eggs are deposited in the tiny venules, they work their way into the adjacent excretory organ to be passed out with host excretions. The passage of the eggs from venule to external environment takes at least six days (Jourdane and Theron 1987).

The eggs need to reach a watery environment to hatch. When water rushes in through the permeable shell of the egg and ruptures it, the tiny larva of the schistosome is released. The egg will not hatch if contact with water is not immediate upon release from the host. Eggs of some species can survive in shaded areas for up to a week before making contact with water.

While water is necessary for the egg to hatch, the temperature, light, and osmotic conditions of the water also have to be right or the egg dies (Jourdane and Theron 1987).

The larva hatching from the egg, known as the miracidium, is covered with tiny hair-like projections that help propel it through the water. The miracidium can easily be confused with tiny, free-living protozoa of similar configuration. The tiny miracidium can swim around 2 mm (about one-tenth of an inch) per second in still waters, and within a few hours it can locate snails up to 16 feet away (Basch 1991).

The tiny larvae are genetically programmed to develop within specific snails. Locating the right snail is not easy, and many of them find themselves in the wrong snail, entrapped within the snail tissue by the host immune response, unable to develop further. About 60 percent of larvae fail to penetrate the appropriate host snail (Jourdane and Theron 1987). Sometimes a wayward neophyte may have just enough genetic variation to match the genetic immunity of a snail outside the acceptable range of its designated host snail. This leads to radiation of the species with the establishment of a new variant of the original strain. Generally, the new snail host is a related species of the original host.

The evolutionary relationships between parasite and snail influence how the miracidium locates the appropriate snail. Some snails stay close to the water surface, sometimes fixed to floating vegetation, while others prefer muddy bottoms or shady banks. The tiny miracidium, programmed to search out the particular niches of their host snails, most likely respond to light and chemical signals. Once they find the snail, they spend some time exploring its surface before penetration. The snail's own secretions aid the process.

Once inside the appropriate snail, the miracidium develops into a sac-like organism called a sporocyst, full of embryonic cells, all of the same sex as the egg that produced them. One snail can be infected by more than one miracidium of opposite sexes, or all of the same sex. The appropriate snail host tolerates the parasites and poses no immunological challenges.

The mobile sporocyst migrates to the snail's digestive gland for further growth and development between the tenth and seventeenth day (Jourdane and Theron 1987). Each embryonic cell develops into a new larval form, the cercaria. Some sporocysts also replicate themselves in daughter sporocysts capable of producing more cercariae and daughter sporocysts of their own. Production of hundreds of cercariae occurs daily throughout most of the snail's life, and the cercariae are shed into the water as free-swimming larvae with long, bifurcated tails.

The cercariae swim around in search of a favorable animal host in the water. The adolescent larva will then penetrate the animal's skin surface and begin the next cycle of development toward adulthood.

Again, the schistosome larvae do not always find a suitable host. The tiny cercaria has only a brief time—five to eight hours—to locate and penetrate its animal host before running out of fuel (Wilson 1987). Unable to feed, they depend on glycogen stores absorbed from the snail during development. No nourishment can be taken from the external environment by the cercaria or the other larval stage, the miracidium. All nourishment for schistosomes comes from the snail and animal host, so the parasite is totally dependent on its hosts for survival. The cercaria must reserve a sufficient amount of fuel for the energy needed to penetrate the skin of the host and make its way into the host circulatory system. Otherwise it will die, as the vast majority of them do.

Desperation toward the end of their fuel supply can drive the tiny larvae to take on any available host. Cercariae in search of wading birds may sometimes take on a human swimmer with this desperation. The swimmer's skin is not receptive to them. The human host's immune response overwhelmingly reacts to the larvae penetrating the skin surface, stopping the larvae dead in their tracks. Sometimes the larvae manage to get under the skin and thrive but fail to get past the skin barrier and die there. This creates a severe skin reaction known as "swimmer's itch." Cercariae frequently meet up with human swimmers in ponds and lakes throughout the world that harbor migrant birds and infected snails. Whenever an inhospitable host is encountered, the little parasites are doomed.

Turbulence, shadows, thermal gradient, and in some cases chemical sheddings of animal hosts in the water attract cercariae. Upon contact with a host, they explore the skin surface until the right chemical substances emitted from skin secretions, combined with their own secretions, enable them to force entry. This process takes about fifteen minutes (Barriga 1981). Once past the outer skin layer, they lose their tails, and the neophytes can no longer tolerate external water sources. They cannot turn back, and in less than an hour, the tiny cercariae transform into another larval form, the schistosomulum (Wilson 1987).

This larval state solves the fuel supply problem by developing a double-layered outer membrane equipped for direct transfer of nutrients from the host's bloodstream. The outer membranous layer also gradually develops the capability of deterring destruction by host killer cells, even when host immunoglobins tag them for destruction. The parasite cloaks itself with the host's own protein molecules, confusing the killer cells even when immunoglobins cling to it.

The newly formed schistosomulum migrates through the deeper layers of skin until it can tap into the circulatory system by way of a capillary or tiny lymph vessel. Within three days of skin penetration, the tiny parasite has been swept away from the skin on a voyage through the bloodstream. The lungs become the first significant stop on this journey. Here the schistosomulum more than doubles its length without significantly altering its total volume. This gives the young fluke the capability of extending and contracting its length to allow for movement along the walls of blood vessels (Wilson 1987).

The circulatory gateway of the liver becomes the next major stop. Here the immature fluke lodges in tiny blood vessels of the liver, begins feeding on red blood cells as soon as the oral sucker develops, and grows into an adult. As the growing fluke increases in size, it moves upstream to larger blood vessels. Within four to six weeks the adult schistosome reaches sexual maturity.

Time to find a mate. The aggressive, mature adult males hang out around the circulatory gateway to the liver, waiting to pick up a female before moving on. This can be a trying situation if only one sex of the schistosome infects the host.

Within most species, females do not complete maturity until they mate with an adult male. Spinster females cannot reach full sexual maturity and are forced to remain in the veins of the liver without a male to carry them away. Once a male takes a female into a copulating embrace, the act stimulates her sexual maturity, and he carries her away from the liver to a place that he chooses for the production of eggs (Basch 1991).

Desperate adult males will grasp anything resembling an adult female, including an immature or smaller male. Sometimes two eager males will clasp the same female, or an overly aggressive male will grab more than one female. They will even take females of differing species if the host is infected with more than one species of schistosomes. This interspecies coupling can trigger the female to sexual maturity and to the reproduction of female eggs that are the exact copy of her—in other words, clones (Basch 1991). Sometimes interspecies mating produces a hybrid, frequently weaker than the parents.

The hybridization between similar species using similar snail strains offers the possibility for creating a new species with increased vigor and potential for causing disease.

Once the male has taken his female within the gynaecophoric canal, he moves out of the liver, using his powerful sucker to haul his mate away with him. Males of different species have varying preferences for where they will migrate. Some prefer the veins draining the intestines, others the veins draining the bladder, and a few that infect some herbivores prefer the veins draining the nose.

The final destination remains home throughout the life of the pair. Here the male constantly shifts his position within the blood vessels, while the female deposits her eggs along the way in tiny venules (Basch 1991). With the reproduction and discharge of eggs from the host, the cycle of schistosome life continues.

Not all of the eggs manage to leave the host tissues. Most of them become trapped in the wall of the organ they try to traverse, while some of them get swept by the bloodstream away from the target organ, and are unable to escape the host's body. The miracidium will mature within the egg, but it dies within a few weeks. The misplaced egg oozes damaging enzymes into adjacent tissues, triggering response from the host immune system. Lymphocytes seal off the damaged area in a tumor-like structure known as a granuloma. Numerous eggs bunched together in one spot within the wall of the associated organ can be obstructive and damaging to the organ. Each species produces its own distinct disease pattern, based on the target organ associated with the trapped eggs (Von Lichtenberg 1987).

The African Invitation

Schistosomes are found throughout the African continent, but only a few species can infect humans. Early hunters and gatherers probably encountered the tiny parasites on occasion whenever they entered ponds, lakes, and slow-draining flood channels contaminated with animal excretions and host snails.

As people began to settle down in villages near slow-moving water sources containing infected snails, the human infection rates increased dramatically. Villagers living around shallow lakes and dependent on fishing became hosts for the more opportunistic species of schistosomes. Fishermen routinely exposed themselves to the cercariae when they waded out into the

water with their fish nets. Early farmers also risked infection through exposure to contaminated water supplying their villages. Most susceptible were
children playing in the water. The more contact with contaminated water, the
greater the risk and the greater the infection. This problem was compounded
with the addition of infected human excretions to the water, either directly or
indirectly by runoff from nearby toilet areas during the rainy season.

The most notorious invitation to the schistosomes occurred along the
banks of the Nile River in Egypt. Meandering through the northeast African
desert from its highland sources far to the south, the Nile fans out into a
marshy delta on the shores of the Mediterranean. The delta itself forms a
haven for snails and schistosomes. Heavy seasonal rains in the southern
highlands annually flood the lower river valley, coursing through the desert.
As the flood waters recede, snail populations explode in the slow-moving
flood channels and flood basins, and so do the schistosome populations.
Animals coming to drink take in and leave behind larvae of the parasites.

The annual floods, bringing both soil nutrients and moisture to the
lower valley, attracted early farmers. Barley and wheat could easily be planted
near flood channels as the flood waters receded. Scattered small farming villages appeared throughout the Nile Valley by 6000 B.C. (Fagan 1996). With
time, domestic cattle were added to the farmsteads, along with donkeys,
sheep, goats, and pigs. The human settlers and their domestic animals replaced
the natural animal hosts to become part of the schistosome life cycle.

Steady population growth increased the demands for cultivated foods,
straining the natural water system. This challenge was met by expanding upon
the natural flood channels and holding basins by digging artificial channels to
direct the flow of water to more areas for cultivation. Early canals consisted
of small earthen networks that did not go far beyond the natural water source.
Most likely each village independently dug and maintained its own network
of local irrigation canals. Canals and holding basins, manmade or natural,
enabled the population of snails and schistosomes to increase and survive.

By the time Egypt became a unified state around 3250 B.C., networks of
irrigation systems and villages covered the Nile Valley. Broad canals and simple earthen ditches carried the flood waters to fields far beyond the natural
flood channels. This vast irrigation network not only supported the large
human population, but also expanded the watery environment of snails and
their schistosome larvae. The great Nile Valley invitation had been accepted,
the schistosomes thrived, and human beings became the preferred animal host.

Schistosomiasis haematobium

Infection with this particular schistosome in Egypt became known as bilharziosis, named after Theodor Bilharz who discovered it in the veins of a man during an autopsy in Cairo in 1851. This disease dates back to antiquity; descriptions of the symptoms and remedies are found in ancient Egyptian papyrus scrolls over 3,500 years old (McElroy and Townsend 1989). The eggs of S. haematobium have also been identified in Egyptian mummy tissue from this same time period (Grove 1980; Millet et al. 1980; Ruffer 1910), confirming the early written descriptions. Most likely the disease dates back even earlier, to the time of the earliest farmers.

S. haematobium has adapted to human beings almost exclusively. Before humans dominated the habitat, the natural hosts had been baboons, vervet, and white-throated guernon monkeys. The Nile rat, drawn to human settlements, also harbors the parasites. Domestic sheep and pigs can also be infected by S. haematobium, helping to maintain the parasites within the human population (Rollinson and Southgate 1987). The snail hosts belong to the Bulinus africanus species, and they prefer quiet waters, generally shaded from the sun, or muddy bottoms. The banks of earthen irrigation ditches and holding ponds with vegetation growing along the sides make ideal habitats for these snails.

The eggs of S. haematobium are deposited in the venules around the bladder of the host, so that the eggs can work through the bladder wall and exit the body with urine. Eggs that cannot find their way out of the host's body become sealed off in granulomas within the bladder wall by the immune system. When infection with S. haematobium is high from frequent exposure to the parasite, increasing the number of adult flukes and the numbers of eggs produced, there is greater risk of harm to the host through formation of massive granulomas.

Children playing and urinating in irrigation ditches and basins make ideal hosts for maintaining a high level of infectious parasites in a village population. They repeatedly get infected until they reach prepubescence, when they obtain a degree of resistance to new infections (Hagen 1987). However, the schistosomes acquired before resistance becomes established continue to produce eggs throughout the life of the adult flukes, and high levels of misplaced eggs continue to invoke the immune system with inflammation and granulomatous responses.

Eggs trapped and attacked by the immune system in the bladder wall cause bleeding into the urine, producing "red urine," and sometimes mild discomfort with urination. The patches of granuloma formed in reaction to the trapped eggs eventually shrink as the encased eggs cease to be active, and the bloody urine ceases, until another lot of trapped eggs activates the process again. Infection resulting in red urine in pubescent children has become so common in some Egyptian villages that it is accepted as normal (Von Lichtenberg 1987).

The remaining adult flukes die off, and the infection ceases as immunity is gained with approaching adulthood. The majority of villagers infected with S. haematobium generally do not show any symptoms beyond red urine in childhood. Their immune systems have learned to resist reinfection from cercariae following the initial infection, and to adjust to the presence of wayward eggs, just as their ancestors' immune systems did in the past. The long association between S. haematobium and village farmers in the Nile Valley, going back over five thousand years, has created a fluctuating equilibrium between them.

However, some villagers can face a risk of serious disease when their immune systems cannot resist reinfection through repeated exposure to cercariae, leading to high numbers of reproducing adult flukes and wayward eggs. The bladder can be so severely affected by encased eggs that it loses its ability to contract and empty. Chronic bladder irritation encourages other pathogens to gain a foothold, causing infections in the bladder or kidneys. Some affected individuals, as they grow older, eventually develop bladder cancer from the chronic irritation (Von Lichtenberg 1987).

Numerous eggs, sometimes numbering in the millions, passing from the bladder into the urethra (the tissue canal leading out of the host's body), can pile up at the junction between the urethra and bladder, and die there. The massive amount of granulomatous tissue created in response to the large number of trapped eggs can obstruct the flow of urine out of the body. Likewise, the tubes leading from the kidneys to the bladder can be blocked by egg clusters at the junction with the bladder, leading to kidney failure. Eggs can also be carried by the bloodstream to other areas within the pelvis or lower abdomen and become entrapped, particularly within the appendix. They can also be carried to the lungs and liver with subsequent formation of granulomas.

Regardless of how long a particular parasite and human population have been living together, there will always be a small percentage of the human population unable to develop resistance or tolerance to the parasite.

Conversely, a small number of variants within the parasite population will always be able to provoke susceptible immune systems. The final consequences in disease terms may be a collision of the two variants, causing severe damage to the host, leading to death.

Trade networks between ancient Egypt and regions within the Middle East, particularly the slave trade, spread *S. haematobium* to kingdoms in the Levant, Mesopotamia, Asia Minor, and the Arabian Peninsula. Trade between the Arabian Peninsula and India also led to a small focus of *S. haematobium* on the west coast of India. Later, Portuguese exploration of the ports of Africa brought a small focus to southern Portugal that no longer exists there. The parasites could only become established in these regions because of the right environment for their needs and the availability of compatible Bulinus host snails.

Schistosomiasis mansoni

Another major complex of African schistosomes belong to the *S. mansoni* species. They are widespread throughout tropical Africa, with wide variation of strains leading to variations in infection. The designated snail hosts belong to the genus *Biomphalara*. The *S. mansoni* cercariae will accept a wide range of animal hosts that have spread the parasite over a range of geographic areas. Baboons appear to be the leading natural reservoir for these parasites (Rollinson and Southgate 1987).

Snail hosts for *S. mansoni* thrive in artificial lakes, ponds, and irrigation ditches, particularly during the dry season when the water becomes stagnant and vegetation grows high (Southgate and Rollinson 1987).

S. mansoni adult flukes migrate to the veins of the host's large intestine. Here the eggs deposited by the females in the venules transcend the intestinal wall, to be carried out of the host's body with feces. Individuals harboring few adult flukes usually show no signs of the infection.

Most individuals heavily infected with *S. mansoni* suffer flu-like symptoms when the eggs are first produced. Fever, chills, sweating, headache, cough, loss of appetite, and diarrhea may last for several weeks (Warren 1975). The immune system, alert to the presence of large numbers of adult flukes, responds with vigor to the foreign enzymes produced by the exploding numbers of trapped eggs appearing at the same time.

S. mansoni adult flukes live a long time, up to twenty or thirty years. The number of trapped eggs produced by one pair of adults over a twenty-year lifespan has been estimated to be at least one million (Warren 1975).

Individuals carrying high fluke burdens suffer chronic disease from over-whelming numbers of eggs trapped in the walls of the large intestine, with some carried by the blood circulation to the liver. The immune system, hyper-sensitive to the eggs, reacts to the eggs before sealing them off in granulomas. The intestinal wall can be covered with granulomas that often cause periodic bleeding. Large numbers of eggs and egg granulomas piling up within the por-tal vein of the liver can lead to fibrous narrowing and blockage of the vein and cirrhosis of the liver. This can also cause back-up pressure on the veins to the esophagus with rupture and bleeding, causing the victim to vomit blood.

Most victims of severe disease caused by *S. mansoni* are young men repeatedly exposed to the infection as boys playing in contaminated water. They often can continue their normal activities of daily life, although inter-rupted by periods of bloody vomiting and abdominal discomfort (Von Lichtenberg 1987).

The slave trade carried *S. mansoni* to the Levant and the Arabian Peninsula. Migrants to Madagascar carried the parasite with them. The slave trade to the New World opened up new horizons for *S. mansoni*, since many slaves carried the parasite with them. Local *Biomphalaria* snail species in Brazil, Surinam, Venezuela, and the Caribbean accepted the parasites. Black rats (*Rattus rattus*) as well as humans maintain the infection in the New World (Rollinson and Southgate 1987).

The Asian Invitation

Rural Asian fishing and farming villagers in regions where schistosomes and their snail hosts abound encountered the same high risks of infection as did their African counterparts. Seasonal flooding of river valleys enticed early farmers to plant their crops of rice in natural marshes left by the receding floods. China's middle Yangtze Valley in Hunan province supported some of the earliest rice farmers, dating back more than nine thousand years, and by 5000 B.C. rice farming communities had spread throughout southern China (Fagan 1996). The raising of water buffalo, pigs, and ducks was added to rice farming. With increasing populations, water management systems were developed to control the flood waters, and by 2000 B.C. state societies thrived throughout Southeast Asia.

The earliest evidence of schistosomes was found in the mummified body of the wife of Litsang, the marquis of Tai, chancellor of the principality of Changsha along the banks of the Yangtze River in Hunan province during the early western Han dynasty. She died 2,100 years ago with the eggs of *Schistosomiasis japonicum* trapped in her liver and lower intestinal wall (Cockburn 1980).

Schistosomiasis japonicum

The most prevalent schistosome found in Asia is *S. japonicum*, which appears to have originated in south China, most likely in the Yangtze Valley in Hunan province. It spread out into other river valleys, and into the delta of the Pearl River that empties into the South China Sea. The development of rice farming and water management systems promoted the growth of the snail hosts that included three genera, *Oncomelania*, *Tricula*, and *Robertsiella* (Southgate and Rollinson 1987). The schistosome can infect a number of wild animals. Human beings and their domesticated cattle, pigs, and dogs replaced the wild animal hosts where farming pushed them out.

Thai and Laotian peoples, the original inhabitants of south China, were pushed into present-day Thailand and Laos by Han Chinese coming into the region from the north around two thousand years ago. They carried the schistosome with them, and infection continues in some areas of both countries. Migrants from south China spread it to the islands of Hainan and Taiwan, parts of Japan, the Philippines, Sri Lanka, and the west coast of Indonesia. Field rats contribute to the maintenance of the infection on Leyte Island in the Philippines (Southgate and Rollinson 1987).

S. Japonicum adult flukes migrate to the veins of the host's small intestine, where the female deposits her eggs in the venules, and the eggs work through the intestinal wall to be excreted along with feces. The eggs can survive for at least a week in shady areas (Jourdane and Theron 1987), making shaded toilet areas near irrigation ditches ideal spots for protecting the eggs until runoff water from rains sweeps them into the canals.

Small numbers of adult flukes generally do not cause any symptoms. Susceptible individuals can develop high numbers of adult worms from repeated exposure to cercariae. Problems begin with the first round of egg laying, which results in huge numbers of eggs trapped in the tissues of the small intestine. The presence of so many adult flukes and the large number of eggs excreting enzymes heightens immune reactions similar to those caused by *S. mansoni*, but more severe (Warren 1975). The infestation causes daily fever, severe bodily discomfort, aching joints, skin rash, indigestion, swollen lymph nodes, and sometimes diarrhea (Von Lichtenberg 1987). This reaction to *S. japonicum* eggs is known as Katayama fever, which lasts for several weeks, and the individual can die from it.

With time the afflicted individual develops serious problems from the large numbers of entrapped eggs and the granulomatous reactions of the immune system. One adult worm pair alone produces at least 10 million trapped eggs within a twenty-year life span. Most of the eggs are trapped in the small intestine. Some eggs transmitted by blood flow to the liver create problems with blocked blood flow in the portal vein similar to those caused by *S. mansoni*. *S. Japonicum* eggs sometimes locate in the brain, where they can cause focal epilepsy (Warren 1975).

CONCLUDING COMMENTS

The snail hosts of schistosomes primarily live in the tropic and associated subtropic zones. Many areas, such as the Nile Valley, undergo wet and dry seasons. The snail populations are discontinuous with the wet and dry climatic cycle (Southgate and Rollinson 1987). During the dry seasons, particularly when temperatures are high, the snail population decreases dramatically. Snail eggs deposited along the drying banks of water channels toward the end of the dry season wait for the floods to come and then recede. They cannot hatch until the flood waters reach them. Therefore, infection by schistosome larvae comes to a standstill. Flood waters sweeping back into the dry water beds bring back the snail population. Schistosome larvae from infected animal or human hosts enter the water via urine or feces, infect the renewed snail population, and restart the cycle of infection between snails and warm-blooded hosts.

This intermittent cycle has long plagued Egyptian farmers dependent on the annual flood waters of the Nile. With the development of artificial water channels, Egyptian farmers unknowingly increased their contact with infected snails. Farmers along the Nile continue to follow the same methods for watering their fields that their ancestors employed for centuries. Children still play in drainage ditches, villagers continue the same practices of toileting in or near the irrigation canals, and the risk of infection by schistosomes following the flood season remains.

Recent changes, following the building of the Aswam Dam in the 1960s, have upset the delicate balance between the flood water cycle and human infection. The annual flooding that farmers have depended on for centuries has been replaced by continuous irrigation water let out by the dam. Flood waters that once swept through the valley now back up behind the dam, with gradual and continuous water release to the farmers. Constant slow movement of water through canals, ditches, and pools year round has altered the ecological system of the snails dramatically. The cycle of drying of water channels with drops in infection alternating with floods and increases in infection has ceased. Infection by the schistosomes now occurs uninterrupted throughout the year. Greater numbers of *S. mansoni*–infected snails can be found in the delta area of the Nile year round, while the numbers of *S. haematobium*–infected snails have been increasing upstream (Grove 1980; Wilkens 1987).

Similar modern water projects in other parts of Africa and elsewhere have affected the nature of schistosome transmission from snail to human host. Wherever climate, human behavior, and snail behavior upgrade transmission, the schistosome populations rise. Increasing movements of infected people throughout the world greatly enhance the spread of schistosomes. An estimated 200 million people worldwide were infected with schistosomes toward the end of the twentieth century (Mott 1987).

Exploding human populations searching for new farm lands in the tropical zones of developing countries run the risk of encountering and spreading schistosomes capable of infecting humans and their domestic animals. Deforestation and the creation of permanent artificial water systems sends an invitation to potential snail hosts, as the invading human population along with their domestic animals replaces the natural animal hosts. Tropical forests of central and west Africa harbor *Schistosome intercalatum*, which is capable of infecting humans and able to hybridize with *S. haematobium*. The *Schistosome mattheei* in South Africa causes severe disease in domestic cattle, sheep, and goats, and it can infect humans. *S. mattheei* can also hybridize with *S. haematobium*. Several other schistosomes throughout Asia can infect humans, including *S. mekongi* in southern Laos and Cambodia (Rollinson and Southgate 1987).

Deforestation in tropical areas, the implementation of artificial water management systems, and human behavior have increased the spread of schistosome infections. The opportunity grows for exchange of genes between different species of schistosomes to create hybrids with the potential to cause greater harm than the parents. The constant stirring of the pot of schistosomes and the crowding out of natural animal hosts by increasing human populations presents a new expansive paradigm for the little blood flukes.

CHAPTER 7

BRAVING NEW WORLDS
Invisible Enemies of Settlers

Paradise Found and Lost

The wanderlust of our ancient hunting and foraging ancestors was not lost with the new age of farming, sedentary villages, and developing civilizations. Social unrest, natural disasters such as floods and drought, pressure on marginal environments, and increasing population densities encouraged people to migrate into new lands. They went looking for fertile soils, plenty of clean water, abundant natural supplementary wild foods, grazing land for domestic animals, and building materials. Many of them settled in areas along trade routes: along rivers, coastal areas, or overland trails. With the establishment of trade links, most people found it desirable to stay linked with them and to participate in the constant flow of trade goods and the exchange of ideas.

The process of humans moving into new areas and settling down attracted local animal and insect pests, while driving out many other creatures unable to tolerate human habitation. With time, the new human community would become tolerant, or less reactive, to any pathogenic microbes associated with the new environment. Endemic diseases result from the adaptation to local pathogens by humans and/or their domestic animals. Sometimes the delicate balance between tolerant hosts and endemic microbes can be upset by malnutrition, famine, or any other form of stress on the immune system that allows local pathogens to gain control.

Wild animals displaced by humans often retreated to nearby wilderness areas. Their local pathogens usually went with them, maintaining their cycles of natural, endemic infections in these wilderness areas without disturbing the nearby human settlements. Human settlers may or may not have been aware of the protection they gained from local diseases by leaving unsettled wilderness belts near human settlements. This is particularly true for infections carried by blood-sucking insects preferring wild animal hosts over human or domestic animal hosts. As long as human beings did not intrude into these wilderness belts, they and their domestic animals remained outside the cycle of infection between natural animal host and insect vector.

The pattern of human immigration into a new area, displacing natural flora and fauna, but retaining areas of undisturbed wilderness, became a common theme throughout the world as human populations increased with the advances of agriculture. This type of human settlement allowed the natural flora and fauna to survive intact while agricultural societies rearranged parts of the environment for their own needs. Both could coexist as long as neither one encroached upon the other.

Wild infections would have been primarily contained in areas left to nature. Occasional human infection by accident could be expected when human beings or their domesticated animals entered these areas. Hunters, honey gatherers, and other adventuresome folk entering the wilderness areas placed themselves at risk. The opposite process also could have happened, with wild animals at risk of infection from domestic animals whenever they entered human habitation areas.

Many wild infections cannot survive in humans, but some can. As long as the wild endemic diseases that can infect humans remain separate from human habitation areas, the human community has no need to develop tolerance or immunity to them, but the risk of serious disease will remain high. Those endemic infectious diseases that have moved in with the settlers will eventually be tolerated within a fluctuating equilibrium, and will cause less severe or mild disease in most individuals growing up with them.

Any upset in the delicate arrangement between human habitations and wilderness areas can lead to disaster. Expanding human populations rapidly invading wilderness areas and destroying the natural flora and fauna leave insect vectors and their parasites no choice but to try subsisting on the invaders. The ravages of war often allow the wilderness to reclaim once cultivated areas, and force humans to seek refuge in areas where they risk exposure to wild diseases. New animal diseases introduced by invaders or traders also can devastate wild animal populations, placing humans and domestic animals at risk from wild infections that lose their natural hosts. Sometimes a variant of a wild disease makes its way into human settlements, causing devastating epidemics. Paradise can quickly be lost.

Avoiding Africa's Fly Belts and the Sleeping Sickness

One of the best examples of how humans have coexisted with wilderness areas can be found in Africa along the heavily infested tsetse fly belts. The tsetse flies (*Glossinae*) are bloodsuckers capable of transmitting various forms of parasitic protozoa, known as trypanosomes, to a variety of wild animals within their range. The cycle of trypanosome infection delivered by the flies to their natural wild animal hosts can be disrupted by human behavior, with the flies transferring the infection to humans and their domestic livestock, especially cattle. Infection with these wild parasites produces a disease complex known in its final stages as sleeping sickness.

The original fly belt extended from the shores of west Africa, along the rim of the Congo basin, into the Great Lakes region of east Africa, extending south along the Rift Valley into the Limpopo basin of Zimbabwe and the Lwangwa Valley of eastern Zambia (Ford 1971). For centuries human activities within the fly belt were limited because of the dreaded trypanosome infections. The fly belt has been modified by weather changes, and by human intervention involving agriculture and cattle raising. Thus it has contracted and expanded throughout time, while remaining a dynamic force within the heart of Africa.

The parasitic nature of trypanosomes may have evolved among leeches, segmented worms belonging to the Annelids, found in the same wet areas as the free-living ancestors of the trypanosomes millennia ago. Leeches may have transmitted the parasites to forest animals and reptiles (Ford 1971), and the blood-sucking tsetses would have picked it up from them. The different internal microenvironments of the flies and each new animal host led to variations in the trypanosomes, which were able to adapt to rapid environmental changes. Interestingly, tsetse flies in general seldom become infected by the parasites—typically, less than 10 percent, or perhaps only 1 percent, of a fly population will be infected (Baker 1974). However, those that become infected transmit the trypanosomes to their hosts with each blood meal.

Trypanosomes invade the fluid pathways of the host's body, the blood, lymph, cerebrospinal fluid, and sometimes fluid surrounding tissue cells. Individual trypanosomes can reduce the threat of host immune responses by chameleon-like transitions that alter their identity at different stages of development in the host. As the host immune system produces appropriate immunoglobins to combat the foreigners, they change by shifting surface proteins, so the immunoglobins cannot recognize them (Graham and Barry 1995; Vanhamme and Pays 1995). New immunoglobins have to be produced to match the new identity, and again and again, the parasite alters its identity, exhausting the B cell response of the host. This also allows other infectious invaders a better chance of survival in the host. The parasites revert back to their original long, undulating forms when ingested by the fly with its blood meal from the infected host (Barriga 1981).

Spread of the parasites depends on the tsetse flies and their habits. Fly habits vary with different geographic regions within the fly belt. The major fly vectors in west Africa, *Glossina palpalis* and *Glossina tachinoides*, inhabit the vegetation along banks of rivers and lakes, as well as coastal mangrove swamps. The major fly vector in east Africa, *Glossina moristans*, inhabits forest fringe, thickets, and wooded savannas. The west African riverine tsetse flies require high humidity and constant warm temperatures, while those in east Africa tolerate more fluctuations in temperature and humidity, as long as periods of extreme cold or dry heat do not occur (Ford 1971).

Warthogs remain the favored natural hosts for the tsetse flies found in the eastern savannas, while tsetses living in wooded areas favor bushbuck (Ford 1971). Other large animals play host to the eastern flies whenever they enter thickets or woods to rest in the shade, or to drink water. The flies prefer animal blood over human blood, and if given a choice, they will feed on animals first. Riverine tsetses have broader tastes, feeding on any available blood source, large or small, including reptiles, especially crocodiles, and amphibians. They seldom venture more than 30 yards from water (Chandler 1945), so they must dine on whatever creature ventures near, including humans. Eastern flies have a habit of following any moving object that crosses their path (including vehicles), hitching rides when they run out of energy. Dark colors attract them and whiteness repels them.

Both male and female tsetse flies suck blood. After gorging on blood meals, they must rest two or three days in the shade while digestion takes place. They prefer to dine in moderately shaded areas where animal hosts tend to drink or rest. The flies will not feed in bright sunlight, and they do not like heavily shaded areas of dense forest.

The females mate only once, soon after they emerge from the pupa state. The male's sperm is stored for continuous fertilization of eggs throughout the female's lifetime. The females give birth to fully developed larvae, one at a time, depositing the young in shaded areas within loose soil or debris. The larvae quickly bury themselves under an inch of cover to complete their development into the pupa stage. The adult emerges in about thirty days, and probably lives less than one year. The newly emerged adult must find its first blood meal within a short time, before its reserves become depleted, or else it will die (Chandler 1945; Ford 1971). This can cause desperation leading to indiscriminate choices of atypical host animals.

Trypanosomes harmful to both human beings and domestic animals belong to the *Trypanosoma brucei* complex, while other complexes affect only domestic and wild animals, rarely infecting humans. The *T. brucei* complex naturally infects most wild animals without harm. African domestic cattle that have grown tolerant to the parasites often act as go-between reservoirs for the parasites, allowing flies that bite both cattle and humans to transfer the infection to humans. Imported cattle breeds do not tolerate the trypanosomes, hence they are vulnerable to devastating disease caused by them. Other introduced domestic animals, including sheep, goats, donkeys, horses, camels, pigs, and dogs, also can be seriously affected by many of the trypanosomes (Beck and Davies 1981).

Two distinct variants of *T. brucei* have had an impact on human populations: *T. gambiense brucei*, transmitted by the riverine tsetses of west Africa, and *T. rhodesiense brucei*, transmitted by the savanna-woodland tsetses of east Africa. Great variation occurs in the expression of disease within both types of infection, depending on the immune responses of the host and the virulence of the trypanosome.

Early hunters and gatherers may have been aware of the dangers posed by the flies, and may have avoided infested areas, following fly-free zones in their wanderings (Lambrecht 1967). Agricultural settlers in west Africa encountered the flies whenever they placed their villages near rivers, streams, lakes or mangrove shores. Even if villages stood well away from these areas, trips to the water's edge for fetching drinking water, bathing, washing, fishing, or just crossing, would have enabled the flies to dine on human blood. Continuous contact with the flies and their trypanosomes for centuries led to a compromise state of fluctuating equilibrium between the human populations and *T. gambiense brucei*. The infection becomes a more protracted, chronic disease than infection with *T. rhodesiense brucei* in the savanna-woodlands of east Africa. *T. gambiense brucei* can also be transferred by the flies between humans in densely populated areas, instead of from animals to humans as is the case with *T. rhodesiense brucei*.

T. rhodesiense brucei has remained a wild infection, primarily confined to its wild animal hosts with sporadic infections in human populations. Early agriculturalists in east Africa tended to farm open savanna areas, clearing away brush along with the wild animal hosts of the tsetses. Watering places also were cleared of brush and so were free of tsetse flies. Wilderness areas between human habitation areas remained untouched, allowing the natural cycle of trypanosome infection to continue undisturbed. Climatic changes around two thousand years ago forced pastoral peoples from dried-up grazing lands in the north to go east and south in search of pasture lands for their cattle (Ford 1971). They invaded the Great Lakes area of east Africa with large herds of cattle, following fly-free corridors created by the farmers (Lambrecht 1967). They found paradise, with good grazing lands free of tsetses surrounded by wilderness zones of savanna woodlands. Many of the pastoral peoples came to rule over the local farming villages near their newly acquired lands. Cattle and people remained free of disease as long as the delicate balance between wilderness areas, human habitation areas, and pasture and farm lands remained undisturbed.

Colonization by Europeans during the nineteenth century upset this delicate balance. First, native cattle herds suffered devastation from 1889 to 1896 with the introduction of the deadly cattle disease known as rinderpest. This highly contagious virus destroyed up to 95 percent of the local cattle herds, wiping out the livelihood of the pastoralists and their hold on the farmers. Rinderpest was also deadly to many wild animals, including the favored host of the tsetse flies, the warthog. Social and environmental disruption followed, with hungry tsetses seeking alternative human hosts to survive. Hardship led to abandonment of farmlands. Brush and savanna woodlands reclaimed these areas, with eventual recovery of wild animal populations and tsetse flies, increasing the fly zones. Later return of farmers to reclaim the land exposed them to the tsetses, creating epidemics of disease from the trypanosomes, until the land was cleared of brush and the wilderness pushed back again (Ford 1971).

The disease produced by *T. gambiense brucei* in west Africa differs from the disease caused by its wild eastern cousin, *T. rhodesiense brucei*. The long association between *T. gambiense brucei* and human populations has mellowed the parasite's effects. Repeated infection with multiple fly bites, however, can worsen the effects of the disease in highly susceptible individuals, leading to a quick death. Some infected individuals show few or no signs of disease for several years (Ford 1971).

The tsetse fly bite causes redness and swelling at the point of entry to the host. This subsides within about three weeks as the parasites transform into trypomastigotes and leave the bite location. High fever accompanies the dispersal of trypomastigotes into the bloodstream. Some individuals also develop a transitory skin rash at this time. The trypomastigotes leave the blood and seek refuge in the lymph system. The parasites attack the lymph system, causing periodic fevers with severe headaches along with night sweats. These symptoms can go on for months or years as the immune system battles the parasites. The chronic infection provokes generalized debility and insomnia, along with puffiness of the eyelids, hands, feet, and ankles. Infected lymph nodes become swollen and tender, especially in the neck. Slave traders learned that swollen neck nodes indicated poor chances of survival. They would sort out affected individuals from those to be shipped out for sale (Ford 1971).

Invasion of the central nervous system signals the last stage of the disease. Constant headache plagues the victim, the energy level drops, and the individual moves with a slow, shuffling gait. There is a tendency to lapse into a sleep-like state during the day, with restlessness at night. Some individuals become psychotic. Tremors develop along with slurred speech, and eventually the individual becomes bed-ridden, dependent on others for care. Coma and death result (Ford 1971).

T. rhodesiense brucei infection develops rapidly, and quickly invades the central nervous system, with mental disorders appearing. Reactions to the fly's bite are also more severe, persisting even when later symptoms appear. Severe fever and chills develop as the parasites invade the blood, and the heart muscle becomes inflamed. Unlike *T. gambiense brucei* infection, *T. rhodesiense brucei* infection has little effect on the lymph system. Most individuals die before severe central nervous symptoms appear. Death within three to nine months of onset usually occurs from heart failure and toxic effects of the parasites (Ford 1971).

Making Room for Chagas' Disease in the New World

Several species of trypanosomes exist in the New World, from the warm southern areas of North America to Argentina and Chile in South America (Chandler 1945). Most New World trypanosomes rarely affect humans; only one species has an impact on human populations, *Trypanosoma cruzi*. Disease caused by *T. cruzi* infection primarily affects rural populations of Central and South America.

Unlike the African trypanosome, which is transmitted by flies, the American trypanosomes developed an association with various species of blood-sucking *Reduvida triatomida* and *Reduvida rhodnius* bugs, better known as kissing bugs or cone-nosed bugs. They feed on a variety of wild animals, and become infected with the trypanosomes during the blood meal, but they do not transmit the parasites when they feed. The trypanosomes go through a series of changes and multiplications in the bug's gut before they are excreted with liquid feces while the bug takes its blood meal. Entry into the host can then be gained through the bite wound (Barriga 1981). The site of the bite often becomes irritated, leading the victim to scratch the area, or if near the eye (a popular bite site), to rub the irritated eye, all of which helps the parasites gain entry into the host. Animals can be infected by licking feces-contaminated body areas or by eating the bugs. Houseflies, bedbugs, and ticks have also been known to become infected from the bugs' feces (Zeledon 1974).

Most kissing bugs are brightly colored. They are very active runners, and they can fly for short distances. They have a small, narrow head; long, four-jointed antennae; and a slender, three-jointed beak bent straight back under the head. Females lay small batches of eggs in the same areas they inhabit. Depending on the temperature, hatching occurs two to three weeks later, and wingless nymphs emerge. Several days after hatching, the nymphs take their first blood meal. Hungry young nymphs often dine on the blood of their siblings. Adult bugs can also suffer from blood-sucking relatives, keeping trypanosome infection within the bug population (Chandler 1945). The life cycle varies among the different species, from five months to two years (Zeledon 1974).

The majority of the bugs prefer to inhabit the burrows and nests of rodents, migratory birds, armadillos, or opossums. Generally they avoid human sites, preferring wild animal hosts and their nests. When human settlers moved into the areas occupied by the bugs and their natural hosts, some of the bugs found that human "nests" were just as cozy as those of their wild animal hosts. Thatched roofs (particularly those made of palm grass) with earthen floors, dark corners, cracks in adobe walls, bedding materials, partitions made of cane or palm grass, and storage areas provided cover and ideal breeding places, with plentiful blood meals around. Bugs that do not like to enter houses will feed on humans sleeping outside or in tents. The bugs feed at night while hosts sleep, and they hide during the day (Chandler 1945). Some species too shy to occupy the houses will venture in at night to feed, attracted by bright lights. They will invade domestic animal shelters, feeding on chickens, pigs, goats, and cattle, and they will feed on the blood of rodents acclimated to human habitats, as well as on dogs and cats. Cats and dogs can also be infected by eating infected rodents. Guinea pigs commonly raised inside the houses of the rural poor for food in the Andes of South America frequently become infected by the bugs. Domestic animals can thus serve as a reservoir for the parasite, maintaining the infection within the household and the village (Barriga 1981; Zeledon 1974).

Warmer temperatures during spring and summer lead to increased activity by the bugs, causing seasonal outbreaks of the infection. Different species of bugs with differing strains of *T. cruzi* have adapted to various geographic regions, producing variations of Chagas' disease (Zeledon 1974).

In most people the immune system responds quickly to the invaders, and they display few or no symptoms of disease. Exposure to *T. cruzi* usually occurs during childhood in endemic areas. The parasites can persist at low levels for life. Sometimes chronic symptoms develop later in adult life if immunity is impaired. Somehow the parasite manages to avoid annihilation by the initial immune response when invading tissue cells, by warding off T cell recognition. Delayed immune response develops in a small percentage of infected individuals, with overreactions to the parasites once it kicks in. This delayed hypersensitivity reaction causes severe symptoms of the disease (Kuhn 1981).

The spindle-shaped parasites can invade a wide variety of cells adjacent to the invasion site, but they prefer muscle cells, especially cardiac muscle cells, nerve cells, and phagocytic cells. Once inside the cell, they change into small, round amastigotes, and multiply until the cell ruptures. The released new parasitic forms, known as trypomastigotes, invade more cells and begin the cycle anew. The disease can be more severe in children, and men suffer worse effects than women. Similarly, male animals suffer more than females. The parasites can also be transmitted from infected pregnant women to their unborn infants through the placenta (Barriga 1981).

The bugs often bite near the eye. Wherever they bite, the entry site for the parasites becomes red and swollen as the immune system reacts. The swollen lesion formed by the inflammatory skin reaction against *T. cruzi* is known as a chagoma and lasts from four to eight weeks. The chagoma turns dark or bluish, and leaves a pigmented scar when it disappears. The parasites multiply within the cells of surrounding tissue and invade associated lymph nodes where they form cyst-like structures called pseudocysts, full of multiplying amastigotes. When the pseudocysts rupture and release the parasites, the immune response causes further inflammatory reaction. This cycle of cell damage, inflammatory response, and release of the parasites into the bloodstream can last from four to twelve weeks before it subsides. The infected individual feels unwell, and exhibits variable fever, loss of appetite, swollen lymph glands, and moderately enlarged liver and spleen. About 5–10 percent of children have low resistance to the infection and die from its effects on the heart or brain, or from secondary pneumonia (Rocha 1975).

Major health problems for most individuals with Chagas' disease come ten to thirty years after infection. Problems arise as the lingering infection progressively invades and destroys significant muscle and nerve cells within the heart and/or digestive system. Twenty to 40 percent of infected people living within endemic areas suffer from the chronic effects of the disease, with or without an initial acute reaction. The heart enlarges, blood clots frequently form in damaged heart muscle, and heart failure occurs. Death occurs immediately from heart failure, from blood clots passing into the lungs, or following chronic heart failure over a period of months or years. Damage to the nerves and muscle fibers of the esophagus and/or colon causes loss of motility. The organs enlarge, being unable to constrict when necessary. The enlarged, dilated esophagus allows food to be regurgitated into the lungs, making it difficult to swallow food, and it also causes pain and night coughing. The greatly enlarged and immobile colon leads to chronic constipation and intestinal obstruction (Rocha 1975).

Chagas' disease was the prime vector-borne disease in the New World until malaria was introduced from the Old World. Evidence of the disease from Precolumbian times has been found in mummies from northern Chile dating to before 500 B.C. (Rothhammer et al. 1985). Recent discovery of *Trypanosoma cruzi* DNA in mummified human tissue from ancient residents along the coasts of southern Peru and northern Chile shows that the disease was endemic to the coastal villages of South America four thousand years ago (Guhl et al. 1997).

Leishmaniases: Old and New World

Small sandflies (*Phlebotomus*), minute midges ranging from 1.5 to 3.5 mm (less than one-fourth inch) in size, inhabit warm and tropical regions in both hemispheres of the globe. They feed on animal blood at night, crawling out of hiding places in loose soil, animal burrows, rock crevices, termite mounds, and other natural moist, dark shelters that protect them from bright sun. Rodents and canines are favored natural animal hosts. Some Mediterranean species prefer geckos. The sandflies have very long legs and narrow wings with limited powers of flight. They can only fly a few inches, more of a hop than flight. Their world is limited to only a few hundred feet, where they breed and cycle through their short lives, usually lasting only a day or two as adults. Females lay their eggs in damp crevices away from the killing effects of sunlight and dryness. They hatch from four to nine days later into tiny caterpillar-like larvae with relatively large heads and brandishing two pair of long bristles held erect and spread out like a fan. Full-grown larvae measure less than 5 mm (one-quarter inch) in length. They require high humidity, and they feed on organic debris, including fecal matter. The larvae pupate after two to eight weeks, and hatch into adults in six to ten days (Chandler 1945). Many species of sandflies transmit protozoan parasites known as leishmaniae.

Human settlers moving into sandfly territory presented new alternatives in sandfly life style. Cool, damp, darkened areas for breeding and resting could easily be found in human habitations, along with new sources of blood meals. Domestic dogs and rodents acclimated to human settlements easily replaced the sandflies' natural wild rodent and canine hosts. Human beings also became victims. Some sandfly species acclimated easily to human settlements, moving into and around houses and hiding in cracks, dark areas, and household debris, while others remained in wild, unsettled regions. People working or traveling in wild areas and staying overnight became subject to sandfly bites, with the risk of infection by the leishmania parasites. Fortunately for many potential human victims, the tiny sandflies cannot tolerate wind or high breezes, so that even a gentle night wind helped people avoid being bitten.

Wherever sandflies exist, some form of the leishmania parasite appears to coexist, suggesting a close evolutionary tie between them and with their natural hosts. This evolutionary bond most likely developed long before the continents split apart. Most of the sandflies and their parasites do not interact with humans. Those that do affect humans appear in a number of variants in both the Old World and New World. Leishmania parasites can be found with their sandfly vectors in the Mediterranean basin, northeastern Africa, the Middle East, southern portions of Central Asia, West Asia, and portions of China (Beck and Davies 1981).

New World leishmania parasites that infect humans range from Mexico to South America with their sandfly vectors. They may have originated in the tropical forests of Mesoamerica and South America, where wild sandflies and their natural rodent hosts exist in abundance. Different geographic regions spawned variants of the parasites, along with different sandfly species or strains in both hemispheres. It has been suggested that early Portuguese and Spanish explorers brought one particular variant, the *L. chagasi* complex, to the New World (Bryceson 1975).

Sandfly bites can be very irritating in themselves, and can be infectious with leishmania parasites. The course of the infection depends on the virulence of the parasite strain or species, and the host immune response. The type of sandfly vector may also contribute to the virulence of the parasites, while the nutritional state and genetics of the host affect the immune response. The parasites are gobbled up by macrophages trying to destroy them, but leishmaniae manage to resist destruction by phagocytosis. Both wandering macrophages and those fixed to loose connective tissue in the skin, the lining of the liver, spleen, lymph glands, and bone marrow attack the parasites (Barriga 1981).

Destruction of the parasites within the macrophages can only occur when the MHC II molecules can pick up the protein fragments (peptides) from the parasites and take them to the surface of the infected cell for CD4 T cells to identify. The CD4 T cells must also receive a signal from the infected macrophage surface to respond to the foreign peptide. With this dual signal, the T cells release a chemical signal in the form of cytokines, especially gamma-interferon, to the infected macrophage that triggers it to destroy the enemy within. Without the second signal from the surface of the infected macrophage, the CD4 T cell cannot respond, and the parasites can take over and reproduce within the macrophage. Even if the dual system works and the

CD4 T cells do respond, if they fail to secrete gamma-interferon with the chemical message to the macrophage, the parasites escape destruction (Paul 1993). Susceptible individuals can be genetically predisposed to this disease in more than one way when proper genetic signals in the immune response repertoire are missing.

The parasites thriving inside macrophages change from mobile, elongated forms known as promastigotes into round or oval forms known as amastigotes. They divide and multiply, greatly expanding the infected cell, until it bursts, releasing the parasites for further invasion of other macrophages (Barriga 1981). The course of the disease will depend upon how the immune system of the host responds to this invasion. Quick action with normal exchange of signals between invaded macrophages and T cells empowers the macrophages to kill the parasite before the infection can be established in the host. Such quick immune responses produce little or no signs of the infection.

Sometimes the parasites manage to invade and reproduce within local macrophage-type cells in the skin immediate to the sandfly bite site, but are contained to that area. Although the parasites manage to survive inside the macrophages, once they are released from the cell, other immune reactions attack them and eventually the infection ends there. This form of the disease, known as the cutaneous form and affecting only the skin, commonly occurs on the face. The bite site becomes reddened and raised within two to eight weeks. Then the center disintegrates into a shallow, ulcerative lesion, and eventually heals in three to twelve months. Immunity to further infection with that particular strain follows (Barriga 1981; Bryceson 1975).

Old World cutaneous forms found in rural areas differ somewhat from the cutaneous form found in cities. People in rural areas have more contact with infected animals, both wild and domestic, and the parasites are easily transferred from animals to humans. The skin lesion remains moist and eventually resolves, leaving a scar. This form of the infection, called leishmania major, generally occurs during childhood in infested villages. Lasting immunity to the local variant of leishmania develops following infection (Beck and Davies 1981; Bryceson 1975).

City areas present a different pattern of infection. Transmission occurs from person to person within the high-density human community. The initial lesion following infection retracts, leaving a central crust, but more lesions in the form of little bumps appear around the edge. Nearby lymph nodes also become infected. This form of leishmania appears to be more virulent, passing from person to person via the sandflies, rather than passing from animals to humans. It takes longer to heal, leaving a depressed, mottled scar, but with lasting immunity. The urban infection, known as *Leishmania tropica* or *L. recidiva*, and the lesion produced by it, referred to as "oriental sore," "Aleppo evil," or "Baghdad (or Deli) boil," became the scourge of Middle Eastern and West Asian cities for centuries. Newcomers could soon be recognized by the presence of newly infected sores (Bryceson 1975; Chandler 1945).

The cutaneous form of infection found in the New World follows a course similar to that of the rural form in the Old World, and it is primarily transmitted by sandflies to humans from wild animals in heavily forested areas. Domesticated dogs and rodents in villages in or near infested forests can also pick up the parasites and carry them into human habitats, where sandflies can transfer them to people. Infection in Central and South America occurs most often in young men working in tropical forests. The parasites found in Central America belong to the *Leishmania mexicana* complex, while the parasite in South America belong to the *Leishmania braziliensis* complex. The Central American form commonly affects the ears (Chiclo's ear) of those who gather chicle (a chewing gum ingredient from sapodilla trees), and the localized infection can become chronic, causing destruction of the ear. The South American form can spread along lymphatic pathways, forming many large ulcerative sores, referred to as *pian bois* (Beck and Davies 1981).

L. braziliensis complex in forested areas of the eastern slopes of the Andes can produce severe disease, known as *espundia*, in highly susceptible individuals. Chronic lesions develop around the nose and mouth. The infection begins with the usual skin lesion caused by the parasite. After the initial lesion heals, the parasites spread into localized macrophage type cells within a few days, or they may wait up to five years to become active. The skin and mucous membranes lining the nose and mouth most often fall victim to the destructive behavior of the growing population of parasites released from adjacent macrophage-type cells. Sometimes the mucous membranes covering the palate and/or throat, the cartilage of the nose, and soft palate suffer from destructive lesions. The lesions start out as tiny, itching spots or swellings, usually on the nose. They progress to reddened sores or blister-like swellings that eventually lead to ulcerations (open sores). This process can go on for years, grossly disfiguring the nose and mouth before healing (Beck and Davies 1981; Bryceson 1975; Chandler 1945). In the Old World, a similar infection of the mucous membranes of the mouth occurs in susceptible individuals living in the Sudan and in Ethiopia (Chandler 1945).

The valleys along the western slopes of the Andes contain a variant of the tropical forest parasites that adapted to dryer conditions on this lee side of the mountains. They cause the disease known as *uta,* producing less destructive, self-healing skin lesions (Bryceson 1975).

Less fortunate individuals with immune systems unable to confine the parasitic infection to the body surface cannot stop it from invading the rest of the body. The parasites invade the liver, spleen, lymph system, and bone marrow. Destructive lesions develop within these organs, and the disease becomes known as visceral leishmaniasis.

This serious form of leishmaniasis is found more often in the Old World than the New World. Following healing of the skin lesion at the bite site in visceral leishmaniasis, the parasites invade internal organs, producing twice daily fever and chills, plus enlarged spleen and lymph nodes. The skin of the hands, feet, and abdomen darkens, giving rise to the common name for the disease, *kala-azar,* meaning "black sickness," in India and the Middle East. Anemia eventually develops, along with cirrhosis of the liver. The individual becomes very sick and emaciated as the disease runs its course, with death occurring in a few months or up to five years later in 90 percent of the cases (Bryceson 1975).

Visceral leishmaniasis in the Old World is caused primarily by the *Leishmania donovani* complex. These parasites may have originated among gerbils and jackals in Central Asia, and spread with the trade routes, primarily through dogs and foxes, to the Indian subcontinent, China, the Middle East, the Mediterranean basin, and northern Africa. Young children in the Mediterranean area have become the most common victims, and for this reason the parasite variant is referred to as *Leishmania infantum* (Bryceson 1975). While domestic dogs and wild canids serve as the reservoir for the disease in most areas of the Old World, human beings act as the reservoir in overcrowded and densely populated areas of the Indian subcontinent (Benenson 1995).

Similar severe visceral infections among individuals with poor immune responses have been identified in South America, especially in northeastern Brazil and the Chaco region of northern Argentina and Paraguay

(Chandler 1945). The disease appears primarily in children, but dogs can also suffer from the disease. This severe form of leishmania in the New World occurs with infection by the *L. chagasi* complex (Bryceson 1975).

Variations in the disease of leishmaniasis, from mild skin lesions to severe visceral involvement, may not reflect different species or strains of the parasites, but more likely represents variations in host response to the infection. Genetics plays the major role in the type of immune response the host will have, while the parasite variant plays a minor role in the disease process. Long-term poor nutrition of the host can weaken the immune response as well, allowing the parasites to gain ground with an otherwise healthy immune response. With an inadequate immune response by the host, the parasite naturally gains virulence.

Flying Worms (Filariae)

Settlers who moved into tropical warm, moist areas, particularly in low-lying river valleys and along sea coasts, ran the risk of encountering flying worms. These slender, thread-like worms, known as filariae, adapted to parasitic life with a unique way of sending their offspring to new animal hosts without exposing them to environmental hazards: they "air mail" them. Female worms infecting the animal host give birth to tiny embryos that move into the blood near skin tissues where a blood-sucking insect, usually a mosquito, picks them up. The embryos, known as microfilaria, penetrate the wall of the insect's stomach to develop into elongated larvae within the thoracic muscles. They eventually move to the insect's mouthparts. When the insect takes its blood meal, the tiny larvae enter through the puncture wound of the bite and into the new animal host, working their way into the lymphatic system.

The adult worms develop in lymph vessels and around regional lymph nodes in the host, while their tiny microfilaria offspring move out of the lymph system into the bloodstream. The insect vectors can only pick them up with their blood meals, so the tiny larvae must be present in the circulating bloodstream near the skin surface at the same time that the vector normally takes its blood meal (Beck and Davies 1981).

The females generally vary in size from 20 mm to 100 mm (three-fourths inch to about 4 inches) in length. The males reach only half the size of the females. Usually only one embryo gets released from the mouthpart of the insect vector at any one time, and it may take many hundreds of insect bites before a male and female adult worm meet and mate. It takes six months to a year for the worms to mature, and some species can live up to seventeen years (Chandler 1945).

The various filariae evolved into parasites millennia ago near fast-moving rivers and streams, and along swampy coastlands in the tropics. The worms adapted to a wide range of mosquito and fly vectors capable of incubating and carrying their young to their animal hosts. Most filariae do not infect humans, but some occasionally do. Early human hunters and foragers probably picked up occasional light infections from the worms, without serious consequences, when they entered the territory of a vector.

The development of agriculture and establishment of human settlements within insect vector territory provided opportunities for some of the filariae to adapt to humans and maintain their numbers within the human population. Repeated infections increased the worm load of the human host, increasing the risk of serious health problems. Settlements established outside but near vector territory also ran the risk of repeated infection with frequent trips through the vector-infested zone.

Most people lightly infected with the filariae in endemic areas show few if any symptoms, as long as they are not malnourished and their immune systems develop tolerance to the small numbers of worms. Infection during childhood generally results in tolerance to filariae, but secondary problems associated with the death of large numbers of worms can arise during adulthood. Some individual immune systems don't allow the tiny worm embryos to develop into mature worms at all, while others react violently to the invading microfilaria. Some individuals infected for the first time, with resulting mature worms, later become sensitized to the immature microfilaria and destroy them, while allowing the initial adult worm population to survive (Ogilvie and McKenzie 1981).

Three species of mosquito-borne filaria worms, *Wuchereria bancrofti*, *Brugia malayi*, and *Brugia timori*, adapted to humans. *Wuchereria bancrofti* adapted entirely to human communities, and requires high-density human populations to survive (Ogilvie and McKenzie 1981). This particular filaria must have established itself early on with human settlements along low-lying sea coasts and in river valleys (Chandler 1945) of tropical Africa where it is endemic today. *Wuchereria bancrofti* spread from Africa with sea trade to coastal areas of Asia, from India to China, the islands of Japan, Taiwan, the

Philippines, and islands in the Pacific. The slave trade brought the worms to the New World in the West Indies, along the coast of South America; at one time they were found in Charleston, South Carolina. The worms can be transmitted by a wide variety of mosquitoes belonging to the genera *Culex*, *Aedes*, *Mansonia*, and *Anopheles*. Most mosquito vectors make their airmail deliveries at night, but in the Pacific islands there is a day-biting species of Anopheles that provides daytime deliveries of the worms (Beck and Davies 1981; Orihel 1985).

While *Wuchereria bancrofti* relies on mosquitoes thriving in high-density urban areas, the *Brugia* species rely on mosquito vectors living in rural areas. *Brugia malayi* is endemic in rice-growing areas and swamps of rural southwest India, Sri Lanka, Southeast Asia, China, South Korea, and Japan. *Brugia timori* live in the rural islands of southeast Indonesia (Benenson 1995; Chandler 1945; Orihel 1985).

First-time filaria infection in adults can lead to severe discomfort with acute reactions to the developing adult worms. The worm-infested lymph vessel or lymph node swells, turns red and tender, and becomes very painful. The groin area is most often affected, particularly the male genitals. Some individuals also have fever, and there may be recurring reactions. Children from endemic areas generally do not have these symptoms when first infected (Benenson 1995; Orihel 1985).

Some adults encountering the microfilaria for the first time become highly sensitive to the tiny embryos circulating through the lymphatics of the lungs. They react with a chronic lung disorder known as tropical eosinophilic lung or Weingarten's syndrome. This disease frequently strikes men entering endemic areas for the first time to work, or as part of a military operation. Coughing and asthmatic-like wheezing develops, mostly at night when the embryos are active. Symptoms can last on and off for weeks or months (Ogilvie and McKenzie 1981).

Serious problems can develop in susceptible individuals growing up in endemic areas with large numbers of worms, particularly *Wuchereria bancrofti*. The adult worms eventually die within chronically inflamed lymphatics, most often located in the groin area and lower extremities. Large numbers of adult worms tend to form a tangled mass in the lymph vessels, and when they die off, the immune system reacts to the mass of dead worms by encasing them with granulomatous tissue. This blocks the flow of lymphatic fluid, creating a back-up of fluid into the affected body part, leading to the disease state known as filarial elephantiasis. Extreme forms of this disorder can produce grotesque enlargements of one or both legs, or the external genitals (Beck and Davies 1981; Orihel 1985).

Some adult filarial worms take up residence in the tissues beneath human skin. The most notorious of these filariae belong to the *Onchocerca volvulus* complex that evolved in west Africa using black flies (*Simuliidae*) as vectors. They adapted to humans settling along the banks of fast-flowing rivers where black flies reside. Like mosquitoes, the female black flies require blood meals for the eggs to mature. The flies breed in large, flowing rivers, and they take shelter from the wind in high grass or vegetation along the river banks. They readily attack humans and animals coming near the river. These filariae spread to parts of central Africa and east into Ethiopia, and from there into Yemen, adapting to different variants of black flies. The slave trade brought the worms to parts of Central and South America. The worms adapted to New World species of black flies breeding in small, rapidly flowing streams between 2,000 and 4,500 feet in elevation. The flies frequent areas in and around coffee fields, and transfer the filariae to field workers (Chandler 1945).

Onchocerca females reach much greater lengths than most filarial worms, ranging from 500 mm to 700 mm (over 2 feet), while the males remain very small, 20–50 mm (1–2 inches) in length. The developing worms crawl about under the skin until they reach maturity and mate. Their movements can cause itching, inflammation, and loss of skin pigment. The females form tangled balls with the males in tissue beneath the skin. The immune system reacts to the mass of worms by imprisoning them within a tough, fibrous tissue nodule about the size of a pea, sometimes larger. These nodules typically form on the trunk, near the junction of long bones, around the pelvic arch, and over ribs, while the head area is commonly affected in Central America. The females can live up to fifteen years and can produce thousands of microfilaria each day; the microfilaria can survive in the human host for one to two years. The microfilaria manage to escape their parent's prison and move close to the skin surface so that the biting fly can pick them up (Chandler 1945).

The most serious complications caused by *Onchocerca volvulus* occur when embryos escape nodules on the head and invade the eye, leading to irritation of the eye tissues. The constant irritation created by the steady stream of microfilaria into the eyes creates a continuous inflammatory response that frequently leads to blindness (Orihel 1985). The inflammatory response can be intensified when large numbers of worms or microfilaria die at once, particularly when they are killed by medications (Ogilvie and McKenzie 1981). High proportions of villagers living near rivers infested with black flies in west Africa have suffered from "river blindness," and many villages have been abandoned for higher ground away from the flying worms (Benenson 1995).

Another filaria, known as Loa loa, also likes to dwell just below the skin. Loa loa is endemic to the rain forests of central and west Africa, where up to 90 percent of people living in some villages can be infected (Benenson 1995). The filariae are transmitted by deer flies or mango flies of the genus *Chrysops* in most areas, while minute nocturnal midges of the genus *Culicoides* transmit the worms in the Cameroons. Dozens of larvae empty from the insect's proboscis during a blood meal, and they file out quickly into the bite wound. The adult worms continuously move about under the skin, traveling up to about half an inch per minute, creating painless swellings as they go. They will creep in and about the eyes, which can be very painful. Trying to remove them surgically will send them scurrying into deeper tissues. The females range from 50 mm to 70 mm (2–3 inches) long and the males reach half that length. Adults can live up to seventeen years, producing microfilaria that move into the bloodstream for easy access to their blood-sucking vectors (Chandler 1945; Orihel 1985).

CONCLUDING COMMENTS

The building of tourist hotels along the edges of game parks creates the risk of sleeping sickness disease for foreign visitors. Local cattle that range on the fringes of the game parks can carry the trypanosome parasites, and tsetse flies feeding on them can transfer the disease to tourists (Goodwin 1974). Political unrest in the Great Lakes region of east Africa and across sub-Saharan Africa raises considerable alarm as wilderness areas and tsetse fly belts are greatly disturbed. The massive movements of refugees and abandonment of farm lands make it easy for tsetse flies and other vectors of disease to extend their range. Modern roads and transport systems bring humans together with infectious trypanosome species, as well as with other wild parasites that otherwise would rarely come into contact with humans and their domestic animals.

Chagas' disease is on the move, with the vector bugs taking up residence on long-distance South American passenger trains, and some species moving into big cities with hordes of immigrant rural poor people (Zeledon 1974). Infection can also be facilitated by contaminated blood transfusions. The opening-up of the Amazon basin to settlers poses the threat of new foci of Chagas' disease as people come into contact with wild reservoirs of the infection. At least eighteen possible triatomic bug species present in the Brazilian Amazon can transmit the disease to humans and their domestic animals (Coura et al. 1994).

Severe epidemics of the visceral form of leishmania infection, Kala-azar, were recorded during the early twentieth century in eastern India, with whole villages being depopulated by the disease in Assam (Chandler 1945). The risk of new epidemics remains among the increasing numbers of urban poor in many large cities of the Old World where outbreaks of the disease have occurred in the past. The disease has also spread farther into Africa, and into south-central Texas in the New World. Recently a new form of the cutaneous type, a raised skin lesion that does not ulcerate, has been spreading throughout Central America (Benenson 1995). The movement of settlers into the Amazon basin, forest cutting, and the building of roads through tropical forests have increased the risks of exposure to the parasites. Infected rural individuals moving to poor urban areas of South American cities raise the risk of urban epidemics.

Increasing high-density urban areas of tropical cities filled with poor people living under unsanitary conditions provide an open invitation to trouble. Vast areas of India are allowing the mosquito vector of the filaria *Wuchereria bancrofti* to breed unhampered in pit latrines and polluted waters of the urban poor. The mosquito vector, *Culex fatigans*, has developed resistance to insecticides, placing a minimum of 400 million people at risk of infection with *Wuchereria bancrofti* in endemic areas (Beck and Davies 1981).

Paradise is lost and found again and again as increasing human populations shift back and forth into more and more wilderness areas, erasing wildlife corridors that had offered protection against wild vector-borne parasites. The balance between rural settlements and wilderness zones is quickly coming to an end, unleashing wild diseases into human populations. Once again, changes in human behavior patterns lead to changes in disease patterns.

CHAPTER 8

DOMESTICATED ANIMALS AND DISEASE

Diseases that can be transmitted to human beings from animals are referred to as *zoonoses*. Most zoonotic diseases result from accidental infections in human beings, and people cannot pass them to other people. Diseases can be transmitted from animals through either direct or indirect contact with an infected animal. Direct contact can occur with infected tissue, milk, secretions, blood, urine, or feces. Indirect infection may arise from blood-sucking insect vectors that transfer infection from animals to humans, through inadvertent contact, by ingestion of substances contaminated by infected animal wastes or tissues, or by breathing in dust particles contaminated with animal infectious waste. Several zoonoses cause equal harm to humans and animals. Some zoonoses rarely harm their natural animal hosts, where they act as commensals, but they become dangerous pathogens to humans and/or other animals (Van der Hoeden 1964).

The reverse case, human diseases infecting animals, can also happen. Depending on the type of disease, the infection can develop into disease or be silent, allowing the infected animal to be a carrier, able to transmit the infection back to humans.

Before people settled in with their Neolithic life styles, they had limited contact with animals, so that there was only sporadic disease transmission from wild animals or pets to humans. When advancing human settlements displaced wild animal populations and replaced them with domesticated farm animals, the rules changed. Daily living with domesticated animals allowed diseases once limited to animals to plague farmers and pastoralists. Human beings and domesticated animals sharing living space soon began sharing microbial parasites.

The domestication of animals played a major role in the cultural evolution of humankind and the biological evolution of human diseases. Many human diseases evolved from animal sources once human beings established continuous contact with the animals through domestication. The shift of diseases from animals to people could only take place when a particular variant of an opportunistic microbe or parasite population could adapt to the human microenvironment, and thus target humans as the desired host with human-to-human transmission. The infection, no longer zoonotic, becomes a human disease. Some herd diseases—that is, infections requiring large numbers of animals for successful transmission—could easily switch from domestic herds to people in crowded towns and cities, to become active human diseases. With larger numbers of people crowding together, epidemics arising from animal origins became commonplace.

Man's Best Friend

The dog became the first animal to associate with humans, most likely beginning as a scavenger of human refuse, and ending up as part of the human household. Dogs and humans have been together for over ten thousand years, since long before the agricultural revolution of the Neolithic.

The wild wolf ancestors of dogs roamed Europe, the Near East, Asia, North America, and Central America. They resembled the wolves of South Asia and the Arabian Peninsula, differing from the wolves of northern Europe and Eurasia of today. Evidence for the earliest domestication of the dog comes from the Near East, where a dog skeleton was buried with a human skeleton between 12,000 and 10,000 years ago (Hemmer 1990). Domesticated dogs followed human beings throughout the world, including the New World and Australia, and various breeds of dogs became established throughout the different geographic regions by 3000 B.C. (Zeuner 1963).

Throughout this long association, both human beings and dogs have adjusted to each other's microbial world. Most of the dog's parasites will not infect humans, and most of the human parasites will not infect dogs, but some instances of crossover infection do occur. Some zoonotic infections derived from dogs, such as dog tapeworms, can occur, but rarely. Dogs can also receive infections, such as with measles and mumps viruses, from humans, and they can in turn infect susceptible children and young adults (Bisseru 1967).

The virus that causes measles strongly resembles the virus that causes distemper in dogs, suggesting that both viruses had a common ancestor. The virus that causes rinderpest disease in cattle also resembles the virus that causes distemper in dogs (T-W-Fiennes 1978b). Perhaps when cattle were domesticated and closely associated with domestic dogs, a variant of the rinderpest virus shifted to dogs, and then a variant of this one shifted to people. This argument can be supported by the fact that measles did not appear in the Americas until European contact in the 1500s. Native Americans were highly susceptible to measles, and therefore their dogs must not have carried the distemper virus, since they lacked association with domestic cattle before European contact.

Dogs play a greater role as a go-between for certain infections harmful to humans. Dogs coming into contact with infected wild animals or other domestic animals can inadvertently bring the infection home. Some zoonotic diseases can infect humans by way of the dog, such as rabies.

Dogs and Rabies

Rabies is the most familiar and most frightening disease a dog can bring home. Rabies primarily infects wild animals, including wolves, jackals, foxes, bears, raccoons, badgers, mongoose, and skunks, but the most constant natural reservoir maintaining rabies in various parts of the world is the bat. All kinds of bats, from insect eaters and fruit eaters to vampire bats, serve as natural hosts of the rabies virus. Diseased bats transmit the virus by attacking other bats or animals when the infection reaches its peak in the nervous system, causing erratic behavior in the bat. Bats can also be infected without having the disease, excreting the virus in feces and urine in caves, or wherever they roost. Evidence shows that the virus can be carried by dust particles and be inhaled when large amounts of bat excreta become disturbed by animals or humans for any length of time (T-W-Fiennes 1978b).

Descriptions of rabies transmitted by dogs appear in ancient literature dating back to 3000 B.C. in India (Ahuja 1958), and 1800 B.C. in Mesopotamia (Kaplan and Koprowski 1980). Doubtless rabies and the recognition of mad dogs as carriers of the disease has haunted human communities for many centuries. Rabies carried by bats, particularly blood-sucking vampire bats, was recorded by early Spanish colonists in Mesoamerica (Kaplan and Koprowski 1980), indicating that the disease existed on both sides of the globe long before Columbus sailed to the New World. The rabies virus most likely evolved with bats.

The rabies rhabdovirus consists of a strand of RNA with a lipid (fat-like substance) covering. Infection can only occur when the virus becomes activated within its target cells, nerve cells (neurons) within nerve endings. The virus usually comes into contact with, and penetrates, damaged nerve endings by way of a bite from an infected animal. The infected animal's saliva contains high amounts of the virus. The virus can also be introduced through a cut or wound coming into contact with the infected animal's saliva, or through the mucous lining of the eye and nose (Swango 1989). Dogs coming into contact with rabid animals become easy targets for the disease.

Where the virus gains entry and how much of the virus gets introduced will determine when the disease begins to take hold. Generally, incubation takes three to eight weeks, but it can vary from one week to one year before symptoms of rabies appear. Once the virus penetrates the nerve endings, it migrates to the spinal cord and brain, where it multiplies rapidly, and then moves outward to all parts of the body, including the salivary glands, where it multiplies in preparation for transmission to a new victim. The infected dog's behavior changes dramatically, and the dog soon takes on the classic drooling, "mad dog" syndrome, followed by paralysis, convulsions, and death. Sometimes the disease takes a different course in the dog, with sluggishness and hiding, just the opposite of the aggressive form (Swango 1989). Rabies remains a true zoonotic disease in humans, following a similar course, and it generally results in death.

Cat Fanciers

Domestic cats made their first appearance around five thousand years ago in Egypt, derived from the local wild cat of the same size. Domestication may have come about when cats became attracted to rodents infesting human settlements. Once the Egyptians domesticated cats, they did not allow them to be exported for more than a thousand years. However, smuggling operations spread the domesticated cat throughout the Mediterranean basin, into Europe and Asia; a fresco of a cat appears in Crete by 1500 B.C., and cats are shown in Chinese art by 1100 B.C. (Beadle 1977).

Cats can be very beneficial by keeping away rodents and wild birds capable of transmitting infectious viruses and parasites to humans and their domestic animals. Sometimes viruses and other parasites infecting the cat's meal infect the cat, and occasionally some of these infections can be transmitted to human beings and other animals. Feline enteritis virus infection in cats has been implicated in some cases of human infectious polyneuritis (inflammation of several nerves) (Bisseru 1967).

Cats and Toxoplasmosis

Toxoplasmosis generally produces mild infection in humans, animals, and birds. Caused by a tiny protozoan, *Toxoplasma gondii*, the parasite has an unusual life cycle tied to cats. The infection occurs worldwide. The reservoir for this parasite exists in rodents, among the cat's favorite victims. Female rodents infected with the parasite can transmit the infection to their unborn young through the placenta, thus maintaining the infection in the rodent population. The cat acquires the infection through a rodent meal, and the parasite sets up shop in the cat's small intestine. Here the parasite undergoes a developmental cycle not found in any other animal (T-W-Fiennes 1978b).

The parasites multiply within the cells of the mucous lining of the cat's intestine. While most of them divide and spread throughout the cat's body, as they do in other animals, some of the protozoa develop into male and female sexual cells (gametes). The male and female gametes unite to form fertilized eggs (zygotes), protected by thin but resilient walls. The eggs leave the cat host with its feces. The fertilized zygote does not become infective until it completes its own development outside the cat's gut. Fortunately for the shed parasitic egg, the cat prefers to bury its feces, protecting the new egg from harm. Within one to four days the zygote divides into halves, with each half developing into four infective sporozoites. The fertilized egg now becomes a sporulated oocyst, protected by a tough outer wall, able to survive in damp soil for up to a year. The infectious oocysts can be carried about to animal food sources on dust particles, earthworms, cockroaches, and flies (T-W-Fiennes 1978).

Ingestion of food contaminated with infective oocysts by other animals or humans allows the parasite to leave the protective egg and enter the cells of the mucous lining of the host intestines. Here it begins to spread by dividing and eventually invades the bloodstream to relocate to other tissue cells, where it continues to proliferate. The parasite invades a wide variety of cells, including skeletal muscle, heart muscle, and nerve cells. The infected cells burst when parasite multiplication peaks, releasing the new parasites to invade adjacent cells, until the immune system manages to stop the proliferation of the parasite within the cells. The parasites stop multiplying but remain infectious by sealing themselves off within a protective cystic wall within the affected tissues, where they can remain viable for years, often lasting for the lifetime of the host. Carnivores eating flesh infected with these cysts can develop the infection as the cysts release the parasites into the gut of the new victim. Humans can acquire the infection in a similar manner by eating undercooked meat from infected sheep, cattle, or pigs (Jones 1975b).

The connection between cats and most human infections became evident in 1970. Infection rates in human populations with cats range from 20 percent to 60 percent (Jones 1975b), and it has been estimated that approximately half of the U.S. population may be infected, most of them without knowing it (Yeager 1985). Wherever cats deposit feces containing the infective oocysts, in soil, sand boxes, or litter boxes, human infection can be possible, except in very cold or hot dry climates. The infective oocysts can be transported by dust particles in the air, by insects, or by dirty human hands to contaminate food, eating utensils, even drinking water, where they can be ingested.

The parasite proceeds to proliferate by dividing until the human immune system stops it, at which time the parasite enters the dormant cyst stage, and the infection becomes silent. As long as the immune system holds the parasite within the capsule walls, the host does not suffer (Yeager 1985). Most infections of older children and adults go unnoticed. Swollen lymph glands, especially in the neck, a low-grade fever, and tiredness may be recognized for a few days or weeks. Individuals with impaired immune systems can develop serious disease as the proliferating parasites cannot be stopped. Organs such as the heart, muscles, and brain can become inflamed with severe tissue damage (Jones 1975b).

The most vulnerable to infection can be the unborn and very young infants. If the mother acquires the infection during pregnancy, she can pass it to her unborn infant through the placenta without displaying any symptoms of the disease. Infection acquired during pregnancy can result in miscarriage or stillbirth, or serious congenital disease. It is also possible that the newborn may show no signs of infection until later. The parasite particularly targets fetal neural cells to cause neural damage. The newborn may be born

with microcephaly (abnormally small head and brain), seizures, inflammation of the brain, mental retardation, or hydrocephaly (enlarged head from
accumulated fluid around the brain). Newborns can also suffer inflamed
lungs, rash, and fever. Some newborns showing no signs of infection at birth
may develop signs of progressive brain damage during the first few months of
life, followed by death. Some infants born without signs of infection can grow
up to adults before developing symptoms, usually when dormant cysts rupture and invade eye tissues, leading to progressive loss of vision (Jones 1975b).

Serious infection can also occur after birth in the young baby. The
baby's immature nervous system appears vulnerable to the parasite.
Convulsions and other neurological symptoms appear, including hydro-
cephalus, and inflammation of the eye tissues. If the baby survives, mental
retardation and impaired vision result (Faust 1951).

Taking Stock

Sheep and goats became the first domesticated stock animals, descended
from wild sheep and goats that ranged in the mountains and high valleys of
southwest Asia (Hemmer 1990). Herding replaced hunting of these animals,
and their docile nature allowed them to be tamed and domesticated. The earliest evidence for domestication of these animals, by 8000 B.C., comes from
the Zagros Mountains of present-day Iran (Clutton-Brock 1981; Fagan 1996;
Hemmer 1990; Zeuner 1963).

The earliest domestic sheep evolved from the wild mouflon sheep
inhabiting the mountains and high valleys of southwest Asia, west of the
Caspian sea to the Gulf of Oman (Hemmer 1990). Docile sheep are easily
managed and can be herded about to seasonal patches of grass from high
mountain valleys to lowland meadows.

Wild ancestors of domestic goats, the highly adaptable bezoars, ranged
from the eastern Mediterranean to southwest Asia and into present-day
Afghanistan. Goats will eat whatever they can find, and they thrive on
thorny scrub that other animals avoid (Hemmer 1990). They can get by with
little food during hard times, and they can survive extremes in temperature.
This made them ideal domestic stock in marginal ecological zones.

Herding sheep and goats required human caretakers to keep the flocks
moving to fresh food sources and water, and to provide protection from
predators. Herding sheep and goats together became a common practice.

Herding of these animals was so successful that it contributed to the expansion of desert lands throughout the Old World. Repeated grazing of the same lands over the centuries by these animals permanently damaged the natural flora. Between the two of them, they pull up plants by the roots and strip away vegetation, facilitating soil erosion. North Africa and the Near East in particular have suffered from centuries of overgrazing by sheep and goats (Clutton-Brock 1981).

Early farmers frequently combined sheep and goat herding with agriculture throughout the Mediterranean basin and southwest Asia. These animals served as walking larders of meat and milk. Both goat and sheep milk were processed into milk products long before cattle became domesticated and were milked. They provided hides for leather, wool for clothing, bones and sinew for tools, tallow for lamplight, and dung for fuel (Clutton-Brock 1981). Some pastoral peoples sustained themselves primarily by herding without agriculture.

Cattle became the next animals to be domesticated. Long-horned wild auroch cattle roamed the forests and meadows of Europe, the Near East, Asia, and north Africa following the retreat of the Ice Age. The earliest evidence for domestication of cattle comes about a thousand years after the domestication of sheep and goats, in Anatolia and the Balkans (Hemmer 1990).

Cattle herds may have grazed freely under the watchful eyes of their new masters, coaxed by salt and water to be near humans (Clutton-Brock 1981), with eventual corraling at times to control their movements. Cattle herding slowly spread throughout the Mediterranean basin, into north Africa, Europe, and Asia. Cattle were a source of meat and bone marrow, as well as hides for clothing; horns, bones, and sinew for tools; hooves for glue; and manure for fertilizer and fuel. They also served as beasts of burden.

Short-horn cattle appeared in Mesopotamia and the Indus Valley of southwest Asia about the same time, around 3000 B.C.. These cattle proved to be more docile than the long-horn breeds, and ideal milk producers. The short-horn appears to have evolved from domestic long-horn breeds somewhere between these two regions, spreading both east and west at the same time with the demands for bovine milk products (Hepstein 1971). Use of milk products from cows opened up a new avenue for transmission of over thirty different animal diseases to humans (Brothwell 1991).

Several breeds of cattle developed from wild long-horn auroch ancestors throughout their original range, with numerous cross-breedings through time. Popular breeds in arid regions included humped cattle, particularly the zebu. Humped cattle appear to have derived from long-horn cattle inhabiting steppe or desert environments of southwest Asia, sometime during the fourth millennium B.C. They drink less water, they have smaller digestive systems, and they have a larger body surface that allows them to be more heat resistant than other cattle. They became incorporated into the livestock of peoples in and around the Indus Valley, southern Mesopotamia, and north Africa (Hepstein 1971).

Cattle diseases intensified in many areas when domestication took place. Controlled herding with restricted land use and close, repetitive association between humans and cattle, and the mixing of cattle with other domestic animals, assured the increase and exchange of many zoonotic diseases. The beef tapeworm became a common parasite in humans with consumption of undercooked meat from infected domestic stock (see chapter 3).

The domestic water buffalo appears to have derived from the wild arnee of India, and was one of the earliest domesticated animals used by the Harapan culture in the Indus Valley (Hepstein 1971). Having evolved from a swamp habitat, these animals needed warm, marshy areas for survival, where most domestic cattle cannot survive. Water buffalo became ideal vehicles for pulling plows in rice fields, and by 5000 B.C. their use with wet rice agriculture spread throughout Southeast Asia (Barnes 1993). The water buffalo was introduced to ancient Sumer in Mesopotamia around 2500 B.C., and later into the Nile Valley of postdynastic Egypt (Hepstein 1971). These animals became subject to diseases transmitted from insect vectors and other domesticated animals. Water buffalo also develop a form of skin leprosy similar to the human form (see chapter 10).

Several varieties of wild pigs could be found throughout Europe, north Africa, and Asia by the end of the Ice Age. The earliest evidence for domestication of pigs shows that they appeared in New Guinea around ten thousand years ago. The only way they could have arrived on this island was by water craft with humans, indicating a long history of domesticated pigs in Southeast Asia. Evidence of pig domestication in Anatolia and the Near East appears around nine thousand years ago, independent of Asian pig domestication. From there, pig domestication spread into Europe and Africa (Hemmer 1990).

Pigs can transmit some parasites to humans, and they act as reservoirs for influenza viruses. *Trichinella spirali* roundworms causing trichinosis can be acquired from pigs by ingesting undercooked pork. The large roundworms,

Ascaris lumbricoides, that infect humans who ingest their eggs from vegetables grown in feces-contaminated soil evolved from the swine *Ascaris suum* when pigs and people crowded together in Neolithic villages (see chapter 4).

The domesticated donkey evolved from the wild ass of north Africa during the fourth millennium B.C., spreading throughout the Mediterranean basin as a beast of burden. Horses remained a hunted animal long after the agricultural revolution began, with domestication coming rather late. They could not easily be tamed. The aggressive nature of stallions in protecting their mares presented a formidable challenge to domestication. Domestication of horses appears to have occurred toward the end of the fourth millennium B.C. from the wild tarpan of the steppes north of the Black and Caspian Seas (Hemmer 1990). They slowly spread southwest into the eastern Mediterranean, and east into Asia, first with chariots, and later as riding horses among nomadic Scythians (Clutton-Brock 1981). Horses were primarily used by the elite and for military purposes. They gave new power and speed to armies in the form of mounted cavalry throughout the Old World (Zeuner 1963).

Horses can be infected with disease agents from other domesticated animals, and they can act as reservoirs for infectious viruses, such as the rhinoviruses, responsible for triggering the common cold in humans, and many of the mosquito-borne arboviruses causing encephalitis in humans.

Reindeer in the north, dromedary camels in the south, and bactrian camels in the east of the Old World also became domesticated by nomadic herdsmen. These animals, plus elephants domesticated in southern Asia, also could be affected by the diseases of domesticated cattle, sheep, and goats.

Early domestication of jungle fowl, ducks, and geese took place in Southeast Asia (Butzer 1964). The red jungle fowl of India, domesticated throughout the Indus Valley by 2000 B.C., spread westward into the eastern Mediterranean, north Africa, and Europe, and eastward into China. Domesticated geese also appeared in the Mediterranean basin and Central Asia (Hyams 1972). Peacocks came under domestication in Asia, while the guinea fowl was domesticated in Africa (Herre 1969). The crowding of fowl together increased their parasite loads, and spillover into human populations became possible. Accumulation of a tiny microorganism, *Chlamydia psittaci*, in feces from infected birds can lead to a lung disease in humans known as psittacosis, when the microorganisms are carried on dust particles and breathed in by bird handlers. Newcastle disease, a virus infection of fowl, is similar to the mumps virus, suggesting that the human virus was derived from the virus infecting fowl (Bisseru 1967).

Attempts to domesticate other animals, such as the hyena, proved unsuccessful because the nature of the animals would not tolerate it. Human beings have always kept a variety of pets, and our ancestors usually acquired pets by capturing them as young animals. Taming pet animals to tolerate humans and their demands does not equate with domestication. However, pet keeping brings animals into close contact with humans that otherwise would not naturally occur. This also brings humans into close contact with their parasites, allowing transfer of opportunistic parasites to humans.

Goats and Brucellosis

Mediterranean goats became natural hosts for a bacterial parasite, *Brucella melitensis*. This relationship probably developed in wild ancestral goats long before domestication. Brucelli have proven to be opportunistic parasitic bacteria, able to adapt to various species of wild mammals, birds, reptiles, amphibians, and even fish when the opportunity arises, and some insects can carry it around (Van der Hoeden 1964). They can also survive for a time outside the host in water and soil, especially damp soil, where they may last for up to seventy-two days. However, direct sunlight kills them within hours (Spink 1956).

Infected animals discharge brucelli in their urine, and infected new mothers emit them through infected vaginal secretions, placental tissues, and milk. First-time mother animals are most susceptible to infection, since the bacteria seek out the mammary glands, placenta, and fluids surrounding the fetus. This frequently leads to spontaneous abortion of the first pregnancy in ungulates. Feeding areas can quickly become contaminated with infective urine and birth discharges, thereby infecting other animals living in the area. They become infected by ingesting soiled plants, or through contact with the mucous covering of the eye. Repeated exposure to contaminated material assures infection with brucelli.

Once the bacteria gain entry to the body through mucous membranes of the mouth, throat, intestine, or eye, macrophage-type cells take them to the nearest lymph node. Here they continue to invade macrophage-type cells and reproduce. If they cannot be stopped by host immune defenses in the lymph node, they eventually reach the bloodstream and are carried throughout the body to other organs containing fixed macrophage-type cells, particularly those located in bone marrow, spleen, liver, kidney, and the reproductive organs. The placental blood vessels and mammary glands of the pregnant female animal are especially targeted (Spink 1956).

Goats have the greatest tolerance for the infection; few goats display serious illness from the brucelli. This makes them ideal carriers of the disease, and with their nomadic habits and frequent urinations, they can saturate the local environment with the bacteria. Sheep herded with goats can easily become infected by eating contaminated grass. Sheep also have great tolerance to the infection. Perhaps the long association between sheep and goats has helped them develop greater tolerance to brucelli. However, both sheep and goats will sicken with the infection when poorly nourished or when their immunity becomes compromised by another disease. Even though spontaneous abortion frequently occurs with first-time mothers, and nursing mothers transmit brucelli in their milk, young kids and lambs appear resistant to the disease (Spink 1956).

Human infection causing brucellosis requires large numbers of brucelli acquired through repeated exposure (Van der Hoeden 1964). Brucelli can survive for days in unpasteurized yogurt and cheese to infect humans. A physician, T. Zammit, discovered this in 1905 on the island of Malta, while investigating the source of brucellosis in British troops stationed there. Once he discovered the source in goat's milk, it was banned from the soldiers' diet. The infection rate within the troops fell to almost zero, while high levels of infection remained within the civilian population (Spink 1956).

Brucellosis can be easily transmitted to human beings through repeated contact with infected animals and their tissues through skin abrasions, or by rubbing the eye while milking, slaughtering, or assisting in birthing, or by handling contaminated material. High levels of contaminated dust can also be dangerous within closed areas, such as slaughterhouses (Spink 1956; Van der Hoeden 1964).

In ancient Greece Hippocrates described symptoms of a disease compatible with the symptoms of brucellosis. The disease has had many names: intermittent fever, undulant fever, Mediterranean fever, Malta fever, Cyprus fever, Neapolitan fever. Until the 1900s brucellosis often became confused with malaria because of similarity of symptoms. The disease has been around for a long time in the Mediterranean, and I have found signs of the disease in a thirteenth-century population ruled by the Franks at ancient Corinth, Greece. The disease leaves telling signs within the vertebrae of the spine of chronically infected individuals.

Brucelli attack humans in the same way as they do animals, except that pregnant women rarely suffer spontaneous abortion. The human placenta does not contain the same substance, erythritol, found in the ungulate placenta that attracts and promotes the growth of brucelli (Knight 1975). Children, like young animals, show much more resistance to the disease than do adults. Brucellosis varies in its manifestation, depending on the individual's immune response and how much of the brucelli gain entry into the host.

Those people blessed with a good immune system may suffer only a mild form of the disease with "flu-like" symptoms usually lasting two or three months. Sometimes these symptoms may last up to a year before complete recovery. About 20 percent of those infected develop more serious disease, and around 2 percent die (Spink 1956; Van der Hoeden 1964). The frequency and severity of brucellosis increases when immunity becomes compromised by poor nutrition. The disease can come on suddenly or gradually, characterized by fever that comes and goes with daily fluctuations, usually high in the evenings with profuse sweating, and falling by morning with cold chills. This can last for years in chronic cases. Napoleon Bonaparte suffered from chronic fevers and other symptoms, diagnosed later (in the 1930s), from tissue samples taken from his body, as having been caused by brucellosis (T-W-Fiennes 1978b).

Other major symptoms of the disease include weakness, headaches, irritability, depression, insomnia, weight loss, and joint pains, especially back pains. Chronic sufferers develop a hypersensitivity to the infection when their immune systems attempt to seal off infected areas with inflammatory reactions that create tumor-like encasing granulomas. These granulomas can damage affected tissues. Granulomas frequently develop within the intervertebral disk and adjacent vertebrae of the back, sometimes in the knee or hip, thus causing excruciating pain. Granulomas develop in the lymph nodes, spleen, and bone marrow, similar to the effects of Hodgkins disease, and brucelli have been implicated in this disease (Spink 1956; Van der Hoeden 1964).

Brucellosis remains a zoonotic disease of people. The disease can also spread to other species of domestic animals, especially cattle. By 1925 it was discovered that the bovine form of the disease, commonly known as Bang's disease, could be transmitted through cow's milk to humans, as well as by contact with infected tissues. Infected cattle suffer a high incidence of spontaneous abortion, thus the variant affecting cattle is called *Brucellosis abortus*. Young calves, like kids and lambs, have high resistance to the infection. The human disease caused by this variant of brucellosis usually does not produce as severe a disease as brucellosis caused by the melitensis variant of goats and sheep (Spink 1956).

Pigs can also be infected, primarily by eating contaminated animal tissues. The variant acquired by pigs goes by the name *Brucellosis suis*. Unlike the young of sheep, goats, and cattle, piglets have more susceptibility to the disease than adult pigs. Boars can transmit the brucelli through semen from infected male reproductive organs (Spink 1956). Infected males of other animal species are also capable of transmitting the disease in a similar manner. Horses can be infected, and dogs have acquired a variant known as *Brucellosis canis*. Humans can acquire infection caused by different brucelli variants of other animals by contact with infected tissues.

Bringing the Cows Home, and Anthrax

One of the most feared diseases, anthrax, long ago developed a relationship with cattle. Anthrax evolved into a very opportunistic microbe targeting herbivores (plant eaters). Besides cattle, the disease can strike other domesticated animals, including horses, camels, and elephants, as well as wild herbivores. Pigs can pick up the disease from eating feed contaminated by anthrax spores. Occasionally humans and other nonherbivore animals can be infected, but the disease primarily attacks domesticated herbivores (Van der Hoeden 1964). Some breeds of herbivores, such as Algerian sheep, possess natural resistance to the disease.

The areas of origin of cattle domestication coincide with the highly endemic areas for anthrax today in Asia, Asia Minor, southern Europe, and north Africa. This strongly suggests that anthrax developed into a greater threat to humans with domestication of cattle.

The parasitic bacteria causing anthrax, *Bacillus anthracis*, does not depend on living animals to spread infection. Dead animals work better, so killing the host becomes an advantage to the bacilli. Instead of passing from one live host to another, this microbe must kill its host before it can pass to another host.

Once the host dies and the bacilli are exposed to oxygen from the air, they promptly develop into highly resistant spores able to survive for months in the dead carcass, and for several years in contaminated soil where they wait for a grazing animal to take them in. Wind and rain help spread the spores, and farmers plowing contaminated fields help move the spores around. Repeated use of grazing lands can produce high levels of infective spores as the disease annually kills and passes through new victims. Contaminated pastures avoided for years remain infective; anthrax spores have been known to remain viable in contaminated pastures for a hundred years (LaForce 1990).

Carnivores killing and eating infected animals usually do not contract the disease because the bacilli, unprotected by the spore coating, are killed by stomach acids. However, dining on dead carcasses with spores present can lead to infection. Animals can sometimes become infected with the spores by contact through cuts or sores, and sometimes from bites of flies that have fed on infected carcasses. Carnivores as well as herbivores can carry the spores around in their fur or hair, after picking them up from rolling in contaminated soil, or from coming into contact with infected carcasses.

Once ingested by the grazing animal, the spores move through the animal's stomach, protected from stomach acids by the spore covering. As they reach the intestine, macrophage-type cells patrolling the mucosal borders engulf the foreigners and take them to the nearest lymph node for interrogation and destruction. The spores resist and transform into replicating bacilli possessing two large plasmids. One plasmid provides a protective capsule for the bacilli, while the other one releases damaging toxins. The bacteria quickly increase and spread though the bloodstream to attack macrophage cells, particularly those fixed to the liver, spleen, lungs, and kidneys. The massacre causes the release of high levels of potent inflammatory agents that damage body tissues along with the bacilli and their toxins. This volatile combination leads to the death of the host. Anthrax bacilli literally disarm and force the host at toxic gunpoint to kill itself. When the dead host tissues fall apart, the anthrax bacilli are exposed to oxygen. This triggers spore formation to protect the bacilli and allow them to wait in a dormant state for the next victim.

The majority of infected animals (80 percent) die from acute septic (poisonous) shock within one or two days. Epidemics killing thousands of domestic cattle, and sometimes sheep, have been recorded for centuries (Top 1955) throughout the Mediterranean region and India (Van der Hoeden 1964).

Anthrax raged through Europe, killing large numbers of livestock and people, from the 1600s to 1800s, until the cause of the disease was finally discovered (Jaax and Fritz 1997).

Humans infection with anthrax primarily comes through contact with animals or animal products contaminated with spores, usually in the form of cutaneous anthrax. The spores gain entry into the body through cuts or abrasions on the skin when a person handles contaminated animal hides, wool, hair, or other animal products. In the past anthrax turned into an occupational disease among individuals working with animal products; it was often referred to as woolsorter disease, rag picker disease, and tanner disease. The skin sore produced by anthrax went by such names as charbon, milzbrand, or malignant pustule. Imported shaving brushes made from animal bristles contaminated with anthrax spores produced panic over an outbreak of cutaneous anthrax during the early 1900s in the United States (Jaax and Fritz 1997).

Once anthrax spores gain entry through a break in the skin, a raised, reddened area appears at the entry site within forty-eight hours. Flu-like symptoms with fever and headache develop as red swelling forms around the entry site. Tissue within the entry site dies, forming a thick black scab that lasts for several weeks before sloughing off and healing. Most human immune systems can seal off and limit the anthrax spore infection to the site of entry. Immune responses in about one in twenty individuals with cutaneous infections, especially those located on the face or neck, cannot contain the spores (Cecil and Loeb 1951), and the infection spreads to the nearest lymph node, where the bacilli multiply and escape into the bloodstream, unchecked and fatal (Jaax and Fritz 1997).

While most human anthrax infections occur through breaks in the skin, on rare occasions infection can be acquired through ingestion of spore-contaminated undercooked meat. The most dreaded form of human infection is through the lungs. Spores can be breathed by people working in closed areas where high numbers of spores contaminate dust particles, usually where hides, wool, or textiles are being processed. However, inhalation anthrax has always been rare throughout human history.

Inhalation anthrax in humans generally proves fatal. The spores arrive in the tiny air ducts of the lungs where macrophages engulf them and carry them to lymph nodes situated between the lungs. The spores transform into the bacilli, and their protective capsule prevents their destruction by phagocytosis in the lymph nodes. As they multiply rapidly within these nodes, hemorrhaging begins in this area between the lungs. The bacilli spill out into the circulatory system producing their toxins. Blood poisoning and tissue destruction follow.

Symptoms develop one to five days after inhaling the spores and are flu-like, including sudden chills, high fever, profuse sweating, headache, and fatigue. Slight nasal stuffiness and dry persistent cough develop with red-dened and swollen mucous membranes of the nose and throat. General uneasiness develops with stiffness of joints and twinges of pain. Within twenty-four hours of release of high levels of toxins and inflammatory agents, tightness in the chest with difficult breathing develops. The skin turns bluish, and breathing becomes very painful. Choking fits develop as the lungs fill with fluid, sometimes producing blood-tinged sputum. Convulsions often develop, and death soon follows in 90 percent of victims. Sometimes symptoms can last up to ten days with delirium and unconsciousness. Heavy doses of infection usually result in rapid collapse and death before severe symptoms can appear (Alibek 1999; Cecil and Loeb 1951).

One of the biggest dangers from anthrax today stems from its potential use as a biological weapon. Massive numbers of refined anthrax spores released into the airways of a community can cripple and kill most of the inhabitants within a few days. The danger was demonstrated in April 1979 when an accident occurred at Military Compound 19, a bacterial warfare manufacturing center in Sverdlovsk in the Soviet Union, east of the Ural mountains. The accident released a cloud of anthrax spores into the atmosphere during the night (Alibek 1999). Winds blew the spores to the southern suburbs of the town, killing as many as a thousand residents (Congressional Subcommittee on Oversight 1980).

No News Is Good News in the New World

While people in the Old World were busy domesticating a wide range of animals, and in the process acquiring new human diseases, New World inhabitants remained sealed off from most of these activities. While the domesticated dog accompanied migrating humans into the New World, no other domesticated animals from the Old World came to the New World until after European conquest.

The llama and alpaca became the only stock animals domesticated in the New World, descendants of wild camelids in the South American Andes.

They served primarily as pack animals and producers of wool. Andean villagers also domesticated guinea pigs and muscovy ducks for food. These animals remained confined to the Andean region of South America, unlike so many domesticated animals in the Old World that spread to many different geographic regions throughout the Eastern Hemisphere. The only other domestication in the New World took place in Mesoamerica with the turkey, which eventually spread into North America.

People in the Old World adjusted to the new diseases derived from their domesticated animals after several centuries of exposure. These new diseases produced a certain amount of fluctuating equilibrium with their human host populations, wherever they became established as endemic infections. Unfortunately, the peoples of the New World, who had no history of exposure to most of the new diseases derived from domestic stock, quickly fell victim to pathogens introduced from the Old World. They succumbed more readily to the diseases brought by the invaders from the Old World than to the invaders themselves when contact between the two hemispheres was established.

CONCLUDING COMMENTS

Animal domestication played a very important role in the evolution of human diseases. Many of the human diseases of today derived from various animals as they became domesticated in the Old World. Crowding animals and people together in closely packed houses and village compounds promoted the transfer of opportunistic infectious microbes to human populations. Trading microbes back and forth between various animals and humans also triggered new strains of infectious pathogens. Many domestic animals, especially the dog, have acted as go-betweens for zoonotic infections from wild animals and birds to humans. Zoonotic infections also have been, and continue to be, a constant threat to humans working closely with domesticated animals.

Most of the devastating diseases that afflicted Native Americans during European conquest of the New World originated among domesticated animals in the Old World. The centuries of isolation from the Old World while animal domestication took place prevented Native Americans from developing tolerance or resistance to the new diseases acquired from those animals.

New human diseases from domesticated animals continue to develop as we introduce domesticated stock to new geographic regions, disrupting local environments. Introducing stock animals to new environments issues an invitation to local opportunistic microbes to develop new tastes, and humans can soon become involved. By mixing different animals, we invite new hybrids of disease agents when the microbe variants from different animals get together.

We also expose domesticated animals to new diseases that can infect human beings when we overmanage local environments and animal feed. Mad cow disease developed from feeding cattle contaminated sheep brains ground up in their feed as a protein source. Humans eating undercooked beef with neural tissue can acquire the disease. Antibiotics added to animal feeds have produced resistant, virulent strains of animal commensals harmful to humans, such as the *E. coli* strain in contaminated beef.

We continue to crowd our animals into limited spaces, creating high concentrations of waste products that overload the immediate environment. Crowding also provides fertile breeding grounds for the development of new strains of old diseases.

Our interaction with domesticated animals will always provide opportunities for the evolution of new diseases from old and new sources, as well as the occasional zoonotic infection. Perhaps it is now time to change how we manage domestic animals to prevent the relentless opportunities for the development of newer strains of old diseases.

CHAPTER 9

COWS, MYCOBACTERIA, AND TUBERCULOSIS

Tuberculosis haunted the industrialized world in epidemic form from the 1600s to the early twentieth century. Its cause was misunderstood, and the disease had the ability to express itself in a wide variety of unrelated symptoms. Together, these factors allowed the disease to spread throughout the world. By the end of the nineteenth century the cause and contagiousness of the disease had been confirmed, and thereafter, wherever public health measures were instituted, tuberculosis began to decline. By the time of World War II modern medicine had developed antimicrobial medications to combat the disease, and with this new arsenal against tuberculosis, the eradication of the disease appeared close at hand. Unfortunately, this scenario was too optimistic, and resilient strains of mycobacteria resistant to medication have contributed to a new world pandemic of tuberculosis. The disease feeds on exploding human populations living in crowded, dirty slums, and populations beset with AIDS. The fear of tuberculosis has returned.

Mycobacteria

The bacteria causing tuberculosis belong to a diverse group of microorganisms known as mycobacteria. Most of them are harmless and thrive on dead or decaying organic material. They participate in nature's recycling program, breaking down organic material and fixing nitrogen (Haas and Haas 1996). Mycobacteria have been active members of microbe communities in soil and water all over the world since organic life evolved eons ago. Many of them operate as opportunistic microbes, able to adapt quickly to changing microenvironments. Some can harmlessly colonize skin or the mucous membranes lining the airways of the lungs and intestinal walls of fish, reptiles, birds, and mammals. This can happen when susceptible hosts ingest contaminated food and/or water, or inhale moist dust particles or water droplets containing the microbes. Usually colonization is short-lived since the host's resident microbes crowd out the mycobacteria, while the host remains unaware of their presence. However, some of the mycobacteria are more successful at colonization than others, able to adhere more readily to mucosal tissue without causing harm to the host (Collins 1996).

Some environmental mycobacteria can establish harmless colonies along the mucous linings of the mouths, throats, bronchials, and intestines of human beings, where they thrive on shed, decaying cells. They can become dangerous if they manage to get past the mucosal barrier and into deeper tissues; this is particularly true for the group known as the *Mycobacteria avium* complex. Fortunately, host resistance factors, alarmed at the intrusion, can destroy them before they get past the submucosal tissues. But hosts with compromised immunity and/or faulty resistance factors can be victimized by the invaders, which can cause serious and often fatal disease in humans and animals (Collins 1996).

Some mycobacteria left free living in the environment to take up full-time parasitic life, adapting their needs to a host's microenvironment, and becoming dependent on host-to-host transmission. Transmission between hosts can be accomplished by inhalation of moist droplets coughed from the bronchials of infected lungs, or through oral contamination with feces containing sheddings from the infected intestine. Sometimes mycobacteria can pass through the kidneys in urine. They also can be carried through the mammary glands of cows into their milk.

Cows and the Mycobacteria of Tuberculosis

The human form of parasitic mycobacterial disease is generally known as *Mycobacterium tuberculosis*. Cattle infected with a similar, related parasitic mycobacteria develop the bovine form of this disease. Numerous variants of these two related strains exist, including *M. africanum*, discovered recently in human inhabitants of South Africa and similar to both the bovine and human forms, and *M. microti*, infecting voles (Adler and Rose 1996; Barrow 1986; Kreiswirth and Moss 1996).

As with all microbes, diversity within each population of mycobacteria allows any one variant represented to become the dominant form as circumstances change. This makes it possible for some parasitic mycobacteria to transfer from one species of host to another, and back again to the original host species. Changing host microenvironments brings a shift in the dominant microbe form, allowing colonization to be successful, while retaining some of the forms capable of colonizing the former host species or another species. Thus, strains within the *Mycobacterium tuberculosis* complex can move back and forth between voles and cattle, and between cattle and humans, with the dominant variant shifting each time.

Voles are natural hosts to the mycobacteria. They survive infection without ill effects (Francis 1958). Transmission of mycobacteria from voles to cattle most likely occurs when cattle ingest grass contaminated with vole droppings. Inhalation of feces-contaminated dust or droplets represents another possible route. Ingested mycobacteria, protected by a fatty (lipid) capsule from stomach acids, pass through cattle guts unharmed to colonize the mucous membrane lining of the intestine. Sometimes they remain in the upper portion of the alimentary canal and colonize the mucous membranes lining the mouth and throat. When inhaled, they can colonize the tiny air sacs in the bronchials of the animal's lungs.

Mycobacterium tuberculosis has the potential to invade the submucosal tissue. If not stopped by the immune system, it can spread throughout the body to other organs, with the lungs the favored target. Nearly all cattle infected with the bovine form eventually develop active lung disease. They can then transmit mycobacteria in droplets coughed from the lungs to other animals nearby (Adler and Rose 1996). The potential for disease in wild cattle tends to be sporadic, since the herds move about from one grazing area to another. Occasional infection would strike vulnerable, weak and sick animals.

Human populations stayed relatively free of tuberculosis caused by this complex of mycobacteria until they domesticated cattle. Sometime following the earliest domestication of cattle, tuberculosis began its long journey through human populations. Cattle restricted in their range, herded repeatedly to the same water sources, or temporarily confined to crowded, makeshift corrals were more likely to be repeatedly exposed to the mycobacteria from infected animals. Since most infected cattle carry the microbes in their lungs, the mycobacteria easily spread by the aerosol route to other animals as they crowd together. Cattle contract the disease more readily when it is transmitted by the aerosol rather than the gastrointestinal route (Francis 1958). Crowding many animals together with even one infectious animal facilitates the spread of the disease, and the incidence of disease among cattle increases in proportion to the density of the cattle herd (Van der Hoeden 1964).

Susceptibility to infection varies among cattle breeds. Zebu cattle show strong resistance to the microbes, while dairy cattle suffer the most. Diseased cattle can also infect other animals when they are brought into close, continuous contact. Water buffalo, elephants, and pigs easily become infected, while sheep are highly resistant. Goats, horses, and camels sometimes acquire the infection. Dogs can be more susceptible to the human strain, while cats appear to be more vulnerable to the bovine strain. Wild animals kept in captivity or closely associated with domestic animals can also become infected (Francis 1958; Van der Hoeden 1964).

Domestication of cattle brought humans into close, repeated contact with infected animals, making it easy for the mycobacteria to jump species and infect humans by the aerosol route. This has always been the most common route of transmission between cattle and humans interacting in close quarters (Francis 1958; Van der Hoeden 1964). Early farmers often lived very close to their cattle, frequently sharing the same living structures.

Early nomadic herdsmen collecting and storing infected cattle dung for fire may have exposed themselves to aerosol dispersal of the mycobacteria from dung dust. Throughout human history ingestion of the bacteria through infected milk products played a much lesser role in transmission to humans than the aerosol route.

Bovine mycobacteria readily adapted to human beings to establish the human strain that could spread from person to person via the aerosol route. Humans can in turn transmit the mycobacteria back to cattle, particularly by way of infected sputum contaminating feed or water.

Tuberculosis: The Human Disease

Mycobacterium tuberculosis can survive for a time outside the host, protected by its complex fatty (lipid) capsule. Depending on the temperature, mycobacteria in sputum can survive for several months in shaded areas. Direct sunlight destroys the microbes quickly, but they can survive within fine droplets and dust particles for several days away from sunlight, and they have been known to survive in sewage for up to two hundred days (Van der Hoeden 1964). The ideal setting outside the host for these microbes lies within dark, manmade structures with poor sanitation and poor ventilation for both human beings and cattle. The greater the concentration of humans and animals within these settings, the greater chance for maintaining the disease within both groups.

Tuberculosis can be expressed in various ways, depending on the route of infection and host immune response. Cows can transmit the mycobacteria through their milk, but the mammary glands are involved in only a small percentage of diseased cows. However, when individuals, usually children, consume infective raw milk from diseased cows, they can develop localized tuberculous lesions within the intestinal tract, with involvement of associated regional lymph nodes. Sometimes the microbes can invade the mucous membranes of the mouth and throat, and infiltrate the cervical lymph nodes of the neck, where they are usually contained by the immune system. Some researchers suggest that acquiring tuberculosis through milk as a child may protect against the pulmonary (lung) form of the disease by conditioning the immune system to respond immediately to aerosol invasion by the microbes (Van der Hoeden 1964).

Pulmonary infection by the aerosol route is the most common form of human infection. Mycobacteria carried in small droplets of moisture enter the airways of the lungs. They end up in the tiny air sacs known as alveoli, where the oxygen breathed in gets absorbed into the bloodstream and carbon dioxide from the blood is expelled. Local macrophage-type cells engulf the invaders and carry them to adjacent lymph nodes in the lungs, where the battle between microbes and host immune cells begins. What happens next depends on the host's genetically engineered immune response.

The lipid cell walls of the mycobacteria can resist enzyme actions designed to destroy foreign pathogens within the enclosed vesicles of the macrophages. This allows the mycobacteria to survive and proliferate within the protective barrier of the macrophage. Once the mycobacteria break out of the cells, they tend to deviate from their classic rod shape into a variety of stealth forms. Variations include colonies of fungi-like creeping spindles, virus-like forms, and large spherical shapes containing numerous microbes. Changing form helps them adapt to different microenvironments within the host, and avoid detection by the immune system as they navigate between and within macrophages. These changes are continual, from one form to another, depending on the circumstances. Stealth forms can also remain dormant for long periods within macrophages, capable of reactivating when the microenvironment of the host becomes more receptive to growth (Mattman 1993).

The best way to beat tuberculosis is by stopping the initial infection within the macrophages. Since the internal enzymes (lysozymes) within the vesicles of the macrophage are not strong enough to kill the microbes, two other potent enzymes, phospholipase C and acid phosphatase, have to be produced to help destroy them (Mattman 1993). Production of these enzymes depends on instructions from CD4 T cells. They receive dual signals, one sent to the surface of the macrophage by MHC molecules carrying peptides from the intruder, and another originating from the infected cell's surface. This dual signal mobilizes the CD4 T cells to stimulate infected macrophages to release the more potent enzymes to destroy the microbes within their vesicles. Most individuals infected with *Mycobacterium tuberculosis* never develop the disease because the initial infection ends with this immediate immune response between CD4 T cells and macrophages.

What happens if infected macrophages cannot deliver one or both of the proper signals to the cell surface, or the T cells do not respond to both signals? The mycobacteria can then proliferate and spread unless inflammatory immune cells manage to surround them with a chemical barrier and seal them within a fibrous capsule known as a tubercle, before they break away from the site of invasion. Sometimes the capsule can be reinforced with calcification or can turn to bone (Ghon foci) to prevent the invaders from escaping. If this back-up system fails, then the invaders escape to spread throughout the host's body.

During the industrial age tuberculosis was rampant throughout Europe. Northern Europeans considered tuberculosis a genetic disease that ran in families, while southern Europeans treated it as a contagious disease. Many elite and famous families in northern Europe harbored the disease, and they romanticized tuberculosis in the literature of the day. By the end of the 1800s tuberculosis was no longer considered a genetic disease, but a contagious one (Dubos and Dubos 1952). Life styles changed, thanks to improved hygiene and sanitation, and by 1900 the disease receded in northern Europe, where it previously had been endemic.

We now know that although tuberculosis represents a contagious disease, the course of infection within the individual depends on genetics.

Studies with mice indicate that a gene within the MHC system of the macrophage regulates the responses to infection by the mycobacteria (Schurr and Skamene 1996). Without this gene, the macrophages fail to signal the CD4 T cells. Yet back-up inflammatory responses by the immune system can still contain the infection unless it is impaired by other disease or poor nutrition. Immune systems with impaired CD4 T cell function, such as those with HIV infection, cannot respond to signals from infected macrophages, and the disease takes over. How the immune system reacts, or fails to react, will determine the course of the disease.

Hypothetically, if twenty healthy, unrelated individuals readily became exposed to one individual with infectious pulmonary tuberculosis, five to ten of them would become infected but only one of them would develop the disease (Adler and Rose 1996). But if these twenty individuals shared a common genetic MHC flaw hampering their ability to fight the disease, or if they were HIV-positive, most of them would develop some form of tuberculosis.

Environmental circumstances dictate the spread of the disease. The incidence of tuberculosis among humans increases in proportion to the density of the human population. Crowded, densely packed communities have greater risk than scattered home sites. Urban areas with poor sanitation run more risk than those with good sanitation. Air quality, ventilation, and humidity serve as influencing factors. Polluted air and poor ventilation enable the disease to spread. Recirculated air can be very dangerous. Infection can spread quickly from a single source under the right conditions.

Wherever tuberculosis is rampant, nearly everyone becomes exposed, but only susceptible individuals develop the disease. The very young, sick, poorly nourished, and fragile elderly with poor immune responses become easy targets for tuberculosis. Some individuals can be infected without overt signs of the disease, developing tuberculosis only later in life. This happens when the back-up inflammatory immune response fails to restrain the microbes within their capsulized prisons, allowing the mycobacteria to reactivate and spread. Such a failure occurs when the immune system has been disturbed by another disease, by nutritional disturbance, or by other stresses on the body.

The expression of the disease depends on how quickly the mycobacteria can reproduce and spread from the initial invasion of the host. If allowed to proliferate within macrophages near the site of entry in the lungs, they can spread quickly through blood and lymph channels to other sites in the lungs and associated lymph nodes. By this time the inflammatory response reaches full gear, isolating the infected sites by sealing them in capsules (tubercles). The inflammatory immune cells, now alert to the invaders, can also act quickly to isolate any new arrivals before they spread. The chemical barrier formed within the enclosing capsule inhibits the functioning of the infected macrophages and the growth of the microbes (Adler and Rose 1996). Most but not all of the mycobacteria die within the enclosures. Altered forms can remain in a dormant state for months or years, waiting for the immune system to let down its guard and allow them to escape and proliferate again. The infection reactivates itself.

Uncontrolled initial infections develop into acute, generalized infections as the mycobacteria enter the bloodstream and spread rapidly throughout the body. Young children and infants with inadequate immune responses can be especially vulnerable to developing this type of acute infection, and about half of those exposed to the disease under the age of three will die from it. This has been called miliary tuberculosis (Baker and Glassroth 1996) because the many tiny lesions spreading throughout the lungs and body resemble millet grains. Fever, wasting, drowsiness, cough, and difficult breathing ensue, followed by eventual death.

Wherever tuberculosis has become endemic, most children are exposed to the disease. Some of those individuals escaping the disease during childhood will develop reactivated infection later, usually during adolescence or early adulthood. Most adult cases of tuberculosis develop from reactivated infections. Sometimes reactivated infection does not develop until old age (Garay 1996). Once reactivated, the disease has the potential to develop into active, contagious pulmonary tuberculosis.

Reactivated infection can eventually be contained again, if the immune system regains control, but often the growth of the imprisoned, revitalized mycobacteria cannot be stopped. The disease waxes and wanes, with long periods of feeling better followed by bouts of suffering (Dubos and Dubos 1952). The mycobacteria proliferate and expand, straining the barriers surrounding them, and creating destructive, abscess-like cavities, known as granulomas, that can damage adjacent blood vessels and other tissues (Lack and Connor 1997). Chronic reactivated disease occurs in 5–10 percent of individuals initially infected with the disease (Kreiswirth and Moss 1996). The tissue destruction caused by reactivated tuberculosis in the lungs results in fever, fatigue, night sweats, and emaciation. This is followed by cough, chest pain, spitting up of blood-tinged phlegm, and hoarseness. Death comes eventually as the lungs deteriorate. In the past, Europeans called chronic pulmonary tuberculosis by such names as phthisis, consumption, or galloping consumption.

Reactivated tuberculosis can spread to other parts of the body and develop into localized chronic granulomas similar to the reactivated destructive lesions found in the lung, as the immune system tries to confine the microbes to the site of infection. The lymph nodes, heart, kidneys, larynx, bones, and joints often are targeted. In the past, the microbes commonly aimed for the larynx. Paganini, the great violinist, died in 1839 following a long battle with tuberculosis that destroyed his larynx and stilled his voice (Dubos and Dubos 1952). Children and young adults become susceptible to chronic middle ear and mastoid infections with mycobacteria, introduced directly by way of the eustachian tubes from the throat, or carried there by the blood circulation. This can lead to severe hearing loss (Mignogna, Garay, and Spiegel 1996).

Localized infection of lymph nodes away from the lungs frequently develops with reactivated infection, particularly within the cervical lymph nodes of the neck. This form of tuberculosis, referred to as scrofula, can usually be found in young adults where tuberculosis has become endemic. Medieval Europeans knew this expression of the disease as the "king's evil" (Morse 1967); the name comes from the common belief that the touch of the ruling monarch would heal the affliction. The infected lymph node enlarges slowly into a painless mass, accompanied by fever, weight loss, fatigue, and sometimes night sweats (Sloane 1996).

Infection of the intestinal tract can happen from directly ingesting contaminated milk from diseased cows, or it can spread from initial infection in the lungs by swallowing infected sputum. Sometimes it can spread from the blood circulation into the intestines. The folds of the ileocecal region of the gut contain an abundance of lymph tissue that becomes the most common site within the gut for microbe colonization. Intestinal tuberculosis can be expressed as a fibrous mass or as scattered small nodules that tend to ulcerate and bleed, similar to the lesions of Chron's disease and colitis. Containment of these lesions by the immune inflammatory response can lead to strictures and bowel obstruction. The mycobacteria often spread to adjacent mesenteric lymph nodes in the abdomen. Symptoms include abdominal discomfort, pain, weight loss, fever, and weakness. Vomiting, diarrhea and constipation can also occur (Lewis and Field 1996).

The most common expression of skeletal tuberculosis occurs in the spine. The disease localizes mostly in the vertebrae of the lower back. The granulomas formed by the disease slowly destroy the infected vertebrae. The damage frequently leads to collapse of the lower spine, producing a distinct angular, hunched back known as Pott's disease. Infection can also localize within the red (hemopoietic) marrow of other bones and adjacent joints, leading to localized swelling, pain, and deformity. Some localized lesions can appear as painless abscesses, often draining pus through tunneled fistulas to the outer skin surface. Children with skeletal tuberculosis often have swollen, destructive lesions in the small bones of the hands and feet. Healing can take place, but often the lesions reactivate when the mycobacteria regenerate.

Occasionally mycobacteria can enter through a break in the skin, producing a chronic, localized skin infection. Occasionally mycobacteria can reach the skin by way of the bloodstream to form skin lesions. Skin infections, referred to as *Lupis vulgaris*, usually derive from butchering and skinning infected animals. Thus, the lesions have been referred to as butcher warts, slaughterer warts, and porter's warts (Bisseru 1967). The skin lesion can take different forms, from a firm nodule to discolored, pimple-like lesions that can transform into an expanding wart-like growth. The lesions may take years to heal (Pomeranz et al. 1996).

Disease from Environmental Mycobacteria

Most people face exposure to many different environmental mycobacteria throughout our lives with few or no consequences. These microbes did not develop into true parasites, and they rarely cause serious infection and disease. The cell walls of environmental mycobacteria lack the complexity of the parasitic forms of the *Mycobacterium tuberculosis* complex, making it easier for the host immune system to deal with them. Occasionally when they encounter a host in poor health with a compromised immune system, mycobacteria colonizing the mucous linings of the mouth, lungs, or intestine can produce disease similar to *M. tuberculosis*. One group of mycobacteria in particular, the *Mycobacteria avium* complex, known to infect birds, can also produce disease in animals and humans (Collins 1996).

Wild birds appear to be naturally infected with the avium mycobacteria, and they spread the microbes through their droppings (Bisseru 1967). The microbes can survive for up to four years in the environment. Cattle infected with avian complex mycobacteria develop more serious disease than from infection by the parasitic *Mycobacterium tuberculosis* complex, with the infection usually confined to the gut (Van der Hoeden 1964).

Infection by environmental mycobacteria does not protect the host from tuberculosis caused by the parasitic *Mycobacterium tuberculosis* complex. An individual can be infected by microbes from both complexes at the same time. Infection caused by environmental mycobacteria indicates that the host's immune system has been severely compromised, allowing a harmless microbe to become a pathogen.

Members of the avium complex exist throughout the world, and are found in soil, dust, chickens, birds, domesticated animals, and fresh and salt water. Inhaling contaminated droplets of moisture can cause lung infection in susceptible individuals. The highest frequencies of human avium infection occur in western Australia and Japan (Rotterdam 1997).

Chronic lung disease from other infections or polluted air boosts the potential for mycobacteria from the avium complex to colonize the lungs and produce lesions similar to pulmonary *M. tuberculosis* (Holzman 1997). The infection can spread to skeletal tissue on rare occasions and can produce lesions similar to those caused by *Mycobacterium tuberculosis*. But most often avium mycobacteria produce isolated lymph node lesions of scrofula, or skin lesions under favorable circumstances, particularly in children (Benenson 1995).

Environmental mycobacteria known as *Mycobacterium ulcerans* frequently cause localized chronic skin ulcers in populations of tropical regions around the world. Tropical Africans refer to the skin lesions as Buruli ulcers. The ulcer begins as a small, hard, painless swelling, sometimes with itching. Depending on host immunity, the sore can fade away at this stage or progress to a large destructive ulcer or multiple ulcers, occasionally affecting underlying bone. The ulcers usually appear on the arms or legs. Most of the ulcers eventually heal after several years of combat with inflammatory responses, but scarring and shrinkage of the affected tissue often leads to crippling and disfigurement (Grange 1980).

The Ancient Trail of Tuberculosis

Human tuberculosis most likely originated during the earliest times of cattle domestication after 7000 B.C., spreading into Europe, north Africa, and Asia at widely different times. The introduction of dairy cattle susceptible to tuberculosis by 3000 B.C. paved the way for greater frequencies of the disease in both cattle and humans. Increasing numbers of diseased animals, crowded and confined in close quarters for milking, together with greater contact with their human caretakers, ensured that the disease remained in densely occupied human communities. Human tuberculosis spread far and wide, often from a single human carrier. The infection, passed from person to person, managed to survive in small but densely crowded human settlements.

Tuberculosis leaves distinct signature lesions on human skeletal remains, as well as on mummified human remains. This allows paleopathologists to trace the spread of the disease through time. The oldest evidence for human tuberculosis comes from human bones at two sites from southwestern Italy associated with domesticated cattle bones, dating to 4000–3520 B.C. (Canci et al. 1996; Formicola et al. 1987). Human tuberculosis spread into northwestern Europe, as evidenced in the skeletal remains of a young woman from Denmark dating between 2500 and 1500 B.C. (Sager et al. 1972), followed by other cases found throughout western Europe (Grmek 1989). The disease has been found in both human mummies and skeletons from ancient Egypt, along with evidence of dairy cattle depicted on tomb walls, from 3700 to 1000 B.C. (Steinbock 1976).

The earliest written references to human tuberculosis comes from Vedic hymns in India around 2000 B.C. (Steinbock 1976), indicating that the disease was present on the Indian subcontinent. Early written records in China dating around 1300 B.C. (Grmek 1989), records in Mesopotamia around 675 B.C., and an account by Hippocrates in Greece around 400 B.C. (Morse 1967) all describe symptoms of tuberculosis. The spread of human tuberculosis into Asia has been documented in the mummified remains of the Marquise of Tai, a middle-aged woman belonging to the ruling elite of the early Western Han dynasty in Changsha, Hunan, China, around 100 B.C. (Cockburn 1980). The disease reached Japan by the protohistoric (Kofun period) (Suzuki 1985) before A.D. 200.

By the beginning of the Middle Ages human tuberculosis had become well known throughout Europe. The disease reached epidemic proportions in crowded villages and cities with poor sanitation, and peaked during the industrial revolution. The disease appears to have been unknown in sub-Saharan Africa until Europeans introduced it (Cockburn 1963).

Native Americans suffered severely from tuberculosis once Europeans conquered their lands and crowded them onto reservations (Cockburn 1963;

Dubos and Dubos 1952). The disease took its toll, aided by poor nutrition, unsanitary conditions, and the stress of confinement. Doctors assumed that the native peoples suffered more than Europeans because they had never been exposed to the disease before European conquest of the Americas. However, ample evidence has been found in ancient Native American human remains to show that human tuberculosis existed in the New World long before European conquest. The earliest example of skeletal tuberculosis comes from Peru, dating around 160 B.C. (Allison et al. 1981). Other cases of tuberculosis have been documented in mummies and skeletons from South America between A.D. 290 and 1500. *Mycobacterium tuberculosis* DNA has been identified in a vertebral lesion dating to A.D. 1000 from northern Chile (Arriaza et al. 1995).

The earliest evidence for human tuberculosis in North America comes from the southwestern United States. The disease existed in prehistoric Puebloan peoples at Mesa Verde in southwestern Colorado, dating from A.D. 750–900 (Miles 1975), and in a small Kayenta village in northeastern Arizona, dating from A.D. 875–975 (Sumner 1985). Other cases of the disease have been reported in prehistoric southwestern village sites dated later, from A.D. 900 to 1500. The Spaniards did not arrive in this area until 1540. I have studied nine prehistoric skeletal collections from this area, finding one or more cases of skeletal tuberculosis in every collection. The prehistoric village of Puye on the west side of the Rio Grande Valley in north-central New Mexico showed 4 percent of the skeletal sample with skeletal tuberculosis between 1300 and 1540. Another village from the same time period, Hawikuh near the Arizona border in New Mexico, showed a 7 percent frequency of the disease. Considering that about 5–7 percent of individuals suffering from tuberculosis develop skeletal lesions (Steinbock 1976), we can tell that the disease was endemic in the prehistoric villages of the American Southwest, as proposed by El-Najjar (1979).

Evidence for the presence of tuberculosis dating from A.D. 1000 has been found in village populations in the southeastern United States, the central Mississippian Valley of the Midwest, and the upper Midwest in North Dakota and southeastern Saskatchewan. The frequency of individuals with bone lesions ranges from 5 percent to 7 percent, indicating that tuberculosis had also reached endemic proportions in these areas (Buikstra and Williams 1991). The widespread distribution of the disease from South America to North America, with the earliest evidence from the south and the later cases in central and eastern North America, raises questions of how, when, and from where human tuberculosis gained entry into the New World. The same questions are raised with the evidence of human tuberculosis in precontact Hawaii (Trembly 1996a).

Disagreement abounds over how tuberculosis became established in the New World. In the previous chapter I stated that most of those diseases derived from domesticated animals in the Old World did not occur in the New World until contact with Europeans. How then did this disease evolving from cattle get to the New World? Some researchers argue that tuberculosis in the Western Hemisphere was caused by environmental mycobacteria (Clark et al. 1987), but the evidence strongly supports *Mycobacteria tuberculosis* as the pathogen, with human-to-human transmission.

Human carriers infected with inactive tuberculosis most likely carried the disease across the ancient land bridge that once connected Siberia with Alaska during some of the last migrations from the Old World to the New World (El Najjar 1979). Likewise, ancient Polynesian settlers no doubt brought the disease to Hawaii. The disease can remain dormant for up to thirty years before reactivating into contagious infection. This would have allowed human carriers plenty of time to deliver the disease to a new location. The infection does not rely on large numbers of people for survival in a community. Family groups crowded into poor shelters can maintain the disease within their ranks for generations.

From whence might these migrants have acquired tuberculosis? Perhaps the earliest domestication or semi-domestication of cattle occurred much earlier than we realize in Central Asia, followed by the development of human tuberculosis. From there domestication of cattle and tuberculosis could have spread both west and east. The original nomadic populations of Central Asia roamed throughout the region for many centuries, with contacts into northern India and the Iranian highlands during the Neolithic. Once tuberculosis had become well established within human populations, it could have spread through human carriers into northeast Asia and into the New World. Archaeological evidence shows mixing of Central Asian populations with eastern Asian populations in the far eastern portion of Central Asia, long before the Mongols began to filter into Central Asia during the second century B.C. (Oshanin 1964). The disease could also have spread into Southeast Asia and eventually into Oceania.

We do not have all the pieces of the puzzle; for instance, there are many pieces missing from Central Asia and other parts of Asia. Still, one thing is certain: *Mycobacterium tuberculosis* had settled into the human population, separated from cattle, long before the last human migrations into the New World.

CONCLUDING COMMENTS

Since the beginning of the industrial age, tuberculosis has killed more people than any other infectious disease in North America and Western Europe, up to the first decade of the twentieth century. Improved sanitation and hygiene measures slowed the spread of the disease and reduced the number of cases dramatically by the end of the nineteenth century. Antimicrobials introduced in the 1950s appeared to eliminate tuberculosis from modernized parts of the world, offering a promise of eradicating the disease worldwide. Unfortunately tuberculosis has regained momentum over the last twenty years with the development of drug-resistant strains. Today tuberculosis kills more people worldwide than any other infectious disease (Lederberg et al. 1992; Weiss 1992).

One out of ten or twelve healthy people infected today develops tuberculosis, and half of those developing the disease die within six months to two years. The increasing presence of drug-resistant strains of tuberculosis, increasing numbers of homeless people and substance abusers, loss of public health measures in many parts of the world, the spread of HIV infection, poverty-induced crowding of people into unsanitary housing with no health care: all provide incentive for the disease to increase and spread (Lederberg et al. 1992; Weiss 1992). Today approximately one-third of the world's population is infected with tuberculosis, with 8 million new infections occurring each year, leading to about 3 million deaths per year from the disease (Collins 1996).

The potential for more deadly strains of *Mycobacterium tuberculosis* to evolve by natural selection amid the chaos produced by human behavior is great. Add to this the rapid modern air transportation of infected carriers to all parts of the globe, and you have a time bomb about to explode.

Tuberculosis caused by environmental mycobacteria, especially the *Avium mycobacterium* complex, once rare, has now become more common than *Mycobacterium tuberculosis* in North America, especially in individuals infected with AIDS. There is some concern that certain strains of this complex, frequently found in drinking water and in aerosol form around showers and water coolers, may become parasitic and establish itself in the human population, and develop into a human disease with human-to-human transmission (Bisseru 1967; Holzman 1997; Wallace 1997). With a large number of immune-compromised individuals suffering from AIDS and lung diseases in the population, the opportunity for environmental strains to become parasitic is greatly enhanced. The story of tuberculosis is far from over.

CHAPTER 10

THE MORAL DISEASE

Leprosy

The mention of leprosy frequently evokes frightening images of dreadfully disfigured, dirty beggars with ugly sores, clothed in rags. This image has been handed down to us from the past when individuals afflicted with leprosy or anything resembling leprosy were feared and shunned. In the Middle Ages in Europe, deeply religious people considered them to have been rightfully afflicted by God for their sins, and they were treated as outcasts. Many people believed the disease to be contagious, both morally and physically. Hence, leprosy became one of the most feared diseases known to humans for centuries, not only for its physical disfigurement, but also for what was believed to be its moral aspect. The severely afflicted leper was considered a moral degenerate, a social outcast. To become a leper was to enter hell and damnation, to be turned away from family, friends, home, and all things familiar, forever.

What Makes a Leper?

The term *leper* was literally translated from the Christian Bible during medieval times in Europe to mean someone suffering from leprosy. However, the term more likely refers to other disfiguring diseases as well as leprosy. The term *leper*, even during medieval times, was applied to anyone with a chronic skin disease. Chronic sores associated with other diseases, such as yaws and syphilis, as well as advanced cases of psoriasis and vitamin-deficient pellagra could easily have fallen under the broad label of leprosy.

Leprosy remained a moral disease in the eyes of most Europeans until 1873, when a Norwegian physician, Dr. A. Hansen, discovered the real cause of the disease (Fine 1982). In recognition of his work, leprosy was renamed Hansen's disease. Regardless of the new medical name, the disease remains best known as leprosy throughout the world.

Microscopic examination of tissue samples from leprosy patients revealed the real culprit to be *Mycobacterium leprae,* cousin to the mycobacterial parasites causing tuberculosis. However, study of this mycobacterium remained elusive until the 1960s because it kept disappearing from the culture dish. Only in the past thirty years or so have we been able to delve into the secret life of this microbe.

Unlike its romanticized cousin, tuberculosis, which often kills its victim, leprosy may appear detestable but is rarely fatal. Leprosy also occurs far less often than tuberculosis. The infection rate for leprosy had been considered quite low until recently. Now we realize that exposure happens far more often than previously thought. Only individuals with susceptible immune systems actually develop the disease, while individuals with active immune resistance deflect the invading microbes with little or no signs of the disease.

The Culprit of Leprosy

Mycobacterium leprae can shed its cell wall and change form to adapt to different microenvironments in a manner similar to *Mycobacterium tuberculosis*. *M. leprae* has greater stealth capabilities than *M. tuberculosis*. This explains why it has been so difficult to culture in laboratories. Actually, the microbe has been growing on culture media in altered form, unrecognized, in laboratories for decades. Stealth forms include branching, fungus-like filaments and large globule forms containing numerous mycobacteria, which can revert to the classic rod shape under favorable conditions. The classic form fails to grow in culture media (Mattman 1992).

How the microbe finds its way into the human host has been a mystery for centuries. Even today, most people around the world remain suspicious of how it is acquired. Scientists cannot even be certain how it got into human populations in the first place.

The closest relative to *M. leprae* is an opportunistic environmental mycobacterium, *Mycobacterium vaccae* (Grange 1980). This mycobacterium, like many other harmless environmental mycobacteria, can take up residence in the human intestinal tract if accidentally ingested. Could one of its more potent variants have gained entry into susceptible individuals and established itself as *Mycobacterium leprae*?

A small percentage of water buffalo show susceptibility to a form of leprosy known as *Lepra bubulorum* (Klos and Lang 1976), first described in 1926 as a form of skin tuberculosis, but very similar to human leprosy. The infection produces multiple raised, hard nodules, 5–60 mm (one-quarter inch to about 2 inches) in diameter, all over the water buffalo's body. The mucous lining of the nose also becomes infected (Francis 1958). Wild rodents throughout the world can be infected with another form of leprosy caused by *Mycobacterium lepramurium* (Grange 1980). Most likely, leprosy-producing mycobacteria, including the human form, arose from opportunistic environmental mycobacteria.

Mycobacterium leprae that infects humans can infect susceptible American armadillos in the wild, indicating that it was introduced to their environment by human beings following European colonization. No evidence of leprosy exists in the Americas before European contact. Infection with *M. leprae* has also been identified in chimpanzees and mangabey monkeys in west Africa (Fine 1982). This raises the question of survival of parasitic *M. leprae* in the environment long enough to infect other hosts.

M. leprae can survive within expelled nasal secretions from infected hosts for days, and under favorable warm, moist conditions, it can last for up to six weeks (Fine 1982; Thangaraj and Yawalkar 1986), and possibly longer. Nasal secretions deposited on the ground, particularly in tropical and subtropical areas, favor the return of the leprae mycobacteria to the environment. Recent studies indicate that leprae mycobacteria can survive in vegetation and soil of boggy moors for indefinite periods (Blake et al. 1987). This suggests that the microbes may be able to revert to environmental forms under favorable conditions, and reenter susceptible host populations when sufficient contact occurs. This may explain why human leprosy occurs mainly in rural areas.

Mycobacterium leprae has become a true human parasite, with human-to-human transfer. The mycobacteria are shed from infected hosts with advanced forms of the disease primarily through moisture droplets from nasal secretions. This mode of transmission is similar to that of tuberculosis mycobacteria coughed up with sputum in advanced forms of pulmonary tuberculosis. Large numbers of leprae mycobacteria can be released into the air by sneezing, up to a distance of 50 cm (20 inches) (Pedley and Geater 1976). Repeated, close contact with infectious individuals, particularly in crowded, unclean households, ensures *M. leprae* of new victims. But only advanced forms of the disease with infectious nasal secretions can be contagious; milder forms of the disease without nasal involvement are not.

Once the mycobacteria gain entry into the lungs of the new host, local phagocytic macrophage-type cells quickly destroy the intruder unless a faulty immune response exists. Some individuals, who are susceptible to both tuberculosis and leprosy, can be infected with both types of mycobacteria at the same time (Gatner et al. 1980). Each type of mycobacteria has its own way of interacting with a host's immunity.

While tuberculosis mycobacteria prefer residing in the host's lungs, leprae mycobacteria prefer the skin and adjacent superficial nerves. Once they enter the body, *M. leprae* migrate through the bloodstream to the skin, mostly on the face, arms, and legs. They prefer the cooler surface areas of the body rather than the deeper, warmer tissues.

Like tuberculosis mycobacteria, leprae mycobacteria thrive within the macrophages, specifically the macrophages located in skin tissues—both fixed macrophages, known as histocytes, and epithelioid types. The mycobacteria escape destruction within the internal vacuoles of the macrophages by moving out of the vacuoles into the cell's cytoplasm (Grange 1980). Leprae mycobacteria can also thrive within the cytoplasm of specialized cells, known as Schwann cells, that integrate with skin nerves and peripheral nerve fibers. Occasionally leprae mycobacteria will invade nerve tissue itself, but damage to the Schwann cells alone disrupts the integrity of the nerve, causing nerve damage.

Different Sores for Different Folks

Leprosy expresses itself in a variety of ways, depending on how the individual host immune system reacts to it. Genetic programming of the immune reaction decides the reactive response to the microbe. Variations in immune responses produce variations of the disease. Most people exposed to the microbes have few, if any signs of the disease, thanks to immediate immune responses. In about 5 percent of infected individuals, leprosy develops from inadequate immune responses. Occasionally small population groups sharing a high frequency of inadequate genetically determined immune responses will exhibit a much higher incidence of leprosy when exposed to the disease. Certain families are prone to develop the disease because they have similar genetic factors combined with continuous close contact with infected family members.

The disease may be limited to one or a few skin lesions, with or without nerve involvement. Sometimes complete healing ensues without medical intervention, or the lesion can progress into a serious disease that takes over the whole body. Skin lesions can vary in size and appearance. Permanent nerve damage may cause crippling deformities of the hands and feet. Severe infectious forms of the disease can also damage the nose, disfiguring the face.

Signs of the disease are slow to appear following infection. Usually it takes about five years for the disease to present itself in susceptible individuals, thanks to the stealth capabilities of the microbes. Sometimes signs of disease can appear as early as three months after infection, or it may take up to forty years before symptoms appear. Perhaps the stealth forms of the mycobacteria remain inactive until more favorable circumstances appear in the microenvironment of the host and trigger them into action. The disease generally appears in people between the ages of ten and twenty, and it affects twice as many males as females (Thangaraj and Yawalkar 1986).

The immune reaction is complex, involving more than one type of immune factor (Grange 1980). Failure in any part of the immune response can result in a wide range of disease expressions. *M. leprae* infection can produce delayed immune reactions, alternating from successful to failed attempts to confine the microbes to one area. Some immune reactions succeed in beating the disease and healing the damage, often after many years. Some individuals become hypersensitive to cytoplasm released by dead mycobacteria, and their immune systems react violently with inflammatory responses similar to a severe allergy attack. This hypersensitive reaction often triggers the most advanced form of the disease.

The primary genetic response to the disease has been identified within the inherent MHC II molecules of the macrophages. Once the macrophages engulf the mycobacteria during phagocytosis, quick action by the MHC II molecules in presenting peptide fragments from the invader on the infected cell's surface can help the macrophage destroy its enemy before it escapes into its cytoplasm. This works if the proper dual signal is sent out, and the CD4 T cells respond with the right chemical signal to the macrophage. But when the CD4 T cells have been programmed to respond with the wrong chemical signal (Paul 1993), or the dual signal from the macrophage does not work, then the infected macrophage is doomed. How the immune system sets other responses into motion to combat the infection will depend on where the breakdown occurs between the macrophages and CD4 T cells. With normal CD4 T cell responses, inflammatory response factors move in to seal off the ineffective macrophages. When the CD4 T cells send the wrong signal, immune inflammatory factors are slow to respond. Delayed action allows the microbes to multiply and spread. However the battle lines are drawn, the hampered immune system tries to stop the spread of the infection, and in the process, affected tissues become damaged.

The wide range of immune responses to *Mycobacterium leprae* infection makes it difficult to determine the presence of the disease. The most telling symptoms include skin disorders accompanied by loss of feeling or sensation, with associated enlarged, tender nerves. The disease frequently begins with one or more discolored spots on the skin. This is known as the intermediate type of leprosy, and most of these spots heal spontaneously. Thus, they often go unrecognized as leprosy. However, some of these intermediate types do develop into other forms of the disease.

The most commonly recognized form of the disease is known as tuberculoid leprosy. The CD4 T cell sends out normal signals to infected epithelioid macrophages in the skin, but the infected cells do not respond as they should. Immediate immune inflammatory reactions confine the infection usually to one, sometimes two or three areas of the skin, along with adjacent nerves. Skin lesions vary. They can be slightly discolored, rough, dry areas with complete or partial loss of sensation. Or they can develop into red or copper-colored, raised areas with depressed centers accompanied by total loss of sensation, local hair growth, and local sweating. Adjacent nerves become thick and hard with rapid nerve damage. The skin lesions themselves contain few mycobacteria.

Lepromatous leprosy represents the most severe form of the disease. With this form of leprosy the CD4 T cell response to infected macrophages is inadequate or suppressed. The mycobacteria rapidly reproduce and escape into the blood circulation and spread throughout the body. The mycobacteria first attack the skin and mucous membranes of the upper respiratory tract, especially the nose, followed by invasion of the lymph nodes, larynx, tooth pulp, eyes, spleen, liver, bone marrow, adrenal glands, muscles, and male testes (Thangaraj and Yawalkar 1986).

Numerous small, discolored blotches cover the skin and develop into red, shiny, raised skin nodules that merge together, with only slight loss of sensation. As the disease progresses, the skin thickens, ear lobes enlarge, nodules cover the face, the lines of the face deepen, the lips often swell, and eyebrows and lashes disappear. Numerous adjacent nerves enlarge, then become soft and tender. As the disease advances, the nerve trunks can be severely damaged, causing localized paralysis as well as loss of sensation. Affected hands and feet become useless, and "claw" deformities result. The loss of sensation leads to damaged fingers and toes. Laryngitis with hoarseness can occur. The male testicles often shrink, and with the loss of testosterone, male breasts often swell. The legs often become swollen with fluid backing up from blocked circulation due to enlarged lymph nodes. Inflammation of the eyes can lead to blindness. Ulcerating lesions teeming with mycobacteria block the nasal passages, causing eventual destruction of the nose and palate. All of the lesions are full of mycobacteria. The victim with inactive immune responses can die from overwhelming infection from leprae and other invading pathogens (Grange 1980; Thangaraj and Yawalkar 1986; Waters 1975).

Genetics affects the expression of leprosy in very different ways. One type of expression of the lepromatous form, known as Lucio leprosy, was first described in Mexico in 1852. This form of leprosy develops, in certain genetic groups of Indians, into a widespread infection throughout the body without producing skin lesions or loss of body hair and eyebrows, and without widespread sensory loss. Some genetically related individuals in India react to M. leprae primarily with localized nerve involvement without skin lesions (Thangaraj and Yawalkar 1986).

Variations of disease expression between the tuberculoid and lepromatous types frequently occur. These borderline types can lean toward one type or the other, often displaying aspects of both.

Hypersensitive reactions with sudden inflammatory responses to dead mycobacteria can be serious with the lepromatous form of the disease. Painful, small red bumps appear within a few hours on the face, arms, legs, and sometimes over most of the body. This outbreak lasts two or three days, accompanied by fever, painful neuritis, and muscle weakness. The bumps turn purple and gradually subside, but they leave dark discolorations on the skin. Sometimes the raised bumps break down into open sores, and occasionally the eyes and male testes become inflamed. The reaction, known as erythema nodusum leprosum, may occur only once, or several times over months or years (Waters 1975).

Less severe, localized hypersensitive reactions occur with tuberculoid and borderline types. The existing leprous skin lesions swell, turn red, often become scaly, and new lesions appear. The lesions can become open sores that heal and leave severe scars. Neuritis (inflamed nerves) may also occur. This localized reaction can last for weeks or months, and it can trigger change in the disease's development (Waters 1975).

Deformities associated with leprosy can develop directly from the microbe-immune reactions. Damage to nerves includes destruction of the nose and palate, and claw hands. Nerve damage leading to sensory loss and paralysis commonly affects the elbow, wrist, knee, ankle, and facial nerve above the cheekbones. Dry skin from the destruction of sweat and oil glands can lead to cracked skin and open sores that easily become infected from other pathogens.

Deformities can also develop secondarily from damage to body parts that have lost sensation and therefore become susceptible to injury. Eyes that lose sensation cannot feel dust particles, and this can lead to corneal abrasions, scarring, and blindness. The soles of feet lacking feeling develop ulcers, particularly below the big toe. Toes and fingers without sensation can easily be damaged and lost (Thangaraj and Yawalkar 1986).

The History of Leprosy

The history of leprosy can be traced through written descriptions of its more severe forms, and through human skeletal remains. Deformities of the nose, palate, hands, and feet leave telling marks on bones, just as tuberculosis does.

The first true description of lepromatous leprosy appeared as *kushtha* in Sanskrit around 600 B.C. Although we do not have any evidence from ancient human remains of the disease from the Indian subcontinent, the early descriptions detailing the effects of the disease indicate that *Mycobacterium leprae* was well known to the ancient human population in this area.

Trade facilitated the spread of the disease to Southeast Asia, where it was first described in China around 400 B.C. (Thangaraj and Yawalkar 1986), and again around 190 B.C. The disease spread from China to Japan, where it became widespread by the eighth century A.D. Leprosy also managed to reach Oceania, where skeletal evidence confirms its appearance in the Mariana Islands of western Micronesia by the ninth century A.D. The disease may have arrived in the islands as early as the first century with the first Chamorro settlers from Southeast Asia (Trembly 1995).

Leprosy apparently spread westward along trade routes much later than it spread eastward. Written descriptions of leprosy in the Mediterranean do not appear until the Roman period during the first century A.D. (Steinbock 1976). Skeletal evidence for the disease follows the Roman occupation of this region, suggesting that Roman legions may have been responsible for spreading the disease throughout the empire.

Some of the earliest evidence for leprosy in the West comes from human skeletal remains buried during the Roman occupation of the Dakhleh oasis in Egypt by A.D. 440 (Molto 1997). Additional skeletal evidence shows up near Aswan in Nubia by A.D. 550 (Moller-Christensen 1967). Leprosy appears in human skeletal remains from a Byzantine monastery in the Jordanian desert around A.D. 600 (Zias 1985). In addition to skeletal deformities of the hands and feet, evidence of the disease came from finding DNA of *Mycobacterium leprae* trapped in the bone material (Rafi et al. 1994).

I found evidence that the disease existed in Roman Corinth between A.D. 300 and 450. Foot bones with characteristic "penciled" deformities caused by leprosy came from a batch of bones representing several commingled burials within a Roman tomb. Evidence for leprosy in human skeletal remains has been found in a Romano-British cemetery at Poundbury Camp, Dorchester, in Britain dating to the mid-fourth century A.D. (Reader 1974). Examples of skeletal evidence for leprosy have also been identified in human remains dating to the fifth and sixth centuries A.D. from Saxon burials in Britain (Steinbock 1976), and from other burials in France (Duvette and Blondiaux 1993).

The spread of leprosy throughout Western Europe may have been accelerated by Christian pilgrims and crusaders returning from the Holy Land from the eleventh to thirteenth centuries. By this time leprosy had become well established in the Middle East and north Africa. The disease quickly became widespread throughout Western Europe. It reached Scandinavia, where more than three hundred examples of leprosy have been recovered from human skeletal remains in leprosy cemeteries dating to the thirteenth century (Moller-Christensen 1967).

Leprosy gradually declined in Europe after the fifteenth century, but small endemic pockets survived for some time in Portugal, Spain, Italy, Greece, southern Russia, Norway, Turkey, and Cyprus (Thangaraj and Yawalkar 1986). Norway provided the last bastion of leprosy in Europe until the late nineteenth century; the last endemic case was recorded in 1950 (Fine 1982).

Spanish, Portuguese, and African slaves repeatedly carried leprosy to South and Central America. European colonists, primarily Norwegians, in the eighteenth and nineteenth centuries brought leprosy to North America where it persisted for decades in susceptible family groups. The disease found its way to Australia during the nineteenth century (Fine 1982).

Leprosy does not appear to extend as far back in human history as its cousin, tuberculosis. While tuberculosis was acquired from cattle, and can return to cattle, leprosy appears to have been acquired from the environment, and it can return to the environment. Both require close, repeated contact with infectious individuals in crowded living areas for human-to-human transfer. Both can survive for a time outside human hosts in expelled sputum or nasal secretions, facilitating the spread of the mycobacteria to others.

CONCLUDING COMMENTS

Most likely the home of leprosy lies on the subcontinent of India, where susceptible families crowded into poor living conditions in early farming villages acquired *Mycobacterium leprae* from a variant of environmental *Mycobacterium vaccae*. The disease may have started out as a harmless microbe living in the mucosal lining of the gut. One of its numbers, more virulent than others, managed to get past the submucosal barrier. Parasitic life inside human skin and adjacent nerves quickly evolved with human-to-human transfer via nasal secretions, allowing leprosy to become a human disease.

Thangaraj and Yawalkar (1986) estimate the global number of leprosy cases in the 1980s at around 15 million, with most cases in South and Southeast Asia. The Indian subcontinent sustains the greatest number of cases. Other highly endemic areas occur in the Philippines, Indonesia, Papua New Guinea, Myanmar (Burma), and Indonesia. Tropical Africa and some Pacific islands also have high numbers of cases. Brazil has the greatest number of cases in the Americas. Scattered endemic cases continue to appear in California, Hawaii, Louisiana, Texas, and Puerto Rico. These infections apparently arise from contaminated environmental sources rather than from human sources. Infected

Asian immigrants have also brought new cases into these regions, and into New York City (Benenson 1995). Infected immigrants have most likely taken their hidden infections with them into Europe and other parts of the world.

For centuries the only control for leprosy was to isolate the afflicted from the rest of society. This may have helped control the disease, but more likely it helped maintain its endemic status. Forcing susceptible individuals infected with similar but different diseases to live with individuals infected with lep- rosy, under dire circumstances, kept the disease around. Families afflicted with the disease, often isolated from society and living in crowded, substandard housing, passed the disease from one generation to another. Leprosy began to lose its endemic foothold in Europe when the standards of living improved, per- sonal as well as community hygiene increased, and the treatment of infected individuals improved. Similar results occurred in the Americas and elsewhere.

Isolation of individuals with leprosy continued into the mid-twentieth century. Infected individuals were forced to live in colonies or leprosarium hospitals outside society. This appeared to be the only effective way to keep the disease from spreading, and it provided supportive care for those individ- uals suffering from the disease. This approach changed with the discovery in the 1940s of a new drug called dapsone that proved to be effective in control- ling the disease (Fine 1982). The drug controlled the progression of the dis- ease, and thus its infectiousness. Infected individuals no longer needed to be isolated from families and society. They could be treated at home without the danger of infecting anyone else. Dapsone treatment for leprosy became universal. Leprosy soon began to fade in many parts of the globe.

Unfortunately, *Mycobacterium leprae* has learned to resist the effects of dapsone, and now other drugs must be taken along with it to control the disease. Treatment must be carried out daily for at least two years until all microbes die (Benenson 1995). Social disruptions in endemic regions, partic- ularly political, can disrupt treatment plans. Devastation from wars, famine, and other causes shuts down health care and public health systems, allow- ing the disease to regroup. Thus, the dangers of leprosy are far from over in this crowded, angry world.

Leprosy thrives primarily as a disease of the rural poor living in crowded households with substandard hygiene, wherever the disease is endemic. Although genetics plays a crucial role in the development of leprosy, human behavior is the key factor in maintaining the disease in communities throughout the world.

CHAPTER 11

THE COMING OF
CIVILIZATION

The coming of civilization brought another major paradigm shift to human cultural evolution. Around ten thousand years ago, the stage was set for the development of civilization, as human beings began to cultivate the land and domesticate animals. Five thousand years later, civilization began to stir.

Civilization: what does the word mean? The dictionary defines it as reaching a relatively high level of development in culture and technology. People involved in agriculture for several centuries managed to tailor domesticated crops and animals to their needs and to invent more efficient ways of farming and water management, such as irrigation. The discovery of metal, the invention of the wheel and the plow, and the use of draft animals radically changed the human way of life in the Old World. These changes quickened the pace of human cultural evolution toward civilization. They also contributed to the evolution of human diseases.

The dictionary also defines civilization as relative to urbanization or city life, and as a stage of cultural development marked by the keeping of written records. Urban cultural development includes organized economic and social cooperation within a governing structure. Government provides infrastructure for urban life and military protection. Wealth is accumulated, allowing for monumental architecture and creative pursuits in science and the arts.

These changes could only take place following development of more refined agricultural methods capable of producing large surpluses of food.

Excess food and manufactured goods opened the door to controlled management, calling for the development of a tracking system for the movement and distribution of these surpluses. Excess food and goods increased trading options for raw materials needed for developing urban industries.

Farming villages grew into market towns with ever increasing use of the environment for agriculture. Emerging markets and trade encouraged specialization in craft skills. As greater numbers of people came together in ever larger towns, changes in social organization were inevitable. Leadership roles expanded with greater centralized authority for increasing management of larger numbers of people, markets, industry, and trade. Roles in society changed with the need for greater specialization, particularly civil and military roles that often intertwined with religious authority. The role of the scribe developed to keep written records of transactions, and new classes of people evolved to fit the changing social structure. Ironically, those involved in agriculture, the motive force for the development of civilization, usually occupied the bottom of the evolving class systems. Moving up the class system depended on knowledge that went beyond farming. Opportunity and greed added to the development of civilization. The stage was set for the rapid changes to come. The centers of early agriculture became the focal regions for human cultural evolution. They evolved into centers of civilization, differing according to local environmental and cultural resources. Trade routes spread new ideas and technology to other regions. They also facilitated the spread of diseases.

The Lands of Plenty

By 5000 B.C. village farming in the flood plains bordering the Tigris and Euphrates Rivers in Mesopotamia (present-day Iraq) began adapting to irrigation farming. Control over water use brought more extensive cultivation of crops that produced large surpluses. These large food surpluses permitted the development of the earliest known civilization, the Sumerian (Adams 1979). The first known cities appeared by 4500 B.C. as large numbers of people became concentrated within and around walled Sumerian enclaves. Most of the citizens farmed the land outside the city, while others took up specialized crafts and sociopolitical roles. The social structure came under governance by a central ruling authority that dictated the rules and requirements for citizenship.

The earliest known form of writing comes from Uruk in southern Mesopotamia, the oldest known city in the world and the home of the epic hero-king Gilgamesh. Farming villages spread out from the city for miles, providing the food surpluses needed to keep it alive. By 3500 B.C. Uruk had become a sophisticated urban center of about fifty thousand people densely packed within its walls; it lasted for four thousand years (Whitehouse and Wilkins 1986).

The Sumerians expanded their trading networks throughout Western Asia, from the Mediterranean Levant to the Persian Gulf, and from the Black Sea area into Afghanistan, to the Nile valley, and extending eastward to the Indus Valley on the western edge of the Indian subcontinent. As trade increased with new ideas and technology, other cities arose within Mesopotamia and along its trade routes. The expanding irrigated fields of the Nile Valley supported the kingdoms of ancient Egypt, while the Indus Valley produced its own remarkable civilization, the Harappan (Whitehouse and Wilkins 1986).

By 2000 B.C. the eastern Mediterranean and Western Asia had been divided into a network of small and large city-states, which competed with each other for control of lucrative trade goods. Iron tools eventually brought in by the Hittites from Anatolia spread throughout the region, replacing tools and weapons of copper and bronze (Fagan 1996). This new, tougher, and longer lasting metal—iron—became the new symbol of power and wealth.

The successful early city-states gave rise to empires that governed large areas and greater numbers of people, and controlled valuable trade routes. The Sumerians were succeeded by the Babylonian, the Assyrian, and the Persian empires. Sea peoples established enclaves along coastal trade routes throughout the Mediterranean, Black Sea, Persian Gulf, and coastal areas throughout Southeast Asia. The Minoans of Crete dominated Mediterranean sea trade by 2000 B.C., followed by the conquering Myceneans from the Greek mainland by 1600 B.C., and the Phoenicians from the Levant by 1200 B.C. (Fagan 1996). The Greek-Roman world evolved from the earlier civilizations of the Mediterranean region and their trading contacts throughout Western Asia.

Chinese legend describes the founding of Chinese civilization in the north of China by the Yellow Emperor Huang Di around 2700 B.C. Archaeological evidence shows increasing population densities in the area by this time, providing support for the development of civilization. The best known early Chinese civilization is the Shang in the lower Yellow River Valley of north China established around 2000 B.C., while the earliest known Chinese city, Erlitou, lies just south of the Yellow River in Henan province (Whitehouse and Wilkins 1986). Many different early civilizations evolved throughout East, Southeast, and Central Asia as trade networks spread throughout the entire region.

While the Roman Empire expanded around the Mediterranean, the large empire of Chandragupta linked the Indus and Ganges Valleys of the Indian subcontinent into one vast empire, and Chin Shih Huang united much of China into a single empire (Fagan 1996). Extensive trade networks reached between them and several other smaller empires and city-states, bringing increasing awareness of each other plus new ideas and technology in the known world of their times.

The New World witnessed a separate evolution of civilization. Focal agricultural centers in Mesoamerica and the Andean region of South America developed separate civilizations with widespread trading networks. The earliest known signs of Mesoamerican civilization appear on the gulf coast of Mexico with the Olmec by 1500 B.C., eventually giving rise to the Mayan and other Mesoamerican civilizations that led to the growth of the Aztec empire. The Andean region of South America began to witness similar development by 2400 B.C. The earliest known sign of civilization there has been found in the Casma Valley on the coast of Peru at Sechin Alto (Fagan 1996). Several independent city-states followed along the coast and in the Andean highlands, culminating in empires dominated by upland peoples that eventually evolved into the well-known Inca empire. The New World civilizations developed metallurgy but not iron. They also lacked the wheel and ox-drawn plow. The llama and alpaca became the only beasts of burden used in the Andes, and were used only as pack animals. The absence of domesticated cattle, horses, donkeys, water buffalo, pigs, sheep, goats, and poultry from American civilizations spared their citizens the many human diseases that evolved from these animals in the Old World.

Opportunity Knocks

The shadow world of human evolution, the world of microbes, achieved new heights with the development of human civilization in the Old World. More people and animals living closely together facilitated the development and spread of old and new human diseases. As cities grew in size, so did the problems of both human and animal waste disposal, creating hotbeds for the development of microbes. Just as early human settlements attracted rodents, birds, and insects, so did cities, but in far greater numbers, adding to the risk of evolving diseases. The larger and more crowded the city and its suburbs, the greater the opportunity for the evolution of human diseases.

Increasing trade routes provided transportation for microbes to new populations, and new epidemics evolved as endemic diseases escaped into new worlds. Many diseases once restricted geographically soon began to spread throughout the Old World. This was particularly true for diseases that evolved from domesticated animals. Epidemics became common throughout the ancient cities of the Old World (McNeil 1976), often sparked by soldiers returning from war, immigrants, traders, pilgrims, and the slave trade.

Successful infection by a pathogenic microbe depends on how it gets transmitted, how quickly it establishes itself in the host, the adaptability of the pathogen, the susceptibility of the host, and favorable environmental conditions. Increasing herd size or density of potentially susceptible hosts increases the chances for infection. Crowding large numbers of susceptible hosts with alterations in the environment can greatly enhance these chances.

Microbes that could not survive in small populations with limited numbers of susceptible hosts gained by the development of civilization with its ever increasing numbers of people crowding into tight confines. These "hit and run," opportunistic pathogens generally originate by jumping species from animal hosts to human hosts with occasional, sporadic infections that quickly fade out in small populations. Small populations cannot maintain the infection as an endemic disease with its rapid action and hunger for new hosts.

"Hit and run" diseases operate as acute infections caused by highly contagious microbe invaders moving rapidly from one victim to another, leaving their victims either dead or immune. The immune response either kills off the microbes or severely limits their proliferation and infective capabilities. Survival of the microbe population within the human population depends upon the introduction of new victims at regular intervals before the cycle of infection completely breaks. For this reason, they are known as density-dependent diseases (Cockburn 1963), or herd diseases, that thrive in urban populations. They depend on the susceptible young of a large host population to remain active. Most of them are transmitted by moist droplets exiting and gaining entry through the respiratory tract. Some can be transmitted through the oral-fecal route.

Even diseases that have existed in human populations for centuries before urbanization act like acute infections in densely populated urban areas. The constant turnover of newborns and influx of nonimmune individuals from outside the city ensure fresh new hosts readily available for infection.

Virulent members of microbe populations that generally cause no harm find opportunities in urban settings to strike out on their own as parasitic forms, gaining dominance in larger numbers of susceptible hosts. This is particularly true of the pathological variants of streptococci, bacteria that usually live quiet lives as commensals on human mucous membranes and skin.

Pathogenic streptococci develop more resilient outer capsules that make it difficult for macrophages to engulf them. They quickly link up with each other to form large mucoid colonies and produce a variety of toxins damaging to host tissues (Stollerman 1975). The virulent strains that turn against the host are known as the hemolytic streptococcal infections; they cause scarlet fever, strep throat, and erysipelas, an acute infection of skin and mucosal membranes. These infections can be explosive and deadly in crowded urban communities.

The risk of urban diseases depends on the density of people and their animals, as well as on the density of scavenger rodents, insect vectors, and birds, and the extent of alterations of the environment. Interaction between rural and urban communities allows the microbes to move back and forth from one environmental setting to another. Early cities with constant interaction between urban and rural environments encouraged rural microbes to become urban microbes. Newcomers from outside the local area who became exposed to the urbanized microbes could then take them home. They also brought in new microbes to add to the mixture of resident city pathogens. Local rural areas also could receive the new microbes from interactions with the city. Cities quickly became the centers of disease, stirring the pot of microbes for the future.

Evolution of Childhood Diseases

The so-called childhood diseases of modern societies are those acute infections that typically strike school-aged children. The crowding of large numbers of children in day care centers, schools, or play areas for long periods of time provides ideal breeding grounds for various contagious diseases, particularly during the winter months. The air within enclosed schools generally gets recycled during cold weather, enabling airborne diseases to be transmitted more readily from host to host. Wherever children congregate for long periods of time, contagious diseases spread readily.

The most common modern diseases of childhood include measles, mumps, rubella (german measles), whooping cough (pertussis), diphtheria, streptococcal infections, chickenpox, and the common cold. Nonimmune adolescents and young adults can also be affected, and the common cold afflicts all ages. Diarrhea from gastrointestinal infections is also common, particularly among very young children and infants. Most of these diseases originated from animal sources and prospered during the development of early civilizations in the Old World.

Measles

Measles (rubeola) operates as a "hit and run" disease caused by an RNA Morbillivirus. Related strains produce distemper in dogs and rinderpest in cattle (Andrewes 1964; Bussell and Karzon 1966; T-W-Fiennes 1978b). This Old World virus did not gain a foothold in human populations until people and dogs began crowding into early cities. The constant flow of newly susceptible human hosts in large urban populations made it possible for this highly contagious virus to jump species from canine hosts. The virus is transmitted by airborne droplets that affect the upper respiratory system, and consequently, infection blankets the exposed population. The virus acts unusually fast, infecting large numbers of new hosts, with a large percentage of exposed individuals developing the disease.

Distemper in dogs can be deadly in half of the dogs infected, particularly in young pups. The infection starts out as an upper respiratory infection, developing into a severe lung infection that often spreads to the brain in the more susceptible canines. Distemper virus is maintained in wild canines, such as the wolf and fox, and in mustelids, such as the ferret, mink, weasel and skunk. When stressed, these animals can develop disease from the infection; otherwise it causes no harm to them (T-W-Fiennes 1978b).

Rinderpest can be deadly to susceptible cattle, racing like wildfire through large herds, quickly destroying up to 95 percent of the animals. Wild ungulants also react to the virus with rinderpest disease. While most breeds of domesticated cattle may succumb to the disease, some breeds have developed resistance to the virus (Bussell and Karzon 1966).

The viral strain causing rinderpest begins with upper respiratory infection and ends by striking the ruminant gut with severe destructive changes, leading to the death of the animal (Bussell and Karzon 1966). Many of the cattle plagues recorded in historical documents most likely resulted from rinderpest epidemics.

Rinderpest virus abounds in secretions from the mouth, nose, eyes, urine, and feces of infected animals (Bussell and Karzon 1966), and it depends on immediate transfer to new hosts since it cannot survive more than a day or so outside the host (Hare 1967). Crowding susceptible animals into pens or corrals promotes the spread of the virus.

While the virus strains that attack dogs and cattle can be deadly, the virus strain causing human measles has evolved into a mild, short-lived urban disease. The disease can be much more serious when a human population is exposed to the virus for the first time, and this suggests that measles began as a more severe infection when first introduced to humans (Benenson 1995). Children between the ages of one and six years are the most commonly affected age group in endemic areas. Those in poor health with chronic malnutrition, especially very young children, suffer a more severe form of the disease that may often be fatal (Morely 1980).

Once the infection gains entry through the upper respiratory system, it affects the mucous membranes and skin by attacking adjacent lymphatic tissue, thriving in lymph cells. Lymphatic tissue of the tonsils and intestinal tract becomes the primary target. A fully activated immune response triggers T cells into explosive reaction against the infected lymph cells. The destruction of infected lymph cells causes damage to adjacent capillaries and leakage of fluid into neighboring tissues. The immune reaction also produces a rash on the mucous membranes and skin.

Runny nose, sneezing, elevated temperature, and cough signal the onset of measles, about ten days after exposure to the virus. Within a few days the mucous membranes and skin briefly become red as the rash appears. Sensitivity to light accompanies irritation of the mucous membranes covering the eyes. The rash first appears in the mouth (koplik spots), followed by a fine, light pink rash on the face, neck, and behind the ears, spreading to the chest, down the trunk, and out along the arms and legs. The skin lesions increase in size, often fusing together in some areas, increasing in color to a dark red and then a brownish color, before fading away as the rash sloughs off. The rash lasts about four to seven days. The virus sheds primarily through the secretions from the nose and mouth during the disease episode. With recovery comes complete immunity to the virus without residual virus carriers. Middle ear infection can follow the attack in young children. Rare cases of pneumonia and inflammatory responses in the brain can occur with poor immune responses (Benenson 1995; Top 1955).

Measles thrives in large urban populations, appearing in cycles about two years apart, with relatively few cases in between. Small cities and rural communities within endemic areas will have sporadic epidemics of measles only when sufficient numbers of susceptible individuals come in contact with the infection. Breaking the cycle of introducing new susceptibles into the population stops the infection (Burnet and White 1972; Top 1955).

It has been difficult to decipher measles in ancient records, because it was often confused with other rash-producing diseases. The Persian physician Rhazes in the ninth century A.D. first differentiated measles from other diseases (Top 1955). Most likely measles gained prominence among the newly forming cities in Western Asia where dogs, cattle, and people mixed in great numbers. The disease was then carried by infected individuals from one city to another along trade routes. Measles reached the New World with the arrival of the Europeans by the sixteenth century, where it had devastating effects on nonimmune Native American populations.

Mumps

Mumps represents an acute infection caused by a virus belonging to the RNA Paramyxoviruses (Benenson 1995). Similar viruses from this group naturally infect wild birds and cause newcastle disease in domestic poultry. Newcastle disease virus invades the bird's respiratory system and spreads to the gastrointestinal tract and central nervous system. Large, crowded flocks of poultry under stress react to the virus with severe symptoms and high death rates (Bisseru 1967). The Paramyxoviruses, like the Morbilliviruses, cannot survive for long outside the host, making them dependent on large numbers for survival. Transmitted by the aerosol route through the respiratory system, they thrive among urban populations. The greater the density of susceptible hosts, the better chances for infection.

Human infection follows a predictable route, within two to three weeks following exposure. The virus invades the upper respiratory system and localizes in the salivary and parotid glands with characteristic swellings of the lower jaw. Sometimes one side becomes affected before the other. The virus can invade the bloodstream to attack other glandular structures in the body, favoring the male testes and female ovaries in adolescents and young adults.

Headache, loss of appetite, chilling, fever, and painful swelling of the affected glands appear and last for eight to ten days. The swellings result from hyperimmune responses to contain and destroy the infected cells within the glands. The older the individual, the more severe the symptoms. The virus begins to shed before symptoms develop, and it continues to shed for over a week following the resolution of symptoms. The disease strikes people mostly between the ages of five and fifteen years. It rarely appears in people younger than four or older than forty. Up to one-third of infections remain silent, with no apparent outward symptoms, although the infected individual is contagious. Immune-compromised individuals can suffer invasion of major glands, or occasionally the virus attacks brain tissue. Severe inflammatory responses follow (Top 1955).

Mumps occurs in cycles about every seven years in large urban populations where the disease has become endemic. Recovery from the disease provides lasting immunity to the virus (Top 1955), so infection remains sporadic until the number of susceptible hosts increases enough to sustain an outbreak. The virus dies out in small populations once it has run its course, but large urban populations always have some susceptible individuals available for maintaining the virus.

The history of mumps has been more easily tracked than the history of measles, because of its characteristic parotid swellings of the lower jaw. Hippocrates described the symptoms of mumps (Cockburn 1963), indicating that the disease was well known in the Mediterranean region by the fifth century B.C. Most likely the disease evolved in Western Asia, perhaps in the Indus Valley, with the crowding of domesticated poultry and people together in the evolving urban civilizations.

Rubella

Rubella (german measles) often gets confused with measles. The small RNA virus causing rubella belongs to the Togaviridae family of viruses, in the genus *Rubivirus* (Benenson 1995). There is no known related animal disease. The rubella virus strikes in a manner similar to measles, by way of aerosol transmission through the respiratory system. This virus also produces a rash. However, about half of the infections in children produce no rash.

Like measles, the infection primarily strikes mucous membranes and skin. The disease begins with headache, low-grade fever, mild runny nose, watery eyes, general discomfort, and swelling of the lymph glands in the neck. Rash may develop after these symptoms become established, resembling the rash of measles. The rash does not cover the entire body at one time, but appears first on the face and neck, fading from there the next day as it appears in turn on the trunk, arms, and legs. It rarely lasts more than three days. The virus begins to shed just as symptoms appear, and continues until complete recovery. The disease lasts only a short time, followed by lasting immunity against the virus. Sometimes infected young adults, especially females, may experience temporary joint inflammation. Individuals with compromised immune responses can suffer middle ear infections and pneumonia (Benenson 1995; Top 1955).

The developing fetus in the first few weeks of pregnancy of young women infected with the virus suffers the most severe effects of rubella. The virus can cross the placental barrier between mother and fetus during the first twelve weeks of rapid fetal development, and can invade fetal tissues. The timing of the viral invasion will determine the type of damage inflicted on the developing fetus. Many infections in the first few weeks of fetal development result in severe malformations that cause fetal death and miscarriage. The virus can inflict damage on whatever organic system shows the most vulnerability at the time of infection. Congenital deafness, mental retardation, microcephaly (abnormally small brain size), heart defects, liver and spleen dysfunction, and bleeding under the skin commonly stem from congenital rubella (Benensen 1995).

The history of rubella is unknown. The disease occurs in sporadic epidemics throughout the world's cities, infecting primarily children, adolescents, and young adults (Top 1955). Chances are the disease established itself within the human population during the development of the first cities in the Old World, since it was unknown to the New World before European contact in the sixteenth century A.D.

Whooping Cough

Whooping cough (pertussis) describes an acute respiratory infection caused by airborne bacteria known as *Bordetella pertussis*, that can survive only a short time outside the host. Sunlight and heat quickly destroy it. Coughing attacks with an inspiratory whooping sound characterize this disease. First recognized in the sixteenth century A.D., whooping cough now occurs throughout the world in large cities. It has no known related animal sources, and the history of the disease remains unknown. The infection prevails more in cities of cold, temperate regions of the world, appearing in cyclic outbreaks every three or four years. Most victims are young children and older infants. Lasting immunity usually follows with recovery (Benenson 1996; Top 1955).

The initial infection attacks the mucous membranes of the throat and the large and small passages (bronchi and bronchioles) into the lungs. During the first week or two of infection a dry cough develops. Eventually, copious amounts of mucous appear as the immune system kicks into high gear in attempts to rid the air passageways of the infection. This creates an irritating sticky mass that triggers sudden, intense coughing spells, particularly at night. The intense coughing does not allow time for the inspiration of air, and when the victim finally gets a break in the coughing to suck in air, the whooping sound associated with the cough can be heard as air rapidly flows over the vocal cords. Coughing can be so severe it causes vomiting. The coughing attacks can last for two to four weeks, exhausting the host and decreasing oxygen flow through the lungs. The face can turn deep red and purple with the coughing fits that last five to ten minutes at a time, while producing copious amounts of thick mucous. Gradually the coughing subsides with recovery, but periodic coughing can occur for months (Benenson 1995; Top 1955).

Young children under three years of age suffering from whooping cough commonly develop pneumonia that can end in death. Emphysema can follow coughing attacks. The tiny air sacs in the lungs become overinflated with air, causing them to lose their elasticity. This makes it difficult to expel air from the lungs, leading to severe lung disease that can be fatal in the very young. They also can suffer from convulsions and middle ear infections from this disease. The pressure inside the chest cavity caused by severe coughing can increase pressure on blood vessels to the head, causing blood vessel breakage and bleeding into the eyes, brain, skin, and mucous membranes (Top 1955). This is a scary disease for young children and infants, and many of them die. Whooping cough epidemics once commonly occurred in modern cities throughout the world before a vaccine was developed to combat the disease.

New World populations did not know this disease before European contact. Thus, an Old World origin during the development of civilization can be hypothesized.

Diphtheria

Diphtheria results from commensal bacteria gone bad. The bacteria belong to a family known as Corynebacteria that occurs not only in humans but also in several animals (Van der Hoeden 1964). The human strain can be transmitted from contaminated human hands to a cow's udder during milking, thus soiling the milk with the pathogen. The milk then becomes the vehicle for transmitting the bacteria to new human hosts, particularly the young. However, most infections travel through direct contact with infective secretions or by aerosol droplets. The bacteria can withstand heat, cold, and drying, and can survive for a short time outside the host. This gives the bacteria a chance to contaminate commonly used objects, plus food and drink. The majority of infections can be harmless, with the bacteria thriving on the mucous membranes of the nose and throat without causing any harm to the host.

Problems arise when the bacteria become infected by a virus (Benenson 1995; Burnet and White 1972). The viral infection induces the bacteria to produce a defensive toxin (poison) against the virus. The toxin discharged by the infected bacteria damages the host's mucous membranes wherever the infected bacteria reside in the throat and nose. With release of the toxin, symptoms gradually develop—moderate rise in temperature, sore throat, and tired feeling—as the immune system reacts to the poisonous substance and attacks the infected bacteria. The toxin can be more dangerous and far more difficult to handle than the infected bacteria; thus, the toxin acts as the primary culprit of diphtheria. Attempts by the immune system to localize the poisonous bacteria produce patches of membrane surrounded by inflammation at the sites of invasion. Temporary paralysis of the affected site follows, and this may interfere with speech and swallowing. The tonsillar area becomes the most common site of invasion. Sometimes the entire mucosal area of the nose and throat becomes infected, or the infection can be limited to just one portion of the nose or throat. Extensive membrane production can extend down the throat into the air passageways of the lungs, inducing deadly suffocation. This used to be common in very young children (Top 1955).

Failure to contain the infection at the site of invasion can allow dissemination of the infected bacteria throughout the body via the circulatory system. The toxin can severely damage peripheral nerves and heart muscle. Respiratory paralysis can result from toxic destruction of motor nerves responsible for intercostal muscle action needed for breathing. The spleen enlarges, the kidneys can suffer, and tiny hemorrhages in the skin and mucous membranes can develop as death approaches. Chances of recovery, with or without permanent disability, improve if survival lasts beyond eight days of serious onset (top 1955).

Toxic Corynebacteria can spread quickly in crowded cities and towns, causing serious epidemics with fatal outcomes for many young children, adolescents, and young adults. Descriptions of the characteristic membranes of the tonsils and throat appear in early written accounts from ancient Babylonia (Wilson 1967), and Hippocrates mentions the temporary paralysis of the throat produced by this disease. Talmudic medical records from A.D. 200–600 mention suffocation by a false membrane (Hare 1967). Such accounts indicate that diphtheria was a serious disease in ancient cities of the Old World.

Chickenpox

Chickenpox (varicella) is an old human disease that benefited from urbanization. This disease, caused by a herpes virus, can survive in small populations by hiding out in nerve endings long after the disease has been resolved. Years may pass before the virus can reactivate as herpes zoster (shingles) that can infect young susceptible individuals. Urbanization increases the numbers of susceptibles on a regular basis, allowing the virus to behave like other acute viral infections and to develop into epidemic proportions.

The infection begins suddenly with a slight fever, mild discomfort, and a generalized skin eruption of small, red bumps that turn into small blister-like, liquid-filled vesicles. They itch like crazy, break, and scab over. The lesions appear in successive crops all over the body, starting with the torso. Highly susceptible individuals develop lesions on the scalp, palms of the hands, soles of the feet, inside the mouth, and sometimes even on the mucous covering of the eyes. The disease process takes from two to four days, sometimes up to seven days, before the lesions begin to fade. The infection is transmitted by direct or indirect contact with leaking vesicles and by airborne droplets carrying the virus from the mouth. Symptoms develop within two to three weeks after exposure. The virus sheds from the victim just before the rash appears and until the last vesicle disappears. Adults and older children suffer more severe chickenpox than younger children (Top 1955), and newborn infants have the highest risk for developing a severe generalized infection, which can be deadly in 30 percent of those exposed to the virus (Benenson 1995).

Herpes zoster consists of painful eruptions of vesicles along infected nerve pathways, similar to the chickenpox vesicles, and just as infectious. The lesions usually confine themselves to one area of the body within a single or associated group of nerve endings (Benenson 1995).

The only inkling we have of chickenpox from the past comes from Rhazes in the ninth century A.D. He mentions a mild form of smallpox that failed to protect the individual from a major outbreak of smallpox (Top 1955). This suggests the mild form was actually chickenpox and unrelated to smallpox. The disease often became confused with the more deadly small-pox infection, making it difficult to trace through time.

The Common Cold

Symptoms of the common cold can be produced by different respiratory viruses. Several such viruses can circulate within a large urban population at the same time, offering a mix of cold infection sources to a variety of suscep-tible individuals. These viruses can be transmitted by airborne droplets or through freshly contaminated hands and objects. They have a short incuba-tion period of one to four days before symptoms develop with inflammatory response by the immune system. They attack the mucous membranes of the nose and throat, producing irritation, runny nose, watery eyes, congestion, sneezing, and coughing to rid the throat of infection debris. The sinuses and middle ear can be involved. Most infections are mild and not life-threatening, but highly susceptible individuals with compromised immunity can develop severe upper respiratory disease. The virus begins to shed before symptoms appear, and it continues shedding after symptoms disappear (Jackson 1975).

The largest number of respiratory viruses causing the common cold come from more than one hundred recognized types of rhinoviruses circu-lating in large urban human populations today (Benenson 1995). The respi-ratory viruses cause acute infections that cannot be maintained in small populations once they have run through all of the susceptible individuals. Infection produces immunity for only the particular viral type responsible. The large numbers of respiratory viruses make it possible for susceptible individuals to have more than one cold every year.

Horses provide the only natural reservoir for rhinoviruses. Wild horse herds coming into contact with other herds roaming the steppes of Central Asia maintained the virus within the horse population (T-W-Fiennes 1978b). Domestication of the horse brought humans into repeated contact with the viruses. The development of civilization throughout Western Asia enabled the viruses to become established in large human populations. Trade routes allowed them to spread throughout the Old World and develop into numer-ous strains.

The common cold viruses apparently evolved in the Old World with the development of civilization. New World populations received the viruses from European contact in the sixteenth century A.D.

CONCLUDING COMMENTS

With the development of civilization, human populations around the world increased dramatically, from an estimated 8 million by 8000 B.C. to around 300 million by A.D. I (Coale 1975). The birth and survival rates of infants increased for many well-fed civilizations with each advancing century. Opportunities for evolving urban diseases and old diseases increased with each successive stage of development. Microbe evolution became intricately bound to human evolution with the urban setting at center stage.

Most of the urban diseases of today, particularly the familiar childhood diseases, have been with us since the beginning of civilization. Most evolved from animal sources involved with the urban revolution. Some developed from old diseases and friendly commensals. All of the familiar urban diseases developed in the Old World. Diseases once confined by geography spread and adapted to other geographic regions by way of trade routes. Epidemics became commonplace among ancient cities, but the New World was not exposed to them until European contact in the sixteenth century A.D.

Despite the widespread use of vaccines in modern populations to prevent the spread of most childhood diseases, they still appear throughout the world. Diphtheria outbreaks have plagued Russia and the Ukraine in recent years (Benenson 1995), and other childhood diseases appear wherever vaccination has been lacking. There are no vaccines to prevent the streptococcal infections and the common cold, and outbreaks appear routinely in urban areas throughout the world.

Vaccination against a certain microbe in some but not all populations leaves the possibility that the targeted microbe population may evolve into a strain resistant to the vaccine. Survival instincts are strong in the microbe world, and adaptation means survival. We can only hope that new strains of familiar microbes will not cause more harm than the old ones.

The dawn of civilization revolutionized human interaction with the microbial world. The lands of plenty with large urban populations provided fertile ground for rapid disease evolution.

CHAPTER 12

SYPHILIS

The Great Change Artist

S yphilis was the most feared venereal disease throughout the civilized world until the mid-1940s when the introduction of penicillin drastically altered the damaging affects and spread of the disease. Prostitution and loose morals came to be identified with the disease by the mid-nineteenth century when the term *syphilis* came into common use (Hudson 1958). The causative agent of the disease remained unknown until 1905 (Sell and Norris 1983), and the mysterious changing nature of the disease finally began to unfold its secrets in the late 1920s.

The Agent

The cause of syphilis was identified as a microscopic bacterial parasite that looks like a tiny worm upon magnification. It belongs to a class of bacteria known as spirochetes. They are slender, cylindrical bacteria that have the ability to move about on their own. Spirochetes occur everywhere in nature, living off dead or decaying organic matter. Some have adapted to parasitic life on living organisms, often as noninvasive commensals, thriving on dead cells shed by the host. Harmless spirochetes thrive in our mouths, clinging to deep mucosal crevices between our teeth and gums. Some cling to mucosal crevices in our lower gut, and open surface wounds invite these little "critters" to dine on dead cells without causing any harm to living cells (Sell and Norris 1983). Sometimes members of harmless colonies of spirochetes in the mouth can contribute to periodontal disease, while some can combine with other bacteria to cause painful lesions in the mouth and throat, and occasionally settle in the lungs, forming abscesses (Manz and Buck 1997).

Three different kinds of spirochetes have become invasive parasites in humans (Eagle 1952). One group, known as Borrelia, can be transmitted by ticks and human body lice, causing intermittent bouts of fever. These illnesses, known as relapsing fevers, include Lyme disease. Another group, known as Leptospira, and carried by rats, can be transmitted through rat-infested waters to cause Weil's disease, with fever and influenza-like symptoms that progress to jaundice. Deadly symptoms can develop in more susceptible individuals (Forbes and Jackson 1993).

Borrelia and Leptospira spirochetes operate as accidental parasites of humans, and people do not directly transmit them to other people. Another group of parasitic spirochetes have become true human parasites, with direct human-to-human transmission. This group is known as Treponema.

Morphologically treponemes resemble commensal spirochetes that live in our mouths, gut, and surface wounds (Kolker et al. 1997). Perhaps at some time in human history members of a certain type of these commensal spirochetes managed to penetrate damaged mucous membranes and/or wounded flesh, to survive within the internal microenvironments of human hosts. Those microbes unable to survive within the host died off. Treponemes infecting humans have also been found in monkeys, baboons, and chimpanzees in west and central Africa, suggesting the human treponemes originated there (Fribourg-Blanc 1972). A similar treponeme, known as *Treponema cuniculi*, adapted to rabbits as an internal parasite, but cannot survive in humans (Hardy 1976).

Ironically, those treponemes that did manage to adapt as internal parasites behave as if they would prefer to be outside the host. They prefer living in tiny blood vessels nourishing mucosal or skin surfaces, and they feed off dead cells like their commensal cousins. Most of them cannot tolerate the higher temperatures of the internal organs very well, so they flee to the cooler parts of the body, particularly the skin, whenever possible. High fevers within the host can be deadly to the treponemes (Eagle 1952; Turner 1970).

Treponema pallidum identifies the treponemes responsible for the disease of syphilis. This treponeme can change its morphology as it moves around to different microenvironments within its host. Similar changes occur among free-living spirochetes that encounter environmental changes. Following their introduction into a host, parasitic treponemes change shape, depending on where they wind up within the body. Infections near the surface more likely consist of the classic, spirochete form. Treponemes carried to deeper, warmer parts of the body usually are small, rounded or granular forms, sometimes serrated, that reproduce by budding. Numerous small forms frequently join to form cysts that clump together and produce large numbers of classic spirochete shapes. All the stealth forms of treponemes can revert to the spirochete form when conditions favor its survival (Delamater et al. 1951; Mattman 1992; Turner 1970).

The treponemes can only enter the host through damaged skin or mucous membranes, gaining access through tiny, broken blood vessels. Intact skin and mucous membranes prevent their entry. They prefer to live outside host cells (Turner 1970) within small blood vessels located where the host body temperature is lowest, and where low levels of oxygen needed for energy are readily available (Rudolph 1981). Soon after entering the host, they can easily move about through circulating blood and lymph fluids, and can seed out to all parts of the body. Some strains manage to survive in deeper, warmer parts of the body, but they become less active at higher than desired internal temperatures. Treponemes cling to the endothelial cells lining the walls of the tiny blood vessels (Kolker et al. 1997), stealing oxygen and feeding off dead host cells, not unlike microscopic worms. There is also evidence that the treponemes may produce and cover themselves with a slimy material to ward off attack from the host immune system (Sell and Norris 1983), which reacts with a generalized inflammatory response to the invasion.

Generally, a healthy immune system can destroy the invaders within several weeks or months. When the host immune system fails to destroy all the treponemes, the survivors alter their form and lie low for months or years without causing any problems, before resurging to cause damage to their host. Parasitic treponemes cannot survive outside the host for very long. They die when dry, and they cannot survive in high or low heat.

The Many Faces of Syphilis

The disease produces diverse symptoms, influenced by climatic factors, human behavior patterns, immune responses, and nutritional status. Poorly nourished individuals generally have poor immune responses to the infection, and they tend to develop more severe manifestations of the disease. Some individuals lack adequate immune responses to syphilis, regardless of nutritional status. Human behavior patterns influence how the disease will be transmitted, and at what age. Climate and humidity help determine where the infection will enter the host, and where it will localize. Several treponemal strains have remarkable abilities to adapt to changing conditions influencing the internal and/or external environment of their host.

When we think of syphilis, we assume it is always transmitted by sexual intercourse. However, the treponemes can also be contracted directly by contact with open sores or by drainage from sores. Touching infected, open sores and scratching or picking at skin scabs with contaminated fingers can cause infection. Kissing, oral sex, and sharing drinking vessels with individuals having open mouth sores can also spread the disease. Flies may carry the treponemes from infected sores to noninfected sores in crowded, dirty households and villages.

The Yaws Version

Geography plays a key role in determining how treponemal infection will be transmitted and how it will develop in the infected host. The treponemes require moisture and warmth to survive. Hence, the tropics provide ideal climatic conditions for the parasitic treponemes. People living in the tropics wear little clothing, and their skin stays generally moist from sweat most of the time. Sweating rids the body of excess heat while cooling the skin. This provides an ideal environment for parasitic treponemes. Abrasions to the skin commonly occur, particularly on arms and legs, where broken skin allows the treponemes to enter and create skin lesions. The lesions can vary from large, ulcerating sores to wart-like growths (Kolker et al. 1997).

This nonvenereal form of treponemal infection in the tropics is commonly known as yaws. Local names for the tropical infection include *frambesia, pian, parangi, patek, buba,* and *bouba.* Yaws infection was considered a separate disease from syphilis before the 1930s, and was believed to be caused by another type of treponemal infection, *Treponema pertenue.* However, it turns out that yaws is caused by strains of the same type of treponeme as syphilis (Kolker et al. 1997; Hudson 1958).

Human behavior plays a key role in determining who becomes infected with the treponemes, and it influences how the disease will develop. Yaws is usually considered a childhood disease, because young children living in poor, rural villages in the tropics commonly contract the disease, which is widespread (endemic). Small children generally go naked or wear very little clothing. Hence, they commonly receive skin abrasions, and close contact with other children during play and in crowded living areas easily spreads the infection. Flies also help distribute the treponemes in these areas. Wherever the disease commonly occurs in rural villages, most of the village population gains exposure to the infection during early childhood. By the time they reach adolescence and adulthood, infected individuals have already developed tolerance or immunity to yaws.

Yaws can be found in tropical Africa, in tropical areas of Latin America, in the Caribbean islands, and in tropical parts of India, Southeast Asia, and the South Pacific islands (Benenson 1995). Yaws has also been found in New Guinea and in tropical areas of Australia. The disease can be limited to one village, while another village nearby escapes the infection. Human behavior patterns in hygiene and personal habits determine the difference. The village whose inhabitants keep clean and practice good hygiene while avoiding contact with infected lesions will not contract the infection.

The Pinta Version

The tropics also serve as home for the pinta version of treponemal infection, which was first described in 1811. Unlike yaws, this infection appears to be caused by less virulent treponemal strains. Pinta produces a milder form of treponemal disease, confined to closed skin lesions resulting in discolored areas of the skin. Like yaws, pinta had previously been considered to have been caused by a different type of treponeme, *Treponema carateum* (Hudson 1958; Kolker et al. 1997).

While yaws primarily affects young children, pinta strikes mostly older children and adolescents, reaching its peak in adulthood. Like yaws, it attacks bare arms and legs, particularly legs and feet. The treponemes, confined within the closed skin lesions, can remain active for up to forty years (Guthe 1975). Infection is transmitted by direct contact with skin lesions that have been irritated by abrasions or scratching. The possibility of reduviid bugs and flies transmitting the treponemes from infected skin to uninfected skin by depositing them at bite sites has also been suggested (Manz and Buck 1997).

Various types of pinta can be found throughout the world, in isolated tropical areas in India, in west Africa, in Indonesia, and in the Pacific islands

(Guthe 1975; Hudson 1958), but it is best known among certain rural villages in Central and South America. This suggests that genetics also play a part in the host response to the infection, with certain village populations responding to the treponemes with pinta-type skin ailments. Different parts of the world have their own names for the disease, many of which mean "spotted disease," for the spotted, discolored skin areas caused by the infection. Some refer to it as "pintide yaws," and north Africans know it as "kabyle leprosy" (Hudson 1958).

Nonvenereal Syphilis

Moving away from tropical regions does not guarantee escape from treponemal infection. While warm, humid climates favor the development of the skin sores of both yaws and pinta, dryer areas of the warm subtropics and deserts force the treponemes to seek out moist parts of the body. The armpits, the genital-anal region, the areas beneath pendulous breasts or behind knees, and the areas around and inside the mouth become prime targets for treponemal infection. Clothing protects the treponemes as well as the human host from hot sunlight.

The treponemes can also survive in temperate climates, seeking out the same warm, moist areas of the body, and protected from the cold by warm clothing and warm houses. Crowded households, poverty, poor hygiene, shared sleeping areas, plus shared drinking vessels and eating utensils, ensure the survival of treponemal infection in endemic areas. Nonvenereal syphilis once was considered to be a separate disease from venereal syphilis until researchers discovered that the same treponeme caused both infections (Hudson 1958).

Once again, like yaws, nonvenereal syphilis is considered a childhood disease. Young children acquire it through direct contact with open sores, or through common drinking vessels and eating utensils contaminated with infective saliva. Flies may also help spread the disease from one sore to another. By the time of adolescence and adulthood, either tolerance or immunity results. As with yaws in the tropics, some villages escape the disease, while others nearby suffer endemic infection. Villages that do not have infections maintain high standards of hygiene and cleanliness, and their inhabitants do not share drinking vessels and eating utensils.

Nonvenereal syphilis also goes by the names of treponarid or endemic syphilis. It thrives in poor, rural areas in semiarid and arid regions of the eastern Mediterranean, the Balkans, Africa, the Arabian Peninsula, Central Asia, Tibet, Mongolia, and Australia (Forbes and Jackson 1993; Guthe 1975; Wilcox 1960) The disease has been common among poor, nomadic Bedouins in the Middle East for centuries (Hudson 1958). Local names for the infection include *bejel* in Iraq and Syria; *bishel, belish,* or *balash* in Saudi Arabia; *frenjak* or *frenga* in Bosnia and Herzegovina; *skerljevo* along the Croatian coast; *njovera* among the Bantu of South Africa; *matsabane* or *khunwane* among the Bangwaketse of South Africa; *dichuchwa, kwatsi,* or *thosola* in southwest Africa; and *irkinja* among Australian aborigines.

Venereal Syphilis

The venereal version of syphilis, once known as "lues," spread throughout the world, not bound to any geographic region or culture. Adults and adolescents not exposed to the nonvenereal forms of treponemal infection during childhood become susceptible to venereal syphilis. The treponemes primarily are transmitted from open sores on genitals or the mouth during sexual contact, or through infected semen, vaginal secretions, and blood. As in nonvenereal syphilis, initial sores develop in warm, moist areas of the body, particularly in the genital-anal region. Unlike the other strains of treponemal infection in children, venereal syphilis strains can lead to more serious disease in the adult, by affecting major organs, such as the brain and heart. Treponemal infection can also be transmitted to unborn infants of women infected during pregnancy; this is known as congenital syphilis.

Different Scenes, Different Patterns of Sores

All manifestations of treponemal infection involve tiny blood vessels within skin and mucous membrane tissue, making it a vascular (blood vessel) disease (Kolker et al. 1997; Rudolph 1981). Once the treponemes enter the host through tiny blood vessels near the skin or mucosal surface, they bind to the endothelial lining of the blood vessel walls. This causes irritation and induces inflammatory immune responses from the host, along with swelling of adjacent lymph nodes. The affected blood vessel becomes inflamed and swollen, as the various inflammatory and phagocytic cells battle the invaders. Fibrous scar tissue forms as the infection abates, thickening affected blood vessel walls. This narrows the inner space (lumen) of the vessels, retarding blood flow to adjacent tissue cells, and depriving them of adequate movement of nutrients and oxygen. Deprived cells sicken and die, and surviving treponemes fill the space, along with combatant immune cells, inflammatory cells, and tissue repair cells, producing lesions in the skin and mucous membranes. With time, healing takes place as the localized invaders are destroyed and a new network of tiny blood vessels forms to supply the injured area. However, scar tissue replaces damaged tissue wherever the battle has been fought.

All versions of treponemal infection share many symptoms, varying primarily in quantity and location of lesions. They all begin with a primary skin or mucosal lesion. The strong need of the invading treponemes for the right level of warmth and moisture remains a driving force for all infections.

Treponemes that gain entry into the host remain in tiny blood vessels at the site of entry. Within a few weeks the primary lesion of treponemal infection develops as the treponemes multiply and the host immune system reacts. The primary skin lesion caused by venereal syphilis, known as a chancre, develops into a relatively pain-free, erosive sore. It drains serous fluid (the watery part of blood and mucous fluid) full of infectious treponemes. The chancre heals on its own within three to six weeks, leaving a thin scar (Rudolph 1981).

The primary skin lesion of nonvenereal syphilis resembles the primary lesion of venereal syphilis. However, most primary lesions of nonvenereal syphilis occur in the mucous membranes of the mouth or throat. They appear as erosive patches, full of treponemes, often covered with a gray membrane. Similar primary lesions of venereal syphilis can appear on mucous membranes of the mouth or throat, or within the female vagina and cervix.

The primary lesion of yaws, often called the "mother yaw," appears at the site of entry on the skin. The warm, moist skin provides the ideal medium for rapid growth of treponemes, creating an elevated sore that may develop a crusted surface. The primary lesion often enlarges to form an ulcerating mass or large wart-like growth, teeming with treponemes. Healing can take weeks or months.

The primary entry point for pinta appears as a small, red, pimple-like raised lesion several weeks after infection takes place. This lesion gradually enlarges over several weeks or months, to become a scaly, discolored patch on the skin surface (Manz and Buck 1997).

Following the appearance of the primary lesion, treponemes can seed out through the circulatory system. This often—particularly with venereal syphilis—provokes generalized immune responses in susceptible inidividu-

als, not unlike allergic responses. Foreign proteins released by dead treponemes assaulted by the immune system most likely trigger the response,
causing fever, swollen lymph glands, and widespread rash that includes the
palms of the hands. Sometimes the rash also develops on the soles of the feet.

Less sensitive individuals will develop new crops of secondary skin
and/or mucosal lesions from treponemes that have spread to other areas outside or adjacent to the primary lesion. Ulcerative lesions may appear on the
tonsils and throat, mainly in venereal and nonvenereal syphilis. Patchy losses
of hair occur in both venereal and nonvenereal syphilis when treponemes
lodge in tiny blood vessels to the scalp. Apparently the scalp area provides a
habitat level of warmth and moisture for treponemes trying to survive in dry
and temperate climates; they rarely affect the scalp of infected individuals in
the tropics. Perhaps scalps in the tropics stay too hot for the treponemes.

Treponemes can lodge in tiny blood vessels passing near skin surfaces
that feed into bones through a dense, fibrous, membrane covering of bones
called the periosteum. Blocked blood flow and inflammatory reactions to the
treponemes irritate the periosteum, causing swelling, tenderness, and bone
pains. The infection most commonly affects the shinbones, or tibiae of the
lower legs. Growing shinbones in children with active treponemal infection
can become bowed sharply forward as a result of altered blood flow and
inflammatory processes of the periosteum. Finger bones in young children
can also become swollen and inflamed.

Pinta, the only expression of treponemal infection limited to the skin,
usually consists of mild, closed lesions. Skin lesions provide the hallmark
of all treponemal infections, but outside of pinta, these lesions can be
quite variable.

Treponemal skin lesions vary from simple, pimple-like bumps on the
skin that end up as ulcerating or erosive lesions, to wart-like growths, to
patches of discolored scaly skin, or spotty loss of pigment. The soles of bare-
foot peoples, and to a lesser degree the palms of their hands, can be affected
by painful, wart-like lesions and greatly thickened surfaces prone to crack-
ing. This happens especially with yaws and nonvenereal syphilis. Variability
of skin lesions results from the host's immune response, the host's nutritional status, invasion and aggravation by other types of bacteria, external
temperature and humidity, hygiene, and life style.

Although the majority of individuals infected by treponemes usually
overcome the disease within several weeks or months with disappearance

of secondary lesions, poor nutrition can delay recovery by compromising the immune response. Most individuals gain immunity following full recovery from secondary lesions.

About one-third of infected individuals (Benenson 1995) will develop tolerance to surviving forms of treponemes that remain hidden within the body after secondary lesions disappear. Treponemes can survive in stealth form, hidden away from the immune system, for the lifetime of the individual who has developed tolerance to them. Most of these individuals never develop any more overt signs of the disease, while about one-third may not be so lucky (Benenson 1995). Such individuals experience months or years of apparent freedom from the disease, but it then reappears, often with more serious lesions than before. These lesions may also disappear in time, yet new lesions again appear months or years later.

The host's immune system, being unable to destroy all of the treponemes, eventually resorts to sealing off the reactivated microbes in yaws, venereal syphilis, and nonvenereal syphilis. Armed inflammatory cells suround them and slowly encase the renegade microbes along with their inflammatory guards within a thick fibrous capsule known as a gumma. Cut off from nutrients and oxygen, both the imprisoned treponemes and their inflammatory cell guards die, creating a central mass of dead cells within the gumma. Gummas can be quite small, or they can reach several centimeters in diameter, appearing alone or in clusters. Gummas can rupture, creating a severe ulcer that invites other bacteria that aggravate the lesion. Adjacent tissue suffers with interruption of blood flow and spillover of the inflammatory response. Healing of the gummas leaves damaging and disfiguring scars, and in the case of venereal syphilis, occasionally the results can be deadly.

Because of its various stealth qualities, treponemal infection can develop into an unrelenting, chronic disease. Gummas in yaws, venereal syphilis, and nonvenereal syphilis can invade the skin, mucous membranes, and bones near the skin surface, often crippling the individual. When treponemal infections attack young children, late crippling lesions may not appear until adolescence or adulthood. The inner portion of long bones can be invaded by treponemes through their blood supply, while the outer portion becomes affected through blood vessels within the periosteal covering. Gummas can develop in the bones, and the bones may thicken from inflammatory reactions. The skull can be affected by gummas developing in overlying periosteal and scalp blood vessels in both venereal and nonvenereal syphilis, while yaws focuses mostly on the frontal bone of the forehead. The roof of the mouth and the nasal floor can be destroyed by gummas forming in the mucous membrane covering them, in yaws and in nonvenereal and venereal syphilis, leading to mutilating lesions of the nose, known as gangosa or goundou (Grin 1956; Guthe 1975).

Pinta, the mildest form of treponemal infection, also can develop into a chronic disease months or years after the initial lesion appears and fades. However, it involves only the skin. No gummas form. Large areas become covered with different phases of discolored lesions that eventually suffer loss of pigment during healing. Pinta skin lesions pass through a variety of colors— slate blue, violet, brown, and white—and the same person can exhibit this variation of colored lesions representing the different phases of the disease. Pinta lesions spread to the forehead, cheeks, ears, the area around the nose, the forearms, the backs of the hands, and the tops of the feet (Guthe 1975).

Treponemal infection sexually transmitted to adults can develop into a more serious chronic disease than can nonvenereal treponemal infection introduced during childhood. Late lesions of nonvenereal syphilis that develop in adolescents and adults following childhood infection generally stay on the skin, mucous membranes, and bones near skin surfaces, including the skull. Treponemal infection sexually acquired during adulthood involves these areas, but venereal syphilis can also spread to other parts of the body. Treponemes may lodge in tiny blood vessels within the covering of the brain, with gummas blocking blood flow to adjacent parts of brain tissue, causing brain damage. Sometimes tiny blood vessels within the covering of the spinal cord may be damaged, resulting in paralysis; the optic nerve may suffer from blocked blood flow to the brain, leading to blindness; the eighth cranial nerve can be damaged, leading to deafness. Even the cardiovascular system can be affected by gummas forming in the ascending aorta, the major blood vessel rising out of the heart. These gummas weaken the blood vessel wall, allowing the aorta to balloon out into a dangerous aneurysm. Gummas can also form in the liver, creating scar tissue that interfers with liver function (Guthe 1975; Kolker et al. 1997).

Congenital Syphilis

Women who contract venereal syphilis just before or during pregnancy can transmit the disease to their unborn infants. The treponemes pass through the

placenta into the bloodstream of the developing fetus. Infections acquired during the first three months of pregnancy usually end in miscarriage or stillbirth.
Fetuses contracting prenatal infection after the fourth month of pregnancy usually survive with congenital syphilis. Depending upon when the fetus contracted infection in utero, the newborn may show either mild or severe
symptoms early in infancy, or the baby may remain relatively healthy and
symptom-free until past the age of two.

Infants with early development of congenital syphilis usually do not
show symptoms until after the third week of life. The baby develops a skin
rash all over the body, including the palms of the hands and soles of the feet.
Lesions containing infectious treponemes develop, mostly on the face, around
the mouth, and in the ano-genital region. The baby develops snuffles from
obstruction of the nose and irritated throat caused by mucosal lesions. The
nose can be permanently damaged, leading to a depressed nasal bridge known
as "saddle nose." The periosteal covering and cartilage ends of the baby's bones
eventually become inflamed and painful. The lungs, spleen, and liver may
become swollen and inflamed as well. About half of infected babies exhibiting early symptoms die. Those that survive overcome the early symptoms, and
healing takes place. Following the same course as other treponemal infections,
resurgent outbreaks of the disease can appear during childhood, exhibiting all
the late lesions known for venereal syphilis. Children born with syphilis can
also display tooth deformities caused by treponemal disturbances during tooth
development. The permanent front teeth can be notched (Hutchinson teeth),
and the bite surfaces of permanent molars may look like mulberries (mulberry
molar) (Eagle 1952; Guthe 1975; Rudolph 1981; Steinbock 1976).

Changeovers

Adults or adolescents can contract treponemal infection for the first time
through breaks in skin or mucosal membranes in the mouth by drinking
from contaminated drinking vessels, by kissing, or by touching infectious
lesions of children who have the nonvenereal form of the disease. Then, any
infectious lesions that appear in the mouth or genital area of the newly
infected adult or adolescent host can be sexually transferred to other adults
or adolescents who have not had the disease.

While nonvenereal syphilis tends to be endemic, venereal syphilis is
sporadic, appearing only when sexually active individuals who have not been

exposed to treponemal infection encounter the disease for the first time. When childhood infection is reduced or eliminated in endemic areas, more adolescents and adults survive to childhood without contracting the disease. However, this turnabout increases their chances for getting venereal syphilis (Guthe and Luger 1957).

Children who have never been exposed to treponemal infection can get nonvenereal syphilis from adults who have venereal syphilis by nonsexual contact with infectious lesions or secretions. In turn, they can spread the nonvenereal form of the disease to other children; as they mature sexually, they will be immune to venereal syphilis. Where poor hygiene, crowding, and poverty prevail, the disease becomes endemic nonvenereal syphilis again (Blount and Holmes 1976; Eisenberg et al. 1949; Wilcox 1960).

The tropics favor the development of more skin lesions and fewer mucosal lesions, since exposed moist skin becomes the ideal habitat for the treponemes. However, when yaws-infected individuals move to a drier and/or cooler environment, the treponemes will retreat to the moister, warmer areas of the body, away from the now exposed dry and cooler skin. The disease takes on more characteristics of nonvenereal syphilis. Upon return to the tropics, the infection will return to exposed, warmer, moist skin areas as yaws (Grin 1956; Hudson 1965: Turner 1970).

The Great Historical Pretense and the Facts

It is commonly taught and believed that Columbus and his sailors brought syphilis to Europe in 1493 from the New World following his discovery of America. The Europeans, having no resistance to the disease, quickly became infected, and syphilis spread throughout Europe within three years. The disease proved deadly for the Europeans, killing many of its victims within weeks. Syphilis settled over Europe like a cloud, raging from one city to the next, until finally, the deadly treponemes reached equilibrium with their new hosts. The epidemic ended by 1530. The venereal syphilis we know today had become firmly established within the human population in a relatively short time (Baker and Armelagos 1988; Crosby 1969; Harrison 1959; Williams 1932).

Numerous historical documents in Europe from the late fifteenth and sixteenth centuries have been cited to verify the appearance of the disease in Europe within two to three years following Columbus's return. Several edicts issued by cities throughout Europe barring those afflicted with this apparent new disease support this hypothesis.

Treponemal infections can leave definitive lesions caused by the late-forming gummas on human long bones, skull, nose, and palate. Congenital syphilis can be recognized by characteristic deformed teeth and damaged bones. Evidence for the disease has been found in prehistoric bones of adults among native peoples from all over the Americas, while the apparent absence of such evidence in Precolumbian European human bones has often been used to support the idea that Columbus's sailors brought the disease from the New World. The lack of any signs of syphilis among thousands of ancient Egyptian human mummies and skeletons further supports the idea of New World origin.

Did Columbus and his sailors really bring syphilis to Europe from the New World?

The term *syphilis* or *lues* was not applied to the venereal form of treponemal infection until the sixteenth century (Ashmead 1901), and the term *syphilis* did not achieve wide useage until around 1850 (Hudson 1958). The historical references to the time of Columbus's return refer to a highly contagious disease or diseases known under various local names, such as *morbum franciscum, malum francium, bubas, the great pox, evil pocks, grosse verole, the French disease, Neapolitan disease,* and *grandgor.*

Ruiz de Isla's description of a "serpentine malady" in Lisbon in 1539 is often cited as evidence for the new disease being syphilis. He describes three stages of a rapidly developing disease he called *morbus gallicus,* beginning with skin sores similar to syphilis, and progressing to a second stage similar to the late stages of syphilis. A third stage quickly followed, producing prolonged illness with fever, sweats, severe weight loss, swellings, diarrhea, jaundice, swollen abdomen, dry and cracked lips, delirium, coma, and death (Hudson 1958). However, this description does not at all fit the behavior of treponemal infection. Syphilis progresses at a slow, steady pace that can continue for months or years without becoming life-threatening. Syphilis rarely kills, and when it does, death occurs many years after the first symptoms appear. Skin lesions similar to those of treponemal infection can appear with a variety of other infections, making it difficult to sort them out from one another in historic descriptions. Syphilis has often been called the great imitator, and even today the disease can be difficult to diagnose without conclusive laboratory tests.

Leprosy had begun to wane in Europe about the time that the new disease or diseases reached their peak. Physicians had finally learned to distinguish between true leprosy and other infectious diseases, and to treat them apropriately. With the number of cases of true leprosy becoming scarce, most asylums designed to house lepers in Europe closed during the fifteenth and early sixteenth centuries. Individuals infected with other, more contagious diseases who had been isolated along with lepers within the asylums were simply released back into society. Most likely syphilis existed among them, according to references to venereal leprosy and hereditary leprosy as early as the thirteenth century. As we now know, venereal syphilis, not leprosy, is transmitted sexually, and also causes congenital syphilis. The skin lesions of syphilis most likely had been confused with the skin lesions of leprosy (Ashmead 1901; Holcomb 1941; Hudson 1968; Steinbock 1976).

By the end of the nineteenth century most medical historians had disavowed the theory that Columbus and his sailors brought venereal syphilis to Europe. In 1894 Dr. Paul Raymond presented evidence for the existence of syphilis in Europe in the Middle Ages, in a paper read to the French Society of Dermatology. He had examined human bones from a medieval cemetery associated with a leprosy asylum, and he identified gummatous lesions on a Templar knight dating before the return of Columbus (Ashmead 1901).

Descriptions fitting nonvenereal syphilis were widespread in Europe by the eighteenth and early nineteenth centuries, with indications that this form of treponemal infection had been endemic in many parts of Europe for some time. Squalid medieval European towns and villages would have served the needs of treponemal infection. Eating utensils and drinking vessels commonly were shared. Children and adults bathed somewhat infrequently at public bathhouses shared by the whole populace. Nudity was not considered improper either inside or outside the bathhouse, and whole families ofen shared sleeping areas, where they slept in the nude, along with any visitors. Travelers staying at roadside inns expected to share beds with other travelers (Cockburn 1963). The disease could easily be passed around under such circumstances. Local names fitting nonvenereal syphilis included *sibbens* in Scotland, *button scurvy* in Ireland, *radesuge* in Norway, *saltfluss* in Sweden, *sypholoid* in Jutland, the *pian de Nerac* in France, and *spirocolon* in Greece (Wilcox 1960).

The nonvenereal form of syphilis disappeared from most of Europe during the first half of the nineteenth century as human behavior patterns changed (Wilcox 1960). Increasing religious influences from the Protestant Reformation and improved living conditions during the Renaissance

discouraged old habits of poor hygiene, nudity, shared utensils, and intimate contacts that promoted infection.

For centuries before 1493 people constantly moved about in the Old
World, shifting diseases, including treponemal infection, from one geographic
region to another. The most logical place of origin for treponemal infection
appears to be tropical west Africa, where the disease survives today in the only
known wild animal reservoir among chimpanzees and monkeys (Fribourg-
Blanc 1972; Guthe 1975).

When the disease moved out of Africa remains to be determined.
Hackett (1963) and Hudson (1968) believe that it spread very early, long before
the Neolithic revolution and the rise of ancient Egyptian civilization along the
Nile. They believe it spread first to the east through the Arabian Peninsula,
and then to Western and Central Asia, crossing the land bridge to the Americas
by 10,000 B.C. Hackett believed pinta to have been the original treponemal
infection that later evolved into the other forms, while Hudson believed yaws
was the original disease, changing with environment and human behavior.

We have no evidence from ancient human remains of treponemal
infection from Africa, including ancient Egypt, but we do have evidence of
the disease from nearby in the Mediterranean basin and the Middle East.
Bone lesions of the disease have been identified at a Greek colony on the gulf
of Tarent, Italy, dating from 580 to 250 B.C. (Henneberg and Henneberg 1993;
Henneberg et al. 1992). Skull lesions on human remains in Zakho in Iraq,
dating to A.D. 500, have been identified as treponemal infection (Guthe and
Wilcox 1954). Evidence for the disease moving into Western Asia has been
recognized in southern India on a human skull dating to the first or second
century B.C. (Rao et al. 1996).

There has been little research on treponemal infections in ancient
bones throughout most of Africa and Asia, leaving plenty of room to debate
the precise routes the disease followed through time. However, lesions suggestive of treponemal infection in human bones dating around two thousand
years ago or before, from the trans-Baikal region in Siberia (Steinbock 1976;
Rokhlin 1965), hint at the movement of the disease across the Bering land
bridge and into the New World.

The earliest bone lesions suggestive of treponemal infection in the
Americas come from human bones around five thousand years old from
Colombia (Burgos et al. 1994). Early cases have also been identified from
northern Chile in South America (Allison and Gerszten 1982: Arriaza 1995;

Rogan and Lentz 1994), and from Kentucky and Florida in North America (Steinbock 1976). Most evidence for treponemal infection in the Americas dates after 300 B.C., and most examples date much later (El-Najjar 1979).

We do know the disease spread much later into Western Europe, possibly as early as the Roman occupation, and then again with returning pilgrims and crusaders from the Holy Land from the eleventh to thirteenth centuries. The disease could also have been introduced with west African slaves brought to Spain and Portugal between 1142 and 1492 (Hudson 1968). Syphilis infection has recently been identified in human skeletal remains from Europe dating before Columbus's voyage (Palfi et al. 1992; Stirland 1993), and around the time of his return (Steinbock 1976; Williams 1932).

Most of the evidence for tropical treponemal yaws infection available on ancient human bones comes from the South Pacific, where archaeologists have unearthed remains as a result of new construction. The disease appeared in the Marianas Islands of Guam, Tinian, and Saipan by the 800s A.D. (Stewart and Spoehr 1952; Trimbly 1996), and remained there until European contact in 1521 (Douglas et al. 1997; Pietrusewsky et al. 1997). Similar evidence for yaws, dating to A.D. 900, comes from Fiji (Anderson 1995), and after A.D. 1250 from the island of Taumako in the Solomon Islands (Buckley 1998), and from Tonga (Pietrusewsky 1969).

The earliest evidence for treponemal infection of human bones in Japan appears during the late Muromachi period by 1520. Historic documents from this time support the skeletal evidence (Suzuki 1984). No such evidence has been reported from New Zealand (Webb 1995).

Treponemal infection has also been identified in human skeletal remains predating European colonization in Australia (Hackett 1976; Webb 1995), among the Motu of Motupore Island just off the south coast of New Guinea, and among the Nebira on the mainland of New Guinea by A.D. 1200. For centuries Macassans from Indonesia had fished for sea cucumbers in the waters between Australia and New Guinea, and they were well known to the Aborigines. Hence, the Macassans may have brought treponemal infection to both New Guinea and Australia (Webb 1995).

CONCLUDING COMMENTS

When we examine all the facts, we can see how the evolution of treponemal infections in all their forms ties into human cultural evolution. Human behavior and climate dictate how the disease is transmitted and how the infection develops. The disease leaves specific markers on human bones that can be traced back through time, allowing us to track its movements with human migrations, and to identify its place of origin. The data gathered so far indicate that the disease may have existed among small groups of hunters and gatherers long before the Neolithic revolution. It began as pinta or tropical yaws, changed to nonvenereal syphilis outside the tropics, then became venereal syphilis, and changed back again as climate and human behavior changed.

Tropical Africa seems the most likely place of origin, with the disease moving with human migrations through the Arabian Peninsula to Asia. Perhaps people migrating through the Iranian plateau and into Central Asia carried the disease to the Lake Baikal region, and from there into the Americas across the Bering land bridge 10,000–8,000 years ago. Later movements of people and trade took the disease to South and Southeast Asia, and eventually into New Guinea, Australia, and the South Pacific islands. Japan did not get the disease until the sixteenth century.

The early civilizations within and adjacent to Mesopotamia may have facilitated the spread of treponemal infection throughout the eastern Mediterranean region. The Greeks may have picked it up from their eastern colonies, and introduced it to other parts of the Mediterranean region. Roman conquests may also have played a role in spreading the infection.

Treponemal infection arrived late in temperate Western Europe, yet no later than the eleventh to thirteenth centuries. Pilgrims and crusaders returning from the eastern Mediterranean brought back the infection, and possibly some infections were brought in earlier with the Roman invasion.

Syphilis and all its variants are still with us, despite intensive campaigns by the World Health Organization and United Nations Children's Fund to eradicate nonvenereal syphilis and yaws during the 1950s and 1960s. Treponemal infections did drop dramatically, but by the 1970s and 1980s the disease regained lost ground in tropical zones where follow-up prevention programs collapsed during social unrest (Manz and Buck 1997). During the mid-1940s penicillin was found to be effective against active, growing treponemes in venereal syphilis, thus drastically reducing the number of active cases of the disease. However, the drug proved to be useless against inactive stealth forms of the disease (Turner 1970), and venereal syphilis continues to circulate throughout the world.

The tremendous amount of social unrest around the world today, with huge numbers of displaced people living in crowded, poor conditions, offers an open invitation to all kinds of disease, including treponemal infection. Pockets of nonvenereal syphilis and yaws continue to exist in various parts of the world, maintaining endemic foci that can feed into venereal syphilis. As long as these treponemal reservoirs exist, venereal syphilis will continue to makes its rounds among human populations.

CHAPTER 13

Memories of Smallpox

The World Health Organization officially declared smallpox eradicated in May 1980. This declaration followed the last known naturally acquired case, identified in Somalia, in east Africa, in October 1977 (Benenson 1981b). WHO closed the book on smallpox through extensive vaccination campaigns and intense epidemiological controls from 1967 to 1977. Since smallpox was no longer considered a threat to humanity, vaccinations against the disease then ceased.

By 1966 the last major endemic areas of smallpox had localized primarily in Western Asia. Countries involved included Bangladesh, India, Nepal, Pakistan, and Afghanistan. Other endemic foci existed in parts of Africa and in Indonesia. By 1976 the last remaining battleground for control of the disease had been confined to rural areas of Ethiopia and Somalia (Hopkins 1983).

The last major outbreak in Europe occurred in the Balkans in 1972, where it was brought in by Muslim pilgrims returning from Mecca (Hopkins 1983). The disease had disappeared from the United States by 1949, and the last known case of smallpox in the Americas occurred in 1971 in Brazil (Benenson 1981b; Cockerell 1997).

The Virus

Smallpox is caused by a virus known as variola, one of many pox viruses that have been infecting a large range of animal species throughout the world for millennia. They represent the largest and most complex of the pathogenic viruses, having a brick-shaped or elliptical classic form consisting of two strands of DNA. Unlike most DNA viruses that replicate within the nucleus of the host cell, pox viruses manage to replicate outside the nucleus within the cytoplasm of the infected cell. The virus sheds its double membranous coat once it gains entry into the host cell, and slowly begins absorbing from the cytoplasm selected nutrients needed for its replication. Replicated forms of the virus appear either as minute masses or as thread-like strands scattered throughout the cytoplasm of the infected cell. Replicating variola viral clusters often enclose any adjacent material, including other viruses such as *Herpes simplex*, within their structures. The viral clusters constantly move about within the cytoplasm as they grow and replicate (Councilman 1970; Woolf 1977).

Variola most likely originated in an animal population, and jumped species when the opportunity presented itself for adapting to human beings. The closest relative to the human virus capable of infecting humans is a similar pox virus found occurring naturally in west African monkeys. Monkey pox can cause sporadic infection in humans. Symptoms of the disease resemble mild forms of smallpox. Occasionally the infection may be transmitted between people, but otherwise human infection primarily derives from close association with infected monkeys (Fenner 1980). Studies of monkey pox virus in nature indicate that squirrels living in great numbers among the oil palms surrounding west African villages also carry the virus, suggesting that they may be the primary reservoir source (Benenson 1995). The strong similarity between the smallpox and monkey pox viruses suggests that the original source for variola may have come from a variant of monkey pox (Kempe 1975).

Variola virus behaves like a "hit and run" pathogen with human-to-human transfer. It not only thrives in large, dense human populations, but it can also be sustained within interacting small, dense rural groups. No carrier state for this virus by an asymptomatic human host exists. Once the virus infects someone, it either overcomes the immune system to produce disease, or perishes from zealous immune attack. The virus can only be transmitted to another person when symptoms of the disease develop (Kempe 1975). The burgeoning virus populace is released through moist droplets from infected upper respiratory passages, from pus-filled skin lesions known as pustules, or from dried scabs falling off healing lesions. With recovery from smallpox comes lifelong immunity to the disease. When the virus runs out of fresh victims, it dies out from the infected population.

The virus causes infection when it enters the airway passages of the host's lungs. Most smallpox infections are acquired through close contact with an infective individual. The virus becomes airborne from infectious mouth and throat lesions coughed or sneezed into the air. Dried scabs and draining skin pustules contaminate bed linens and soiled clothing with the virus. Handling of the material can easily disperse the virus into the air. The virus can survive in suspended animation within the dust of dried scabs for years, perhaps even centuries, if left away from sunlight and extreme temperatures (Henig 1993). Flies have been suspected of transmitting the virus from draining skin pustules to the nasal region in some cases (Dixon 1962). However the virus gets dispersed, infection requires close contact with the virus. Because the virus is sensitive to sunlight and extreme temperatures, it cannot travel far on its own outside a host.

Like other pathogens, variola virus existed as many different strains throughout the world, with varying degrees of virulence producing severe to mild forms of the disease. Mild and severe forms of smallpox often existed together within the same population (Fenner 1980; Hopkins 1983).

The Disease

Once the virus gains entry through the lungs, it enters nearby lymph nodes where it silently multiplies in lymphatic cells before being dispersed through the bloodstream. This serves as the incubation period, usually lasting from ten to fourteen days. Symptoms of the disease begin when the virus spreads throughout the bloodstream to targeted epithelial cells. These cells form the outer layer of skin, the surface layer of mucous membranes of the mouth, nose, and throat, and serous membranes lining internal organs (Kempe 1975). Infected individuals unknowingly carry the virus around during the incubation period, but they do not become contagious until smallpox lesions develop in endothelial tissues.

The immune inflammatory response of the host, as well as direct injury to targeted cells by the virus, triggers symptoms of the disease (Cockerell 1997). Infected cells swell and die from the ravages of the replicating virus. This creates a degenerating lesion accompanied by inflammation as the immune system sets to work repairing the damage and containing the infection (Blank and Rake 1955).

Inflammatory cells isolate the lesion from the underlying layer of tissue, and repair of the damaged area takes about two weeks. The lesions contain dead and living virus and embattled immune cells mixed with leaking serous fluid. As tissue within the lesion dies, the lesion sloughs off, leaving regenerated tissue beneath it (Blank and Rake 1955). Skin lesions dry out following rupture, producing dark scabs containing virus, which later fall off. Mucosal lesions in the mouth remain moist, infecting saliva and mucous secretions with live virus.

In some individuals the immune system attacks and destroys the virus before it can disperse throughout the bloodstream. Those individuals may suffer a fever, but no other symptoms (Dixon 1962). In most cases of infection, the virus manages to spread throughout the body before the immune system reacts. Delayed immune responses battle the disease for days. Some unfortunate individuals cannot muster enough immune response, and they suffer a terrible death as the virus takes over their body.

As virus courses through the bloodstream, the disease begins quickly as a generalized illness with fever, severe frontal headache, aching muscles and joints, severe backache, and sometimes nausea and vomiting. This phase of the disease lasts four to six days, and is often mistaken for dengue fever (Kempe 1975).

Individuals lacking any appropriate immune response die within twenty-four to thirty-six hours following the dissemination of the virus through the bloodstream. If they can survive the first forty-eight hours, the face, arms, trunk, and thighs turn red as the virus finally gains control over the body. After three days the face becomes mask-like. They toss and turn, become indifferent, cry out at intervals with agonizing pain in the chest, back, and abdomen. The pain comes from internal bleeding as lesions multiply and coalesce within serous membranes covering internal organs. Areas of the skin and mucous membranes of the mouth turn blue-black with subsurface bleeding. Death occurs within forty-eight hours after bleeding begins (Dixon 1962).

Poor immune responses with inadequate control of the infection can also produce deadly forms of the disease. Raised, pinpoint hemorrhages can appear on the face, neck, upper chest, back, and upper arms within a few days of the onset of symptoms, along with mucosal lesions within the mouth and throat. The individual becomes overly anxious and exhibits a peculiar alertness. The lesions on the face coalesce, forming bright red areas that look like severe sunburn or scalding. Bleeding from the nose and corners of swollen lips can occur. By the seventh to eighth day increasing numbers of lesions in the mouth and throat make swallowing and talking difficult. Drowsiness sets in during daylight hours, with restlessness at night. By the tenth day fluid-filled, blister-like lesions blanket the trunk and arms, with some bleeding into the lesions. Bleeding occurs internally, and an odd, sickly smell characteristic of smallpox gradually develops. Skin lesions coalesce on the body to form large scalded-like areas that tend to rub off painfully with friction from bed linens. Death usually occurs between the eighth and fifteenth day. Only about 20–30 percent of individuals with poor immune responses survive the disease, and burn-like, disfiguring scars replace the smallpox lesions (Dixon 1962).

Most delayed immune responses to the virus follow a general course of predictable phases of the disease, with recovery in the majority of individuals. Following the initial phase associated with the dispersal of the virus through the bloodstream, the individual usually feels better and wants to get back to normal activities of daily life. However, the disease is just getting started. Following a lull of about three days, a rash of pale red, round spots the size of pinheads appears on the face, neck, chest, forearms, and back, then spreads to the scalp, palms of the hands, legs, and soles of the feet. Ulcerating lesions form in the mouth and throat, producing the characteristic odor of smallpox. Lesions develop on serous membranes of internal organs. Ulcerating lesions can also form on the mucous covering of the nose, eye, vagina, and urethral opening from the bladder. Within twenty-four hours the rash increases in size and numbers, changing to raised, red blotches known as papules. By the third to fifth day after the onset of the rash, most of the body is covered by papules that quickly become filled with fluid and pus, turning into pustules as large as half an inch in diameter, and teeming with virus. The pustules at first appear pearly gray, changing to yellow. The face becomes swollen and mask-like, with large numbers of coalescing lesions. Between the eighth and tenth day following the onset of the rash, the pustules begin to collapse and rupture over a course of two to three days. The pustular contents dry on the surface of the skin lesions, forming a hard, dried, dark crust. Mucous lesions in the mouth and throat, and serous membrane lesions heal. By the fourteenth day the scabs come off the face, then the body, by the hundreds, for about six days, except for those deeply seeded in the calluses of hands and feet, which gradually get pushed out over time. The skin beneath the scabs grows fine and silvery, shedding every four to six days for about a month, then is slowly replaced by a pitting scar. Permanent hair loss commonly occurs, with scarring of hair follicles. Eyebrows and eyelashes may also be lost (Dixon 1962; Wilkinson 1959).

Milder forms of smallpox occur with less virulent strains of variola virus, which often circulate alongside infection by more virulent strains. These forms are referred to as variola minor, alastrim, kaffir pox, or amaas. Skin lesions in these forms tend to be fewer in number and smaller, with early scabbing, and the disease results in fewer deaths (Benenson 1981b).

Pregnant women infected with smallpox tend to exhibit more severe, hemorrhagic forms of the disease. The serous membranes covering the placenta attract the virus. Infection during the early months of pregnancy often causes spontaneous abortion, and about half of pregnant women infected during the later part of their pregnancies lose their babies (Dixon 1962).

Poor diets and secondary infection from bacteria, especially staphylococcus and streptococcus (Kempe 1975), contributed to the severity of smallpox, particularly in poor, rural areas. Secondary bacterial infection of the eyes with mild forms of the smallpox often left its victim blind. Young children in poor regions were prone to secondary infection, and a small percentage developed bone infections, especially near the wrists, elbows, knees, and ankles (Dixon 1962). Smallpox often became confused with severe forms of chickenpox and measles, and the disease frequently was misdiagnosed until it was too late to isolate the infected individual from others (Wilkinson 1959).

The overall death rate from an epidemic of major smallpox generally fluctuated between 30 percent and 50 percent (Wilkinsin 1959), while the death rate for strains producing minor versions of smallpox ranged from 1 percent to 10 percent, depending on the strain. The death toll from severe, hemorrhagic forms of smallpox reached almost 100 percent (Benenson 1981b).

The Trail of Smallpox

Sub-Saharan Africa seems the most likely place of origin for the human variola virus, where it probably evolved from monkey pox. Once established as a human virus, it spread to distant locations during the long incubation phase within its victims, as infected people passed the infection to fellow travelers along the way. Repeated epidemics introduced the virus several times to other regions. The African slave trade, begun more than a millennium ago, acted as a conduit for the transmission of smallpox.

By 2500 B.C. ancient trade routes, wars, migrations, and pilgrimages, with returning soldiers, merchants, travelers, and explorers, had already helped the virus spread throughout the ancient world. As city-states grew along trade routes, the large urban populations became ideal breeding grounds for repeated epidemics of smallpox.

The virus moved from the Nile Valley to ancient cities in Mesopotamia, the Iranian plateau region, up to the Black Sea and into Central and Western Asia, including the Indus Valley of present-day Pakistan. The virus traveled not only within its victims, but also in dried scabs caught in contaminated clothing and cotton cargo packed in caravans moving across great distances. Early sea trade from the Persian Gulf, following the coasts of Arabia, Persia, and India, and eventually China, may also have played a part in the delivery of the virus to Asia.

The earliest evidence for the presence of smallpox appears in three mummified human bodies from ancient Egypt, dating from about 1570–1085 B.C., including the mummy of the pharaoh Ramses V. The pharaoh died from the disease in his early thirties in 1157 B.C. His face shows evidence of swelling and pustules (Dixon 1962; Hopkins 1983). Microscopic examination of the lesions revealed virus-like particles typical of smallpox, and fragments of scabs had some reaction to smallpox antibody (Sandison and Tapp 1998).

The Hittites of Anatolia described a mysterious epidemic disease attacking them following wars with Egyptian armies in what is now northern Syria in the mid-fourteenth century B.C. The disease spread from Egyptian captives, killing many soldiers and civilians, and raged for at least twenty years among the Hittites (Hopkins 1983). We can only speculate that it was smallpox.

One of the oldest Sanskrit medical texts, the Susruta Aamhita, written by a Hindu physician before the fifth century A.D., describes smallpox and indicates the disease may have existed in ancient India by 1500 B.C. (Hopkins 1983). Ayurvedic physicians translated descriptions of smallpox written around 1000 B.C. from Sanskrit and Pali into Sinhalese on the island now known as Sri Lanka (Cockburn 1963). Brahmin priests conducted temple services and prayers to a smallpox goddess during the last millennium B.C. (Hopkins 1983).

Smallpox reached China around 250 B.C. with invasion by the Huns from Central Asia, and it quickly spread throughout northern China. Smallpox attacked the Han Chinese army of Emperor Kwang Wu Ti in A.D. 48–49 while they fought Wuling tribes in what is now Hunan province in the southern part of China. The disease came from Central Asia, and it may have spread from there along the "Burma road" into Southeast Asia (Hopkins 1983). Smallpox became well established in China, and was thoroughly described by a physician of the Chin dynasty early in the fourth century A.D. (Cockburn 1963). Smallpox arrived in Japan along with Buddhism in the sixth century A.D. (Hopkins 1983).

Neither ancient Greek nor Roman texts contain any clear written descriptions of smallpox, despite the numerous epidemics that they recorded. However, evidence for the disease is cited among soldiers from Carthage on the Mediterranean shores of North Africa in 395 B.C. Carthage had sent its military forces to the island of Sicily to attack the city of Syracuse. During the siege, many soldiers in the Carthaginian army fell ill, covered with pustules, and many died, forcing the army to retreat (Hopkins 1983).

Alexander the Great reached the lower Indus Valley by 327 B.C., where his army became infected with a disease that the Roman historian Rufus describes as a scab attacking their bodies and spreading contagion. The disease burned out before they made their return journey to the West (Dixon 1962; Hopkins 1983).

Symptoms of smallpox fit descriptions of a disease that struck Abyssinian soldiers from the Axum kingdom of present-day Ethiopia when they attacked Mecca during the Elephant War of A.D. 569. The disease spread throughout the Arabian tribes when Muhammad united them in the seventh century. The physician Rhazes from Baghdad in the tenth century recorded the epidemic resulting from the Elephant War, and he became the first writer to provide a comprehensive diagnosis of smallpox (Cockburn 1963; Dixon 1962; Hopkins 1983).

The first description of smallpox in Western Europe comes from Bishop Gregory of Tours, France, in A.D. 581. He writes that the disease spread across southern France and northern Italy. Islamic armies in A.D. 622 spread the disease from an outbreak in the city of Alexandria, Egypt, across north Africa, into Spain, Portugal, and France (Cockburn 1963; Dixon 1962: Hopkins 1983).

Smallpox gradually and sporadically spread throughout Western Europe. Epidemics were reported in Ireland between 675 and 778, and in Flanders in 961. Pilgrims and crusaders reintroduced smallpox to Western Europe with their return from the Middle East. By the end of the twelfth century smallpox had become well known throughout continental Western Europe (Dixon 1962; Hopkins 1983).

Smallpox arrived in Iceland by way of a Danish ship in 1241, killing 20,000 people there. More outbreaks in Iceland followed in 1257 and 1291.

Returning crusaders under Edward I brought smallpox to England in 1300. An epidemic brought from Iceland hit Greenland in 1430. By the sixteenth century smallpox was entrenched throughout Europe except for Russia, where the disease finally gained a foothold in the early seventeenth century (Dixon 1962; Hopkins 1983).

Smallpox haunted the ports of Spain, and Spaniards exported it to the West Indies of the New World in 1507. Chained infections on board ship, plus scab-contaminated clothing and cotton, allowed the virus safe passage to the New World (Benenson 1981b; Dixon 1962). The virus also arrived with black slaves acquired by the Spanish from the west African coast to work in the mines of Hispaniola (now Cuba) as early as 1510 (Stearn and Stearn 1945). Hispaniola quickly became a breeding ground for smallpox.

The disease soon reached the mainland of Mexico in Yucatán, clearing the way for the conquering Spaniards. Cortés arrived in Campoula near present-day Vera Cruz in 1519, where he was soon joined by another group of Spaniards with a black slave carrying the infection. Smallpox raced ahead of the conquistadors, terrorizing and killing many tribal leaders, and eventually half the native population of Mexico. This enabled Cortés with fewer than five hundred men to conquer the great Aztec empire in 1521 (Hopkins 1983; Stearn and Stearn 1945).

Smallpox, along with other Old World diseases, marched ahead of the conquering Spaniards throughout Latin America, paving the way for conquest. Disease wiped out cities along the Peruvian coast, and upset the ruling Incas in the highlands. Pizarro arrived in Inca territory in 1532 amid chaos created by disease and civil war. The African slave trade kept feeding the epidemics that raged for years throughout Latin America, making it possible for Spain and Portugal to easily take control (Hopkins 1983).

Smallpox did not spare North America. European colonists, particularly colonists from England where smallpox continued to run rampant, brought the disease to the shores of North America. Smallpox epidemics occurred off and on, and many ships came under quarantine if suspected of carrying smallpox. However, clothing and bales of cotton contaminated with smallpox scabs often came ashore from these ships. The introduction of black slaves infected with the disease also contributed to the epidemics.

By the end of the seventeenth century, smallpox began its march westward. In the north of Canada, Jesuit priests and the fur trade companies unknowingly helped spread the disease to local native tribes. By 1731 smallpox had become widespread among the colonies and Native American settlements. Smallpox infection on occasion was deliberately introduced to tribes resisting colonial rule by gifts of blankets from the sickbeds of smallpox victims (Hopkins 1983; Stearn and Stearn 1945).

Cotton workers and cloth mill workers infected with smallpox contributed to the spread of the disease. Both the habit of joining broken cotton fibers by moistening hands with saliva and the presence of sloughing scabs from workers recovering from the disease contaminated cotton and cloth. Traffic in rags made from old clothing, some contaminated with the virus, baled and stored for paper mills, also helped spread the disease. The virus survived in dry state for months or years in warehouses and in the hulls of cargo ships (Dixon 1962). By the nineteenth century ships carrying contaminated cotton bales, rags, clothing, and cloth, as well as chain infections among the crew and passengers, had carried smallpox all over the world.

Desperate Measures

Smallpox could not be readily distinguished from measles and chickenpox in the European community until Sydenham sorted out the differences in the 1660s. However, confusion remained until the end of the eighteenth century, as smallpox struck almost every family, rich and poor alike (Wilkinsin 1959).

While Europe was struggling with this new disease, along with many other epidemic diseases that had been introduced from outside the continent, much of Asia had long been acquainted with smallpox and also the idea of inoculation against it. The idea of inoculation appears to have evolved in India among ancient Brahman priests worshiping the goddess dedicated to smallpox. They noticed that not all smallpox victims suffered to the same degree, some having only the mild form of the disease. By carefully selecting dried scabs from victims recovering from mild smallpox, they could simulate the natural transfer of the virus by placing fragments of these dried scabs in the noses of individuals previously untouched by the disease. The resulting, milder form of smallpox protected the inoculated individual against the more severe form of the disease. Each spring the priests would wander through the countryside inoculating young children. Buddhist priests and nuns continued the ancient tradition of inoculation, and carried the practice into Central Asia and China. Records dating from around 590 B.C. from the Sung dynastic period in China describe this method of inoculation introduced by a Buddhist nun from Tibet (Dixon 1962; Hopkins 1983).

Later, another form of inoculation appeared, in which wet drainage from the skin pustules of a victim with the mild form of the disease replaced dried scabs. Inoculation was achieved by inserting the draining pus under the skin of uninfected individuals. This form of inoculation using pus known as "lymph" from smallpox lesions spread into Persia and Anatolia via trade routes from India and Central Asia, reaching Constantinople no later than the seventeenth century (Hopkins 1983).

Apparently this form of inoculation was also known in west Africa. Cotton Mather, Boston colonist, learned about it from a black slave in 1706, and he encouraged the colonists to use it. George Washington had his revolutionary army inoculated in 1777, following bouts of smallpox. Peasants in some parts of Europe also used this technique (Hopkins 1983).

European physicians were aware of this inoculation method, but they resisted using it. Lady Mary Wortley Montague, wife of a British ambassador to Turkey during the early part of the eighteenth century, learned about inoculation while living with her husband in Constantinople. Having survived smallpox herself with terrible scarring, she vowed to use inoculation on her children to spare them the horrors of the disease. Upon her return to London in 1721 she introduced the idea of inoculation to the British court. However, fear of smallpox was so great that few dared risk it (Benenson 1981b; Hopkins 1983).

Meanwhile, rumor spread throughout Europe about how milkmaids infected with cowpox went unscathed during smallpox epidemics. Dairy farmers began to use the cowpox to inoculate their children. Physicians learned of this through reports by an English physician in 1765 and a German physician in 1769, to no avail. Finally, in 1798 an English physician named Edward Jenner published a paper on the effectiveness and safety of cowpox as a vaccine for smallpox. Although English physicians were slow to pick up on the idea, the rest of Europe quickly began to use cowpox vaccines to prevent smallpox (Dixon 1962; Hopkins 1983).

Regardless of inoculation source, a great deal of controversy over the use of inoculation existed in Europe. Questions arose over its safety, the resulting immunization, and whether or not it could be considered religiously correct to interfere with God's just course. Safety was a valid concern, particularly with inoculations often performed haphazardly with little skill, and the "lymph" itself often too potent, or contaminated. Discretion was not always used to obtain the "lymph" for inoculation. The more inexperienced inoculators often obtained pus from victims suffering from major forms of smallpox instead of from victims with minor forms of the disease. Cowpox "lymph" often contained other pathogens, or actually consisted of some other cow pustule infection. Adverse reactions to the foreign substance also caused problems.

For many years following the introduction of cowpox vaccines, practitioners were unaware that the immunization might weaken and revaccination might be required to prevent recurring epidemics. Vaccinated individuals with waning protection could still become infected with the virus, developing mild or modified smallpox that often went undiagnosed, leaving them free to infect others.

Alarmed over the continuous downward spiral of the native populations in their New World colonies, the Spaniards took action in 1803 under the mandate of King Carlos IV to use Jenner's vaccine to inoculate people in the colonies. Transporting and maintaining Jenner's live vaccine across the Atlantic created a problem. They selected orphaned children to carry the vaccine via arm-to-arm transfer throughout the long voyage and the journeys throughout the colonies in order to dispense the vaccine from their active inoculations. Eventually, a cowherd infected with cowpox was found in New Spain that could be used to produce and maintain vaccine by inoculating calves. The Spaniards did the same thing for the Philippines and two Chinese port cities (Hopkins 1983).

Unsuccessful attempts to transport Jenner's vaccine from Europe to the United States gave rise to a new idea for getting the vaccine across the Atlantic. President Jefferson ordered the vaccine delivered in small, corked vials immersed in water. This approach succeeded, and vaccination soon became widely used throughout Euro-American communities. Eventually a source of cowpox turned up in a cowherd on a farm in Pennsylvania. By the end of the nineteenth century attention turned to inoculating Native Americans following several smallpox epidemics on reservations (Hopkins 1983).

During the 1920s a dried vaccine had been developed, but the quality varied and it proved hard to reconstitute. Finally, in 1949 a freeze-drying method was developed to preserve the vaccine without refrigeration, and it came into use by 1954 (Hopkins 1983).

By the early nineteenth century smallpox vaccination had been accepted throughout Europe, and it spread through the civilized world. By the end of the nineteenth century the safety of vaccines had greatly improved. Better understanding of the effectiveness of isolation and routine vaccinations soon put the disease in decline wherever these methods were practiced. After eradication in 1980, vaccination no longer seemed to matter (Cockerell 1997).

Cowpox

Just how cowpox protected against smallpox remained a mystery until the end of the nineteenth century. Nash described the amazing natural history of cowpox in 1781, supporting its use for inoculation over the use of smallpox from victims. He noticed that cows only had the disease once, and that the infection spread to other cows on milkmaids' hands. Jenner had taken "lymph" from a lesion on the hand of a milkmaid to use for his famous inoculation (Dixon 1962).

In actuality, the milkmaids provided the original source of the infection, not the cows. Smallpox lesions commonly appear on the palms of the victim's hands, and they are the last to heal. Thus, those milkmaids recovering from smallpox with lesions on their hands first infected the cow's udder through abrasions, similar to inoculation. The resulting localized lesions, not unlike the local lesions of smallpox inoculation, in turn infected the hands of milkmaids who had not had smallpox, somewhat like reverse inoculation (Dixon 1962). The potency of the virus weakened when implanted in cow tissue, as it adapted to the new microenvironment. The more potent variants within the virus population that thrived in human tissue could not survive in cow tissue, leaving less potent variants within the virus population adapting to the cow. When the less potent virus passed back to humans, it offered little threat of serious disease, but it enabled the immune system to arm itself against attack by the more potent variants of smallpox.

The Hybrid Virus

With the passage of smallpox to cows and calves and back to humans, the modified virus began to take on its own characteristics. By the end of the nineteenth century, the virus had been passed through a variety of laboratory animals in the production of vaccine. This produced a hybrid of the original smallpox virus known as *Vaccinia virus*, first noticed by Buist in 1887. This laboratory-bred hybrid virus produced the same protection as cowpox, and it soon became the only vaccine used for inoculation. Even with this weakened hybrid virus, some dangers remain for adverse reactions from inoculation with the foreign substrate and weak or compromised immune systems unable to react sufficiently to the vaccine. *Vaccinia virus* can be stored easily almost indefinitely, either refrigerated or freeze-dried (Downies 1959).

The World Health Organization set aside enough vaccine from *Vaccinia virus* in freeze-dried storage in 1980 for 200 million inoculations, as a precaution against the accidental or intentional reintroduction of smallpox (Benenson 1981b).

CONCLUDING COMMENTS

Smallpox joined the number of devastating diseases that had an impact on developing civilizations throughout the world, altering the course of history in many instances. Smallpox epidemics toppled great leaders and stopped whole armies in their tracks. The fear of disfigurement from smallpox scars, as well as the dreaded disease itself, haunted many generations. People frantically searched for remedies and found that inoculation could ward off the drastic effects of the disease.

More than sixty laboratories around the world held samples of smallpox virus in 1977 (Benenson 1981b). Following the WHO eradication program, only two laboratories with high security were legally allowed by the world community to hold samples of several strains of variola virus as reference material, in case the disease should ever reappear. The virus samples were assigned to the Centers for Disease Control (CDC) in Atlanta, Georgia, and the State Research Center of Virology and Biotechnology in Koltsovo, Novosibirsk Region, Russia. Some of the major strains represented in these samples have been "fingerprinted" by mapping their DNA sequences. DNA fragments of several strains have been studied and cloned, and work continues on the development of a specific blood test for diagnosing the disease in its early stages (Benenson 1995).

Laboratory accidents have occurred in the past. One such accident in England in 1973 exposed a medical technician to the virus. The infection went undetected and was passed on to two other people who died from it. Another accident in 1978 infected a medical laboratory photographer in Birmingham, England, who was taking pictures. She contracted the virus by way of a ventilation duct from the laboratory working on smallpox. Before it could be diagnosed, she passed it to her mother who died from it. The scientist working in the smallpox laboratory committed suicide over it (Henig 1993).

Have we seen the last of smallpox? Probably not. Stocks of vaccine exist—just in case. For fifty years the Soviets developed tons of smallpox virus to use as biological weapons despite international agreements not to do so. The Soviets also developed a more virulent strain of variola with a shorter incubation period.

Military experts have reason to believe that clandestine laboratories exist in several places, with the goal of developing variola into a biological weapon, particularly for use in terrorist attacks. *Vaccinia virus* itself could pose a threat if misused. While this hybrid virus may be used to carry "lab designer" vaccines to prevent other diseases, the Soviets have attempted to turn it into a potent killer by combining it with ebola virus (Alibek 1999; Benenson 1995).

We now have a whole global generation born since the WHO eradication program of smallpox and the discontinuation of vaccinations. Their vulnerability has been noted by terrorists and rogue governments. Even older individuals vaccinated before eradication could be vulnerable to smallpox infection with waning resistance. Modern doctors will have difficulty diagnosing smallpox. It was difficult enough to recognize in the past, and often not correctly diagnosed until too late. Early symptoms vary and can be hard to link to smallpox (Benenson 1981b).

The possibility that natural smallpox still exists hidden away in some remote populations, or hidden in dry state from old scabs in a secluded area cannot be overlooked. Furthermore, under the right conditions a new smallpox strain could spin off from a potent strain of monkey pox (Fenner 1980). However, the greatest danger from resurgence of smallpox lies in clandestine laboratories. The danger of smallpox use in biological warfare is so great that some countries are returning to vaccination of military and medical personnel.

CHAPTER 14

PESTILENCE, PLAGUE, AND RATS

References to pestilence and plague epidemics appear frequently in historic documents, beginning with the early civilizations of the Old World. Epidemics of various infectious diseases became commonplace throughout Europe, Asia, and north Africa by the Middle Ages. The word *pestilence* refers to any epidemic contagious disease. Similarly, the term *plague* was applied to any widespread contagious disease that caused a high death rate. However, today this term denotes a specific disease.

Our history books teach that the plague ravaged medieval Europe, killing much of its population while spreading fear and panic everywhere, and that the disease engendered many cultural changes in Europe. During the Middle Ages the disease was simply referred to as the pestilence (Gottfried 1983). Some people called it the bubonic plague for the prominent sores, known as buboes, associated with the disease. Scandinavian historians applied the term "Black Death" to the plague long after the epidemics had dissipated in Europe. This was an attempt to distinguish this deadly infection from many other infectious epidemics that affected medieval Europe, and had nothing to do with the color black (Herlihy 1997).

The cause of the disease remained unknown until the end of the nineteenth century. The Swiss microbiologist, Alexandre Yersin, discovered the cause in 1894 when he was called from service in the French colony of Indochina to Hong Kong during the last major plague pandemic. He named the bacteria causing the disease *Pasteurella pestis* after the Pasteur Institute

237

in Paris where he had been educated. The bacteria was later renamed *Yersinia pestis* for his discovery (Herlihy 1997).

The last plague pandemic (worldwide epidemic) had originated in Yunnan province of southwest China with the rebellion of the Muslim Hui in 1866. The disease had been smoldering among wild rodents for some time, and during the revolt it spilled over into domestic rats and the human population. Refugees and rats as they fled carried the disease to the city of Kunming in southeast Yunnan province. From there it spread eastward to Guangzhou (Canton) in 1894, and down the Pearl River to Hong Kong. From Hong Kong, infected rats boarding ships spread the disease to other port cities throughout the world. The disease spread like wildfire from the large port cities of Bombay and Calcutta in 1896, causing more than 10 million deaths in India during the next twenty years. The plague reached ports in Japan and the Philippines in 1897, and ports in Australia, Hawaii, Central America, and South America by 1899. Plague reached San Francisco in 1900, Singapore in 1901, Bangkok by 1904, Java in 1910, New Orleans in 1914, and ports in Texas and Florida by 1922 (Benenson 1981b; Cloudsley-Thompson 1976).

The role that rats and their fleas played in the plague epidemics was not discovered until the early twentieth century, despite earlier observations of sick and dying rats found wherever plague erupted. Once rats had been identified as the major carriers of the disease, people in towns and cities took measures to eliminate them, and port cities worked at preventing them from climbing on board ships at dock (Burnet and White 1972). The last great plague pandemic finally abated wherever rat control had been implemented by the 1950s.

Before the pandemic ended, the infection had been introduced to wild rodents coming into contact with infected rats in various parts of the world. The plague bacteria are now maintained in wild rodent reservoirs in the western United States; large areas of South America; north-central, eastern, and southern Africa; and Central and Southeast Asia (Benenson 1995).

Rats Take Over the World

Rats are opportunists, able to adapt to changes in climate and habitat. The domestic rats that we know—the ones that roam our cities, towns, and farms—came with civilization and commerce. Before civilization, these familiar rats had been confined to wilderness areas in Central and South

Asia. In the wild, nature held rat populations in check, keeping their numbers in balance with the availability of food and the numbers of predators. When food would become plentiful, rat populations would explode, and when the food supply dwindled, the rats would swarm to find food. If no food could be found, they turned to cannibalizing each other (Hendrickson 1983).

The rats took advantage of human intrusions into their territory by scavenging grain crops and food supplies, and as the number of human intrusions increased, rats adapted to people and followed them to other locations. Rats moved with the advances in civilization, and the increases in commerce and trade throughout Asia and the rest of the Old World. They packed up with cargo moving along trade routes, followed armies and migrant camps, and boarded cargo carrying ships for far ports.

As human populations increased, so did rat populations. By the early Middle Ages, black rats had succeeded in taking over Europe, the Middle East, north Africa, and most of Asia. Black rats reached the New World in the 1500s the same way they had been introduced to the homelands of the colonists, by ship. They invaded Australia with the convicts sent there from England, and they found South Africa with the European settlers. Captain Cook and other explorers introduced the black rat to most of the Polynesian Islands (Hendrickson 1983). By the early nineteenth century, rats had taken over the world.

Rats are smart, cunning, fearless, and curious creatures. They also can be quite vicious. When cornered, a rat will fight to the death. Rats are clean animals. They constantly groom themselves and bathe when water is available, being good swimmers. They are strong and agile; being able climbers, they can jump up 2–3 feet; and they can squeeze through small openings. Being omnivorous with voracious appetites, they will eat just about anything, eating an amount equal to as much as one-third of their body weight each day. One thing that they will not eat is white flour, because it lacks needed nutrients. They hoard food, and prefer to dine in secrecy. Their favorite foods include grains and meat. They love marine foods, and they often fish for small fish and gather shellfish in coastal settings. They hunt small animals, domestic fowl, and wild ground birds, and they steal bird eggs. Hungry rats will attack the newborn of large animals such as pigs, and will take on a sick or dying adult, even helpless, dying humans. They also attack human infants when they find one left alone. When food becomes scarce, they can survive up to fourteen days without eating. They do need up to an ounce of drinking water a day, and usually build their nests not too far from water and food supplies (Hendrickson 1983).

Rats are prolific breeders. Females carry their young for twenty-two days, and mate again within forty-eight hours after giving birth. They breed all year round. One female can have up to sixteen litters per year, with six to twelve young in each litter, weaning them in four to five weeks. Rats reach breeding age by two to three months, and most rats have a lifetime of six months to one year in the wild. However, some can survive for as long as five years, and up to seven years in captivity. The young do not have an easy life, and many of them do not survive. Disturbed females will often kill and eat their own young. Baby rats are born helpless, blind, deaf, and naked, vulnerable to severe temperature changes, environmental upsets, and predators. Rats tend to congregate in large packs, and the females share the care of their young, keeping adults in constant attendance to protect them from danger (Hendrickson 1983).

Gnawing constitutes a do-or-die activity for rats. They begin gnawing as soon as the incisor teeth erupt at around eight days of age. This constant activity continues throughout the rat's life, keeping the ever growing incisors from locking together or pushing through the brain. Damage from rat gnawing can be costly, as when they gnaw through insulated wires, thereby causing fires. Wooden structures, concrete block structures, and thin metal containers can be damaged by the gnawing rodents (Hendrickson 1983).

The black rat, *Rattus rattus*, became the major carrier of the plague throughout the world. The color of this rat actually varies from gray to brown as well as black. It has been called the roof rat, ship rat, Alexandrine rat, Sicilian rat, fruit rat, corn rat, and tree rat. The black rat originally lived in trees in South Asia, and adapted to early farming settlements. The black rat is not shy, so it was able to coexist with humans without fear. They followed trade routes throughout Asia and westward into the Mediterranean region with the advances of civilization. Black rats fall back on their tree-dwelling instincts among human settlements, preferring to live in the upper portions of buildings, in attics, or between walls and upper level floors (Hendrickson 1983).

The brown rat, *Rattus norvegicus*, can also carry the plague, but will be less likely to pass the disease on to humans because of its aversion to people. The brown rat, larger than the black rat, is also known as the Norway rat, gray rat, house rat, wanderette (migratory) rat, surmolot, earth rat, alley rat, water rat, barn rat, dump rat, river rat, wharf rat, and sewer rat. Unlike the black rat, the brown rat prefers to be underground near water, such as sewers. The brown rat appears to have originated in Mongolia and northern China, where it burrows underground along stream banks. Packs of brown rats can create intricate underground burrows as long as a city block, as much as 5 feet deep, with a series of passageways, nests, and food caches (Hendrickson 1983).

The brown rat also followed the trade routes out of Asia, coming into Europe from Central Asia in great hordes during the late seventeenth century. They swam across the Volga River by the thousands when food supplies diminished. They soon became the dominant rat throughout Europe, and eventually much of the world as they boarded ships for distant places (Hendrickson 1983).

Brown rats and black rats are mortal enemies, and they do not crossbreed. They can share the same manmade structure as long as they remain apart, with the black rat living in the upper levels and the brown rat seeking the lower portions of the same structure, such as the basement or sewer (Hendrickson 1983). But if they cross paths, war breaks out, with the larger and more ferocious brown rat the winner.

Rat Fleas and Yersinia pestis

Fleas that infest rodents, including the black and brown rat, can act as vectors for diseases infecting the rodents. The bacteria *Yersinia pestis* that causes plague naturally infects several wild rodents not related to the black and brown rats. They maintain reservoirs of the bacteria with chronic infections that seldom kill their natural hosts. Fleas that flourish in these rodent populations become the vectors for the infection, transferring the bacteria from rodent to rodent, and to any intruder, such as the black or brown rat, that happens to poke around or take over the rodent burrow, or dine on rodents infested with the fleas. Both the black and brown rat are susceptible to the bacteria, and most of them die from the disease.

More than two hundred flea species and subspecies can transmit plague bacteria, including the human flea (*Polex irritans*), the dog flea (*Ctenocephalides canis*), and the northern rat flea (*Nosopsyllus fascitis*) that infests rats, mice, and a variety of small animals in Europe and North America. The most commonly known vector of human plague is the oriental rat flea, *Xenopsylla cheopis*. Another rat flea, *Xenopsylla basil-iensis*, serves as the predominant human plague vector in parts of Africa, and this flea has spread with rats to India and South America (James and Harwood 1969).

Fleas are tiny, wingless, blood-sucking insects with long legs that propel them through the hairs on the host's body. Fleas do not remain loyal to a specific host, and they readily jump species when the opportunity arises. Adult fleas may spend most of their lives on a single host animal, or move to another host when the animals crowd together. The females drop their eggs to the ground, usually in the nesting place of the host animal, where the eggs hatch and the larvae feed on organic trash. The body temperature of the host animal is generally too warm for the young larvae to hatch. The larvae prefer temperatures of 65–80°F (18–20°C) with high humidity, and these conditions often exist in rodent burrows. Egg incubation can be inhibited by extremes in temperature and by low humidity. The larvae pupate anywhere from one week to as long as a year, depending on environmental conditions. Adults can survive for a year or more under favorable circumstances. Newly emerging adult fleas can remain inactive until the presence of a host activates them, and adults can survive long periods of starvation in the absence of a host, within the safety of rodent burrows. *Yersinia pestis* residing within infected adult fleas can also endure while the flea waits for its next blood meal (Beaver and Jung 1985; James and Harwood 1969). If the host animal dies, the infected flea can wait for weeks, sometimes months, for its next victim.

When a flea takes its blood meal, it ingests any bacteria circulating in the host's blood. The bacteria then multiply within the flea's gut, forming a gelatinous mass that blocks the long, narrow opening to the gut. As the infected flea feeds on a new host, it regurgitates ingested blood back into the bite site along with the bacteria. The frantic flea repeatedly tries to feed, thus flushing the bacteria into the puncture wound of the host. The build-up of a gelatinous bacterial mass causing regurgitation does not occur in all species and subspecies of infected fleas, which reduces the chances of flea bites infecting a new host. However, bacteria contained in the flea feces deposited at the bite site, or released from crushed fleas over a bite site can produce infection (Beaver and Jung 1985; James and Harwood 1969).

The oriental rat flea, *Xenopsylla cheopis*, is highly susceptible to the gelatinous build-up of bacterial blockage and regurgitation. Thus, these fleas are very efficient transmitters of *Yersinia pestis* (James and Harwood 1969).

The primary natural host of the oriental rat flea is the domesticated black rat, *Rattus rattus*. It is the major rodent responsible for the plague epidemics that have ravaged the world.

Yersinia pestis belongs to the enterobacteriacene family of bacteria, which includes a number of bacteria causing intestinal infections. They all share similar genes that code for specialized sets of proteins to help protect them from the immune system of the host (Barinaga 1996). The bacteria lack protection from a capsule when they enter the host bloodstream, making them vulnerable to deadly phagocytosis by polymorphonuclear white blood cells. However, when monocytic or macrophage cells take up *Yersinia pestis*, the biochemistry within these cells triggers the bacteria to develop insulating capsules resistant to destruction (Benenson 1981). The cell wall of the bacteria also directs the macrophage to produce a variety of tissue-damaging proteins to protect it from the host's immune system, and to create a more sustainable microenvironment for bacterial growth. Capillary blood and lymph flow increases with a build-up of fluid around infected cells, thus promoting the spread of infected cells to nearby lymph nodes (Smith and Reisner 1997).

The Disease

The bacteria multiply at the site of entry into the host, where frequently a small pustule or blister-like lesion appears. When the infection spreads to the nearest lymph nodes, cells within the lymph nodes die from the assault. Invasion of lymph nodes trigger marked inflammatory reactions within the surrounding tissue, creating a swollen lesion known as a bubo. *Yersinia pestis* spreads to other adjacent lymph nodes and into the bloodstream to the spleen, liver, and distant lymph nodes. The damaging proteins wreak havoc in these organs and poison the blood. Infected macrophages may also lodge in the lungs, producing pneumonia (Benenson 1981).

The progress and outcome of the disease depend on how the host acquired the infection, and the host's immune response to *Yersinia pestis*. The most common form of the plague is bubonic plague, caused by an infected flea bite. Two to four days following the flea bite, the victim experiences a sudden attack of chills with high fever, headache, rapid heart beat and breathing, anxiety, scanty production of urine, and the appearances of the first buboes near the bite site. Fleas tend to bite more often near the groin area of adults, and more often near the neck region and armpits of children, leading to swollen, infected lymph nodes in these regions. Sharp, stabbing pains ensue, with the appearance of hot, purple buboes that remain tender and excruciatingly painful. Buboes usually reach up to 2 inches (5cm) in diameter, and may enlarge up to almost 4 inches (10 cm) in diameter (Smith and Reiser 1997). Buboes may rupture and drain spontaneously.

About 40–50 percent of individuals infected by fleas develop only a few localized, small buboes with few symptoms and full recovery. The remaining 50–60 percent of bubonic plague victims die from the disease (Benenson 1995). Once the infection spreads beyond the region of the bite site, the dangers of this disease increase. Failure of the lymph cells to contain the disease allows the bacteria to spread by way of the bloodstream, damaging and poisoning the blood, liver, spleen, and lungs, causing internal bleeding and death.

When *Yersinia pestis* invades the lungs and reaches tiny air sacs, the bacteria gain the opportunity to become airborne when the victim coughs. This allows the infection to be transmitted from one host to another, bypassing introduction through flea bites. Inhaled bacteria rapidly spread through the lymph channels of the lungs. Sudden chills and high fever develop within two to three days, along with difficult breathing and severe coughing. Other symptoms include severe headache, rapid pulse, flushed and bloated face, bloodshot eyes, and semiconsciousness or delirium. Coughing produces a watery, frothy sputum as well as bloody sputum, teeming with infective bacteria. The walls of the tiny air sacs in the lungs break down and hemorrhage, and the poisons released by infected cells spread to the heart, causing left-sided heart failure with fluid backing up into the lungs, ending in death. Victims of pneumonic plague do not survive without immediate modern medical treatment (Benenson 1981b; Smith and Reisner 1997).

Some individuals exposed to pneumonic plague do not develop plague-induced pneumonia, but instead develop localized throat or tonsilar infections with or without symptoms. Crushing infected fleas between the teeth can produce similar localized lesions. Sometimes these localized infections can progress to the regional lymph nodes in the neck, or the infection can spread throughout the body (Benenson 1981b; Smith and Reisner 1997).

Origin and Spread: The Great Rat Migrations

Yersinia pestis began as a natural infection of wild rodents in Central Asia, from the Ustyurt Plateau bordering the Caspian Sea on the west, to the

Mongolian Plateau to the east. From this broad area the infection spread along with wild rodent migrations to adjacent regions. The tarbagan, a large marmot-like rodent, susliks (ground squirrels), gerbils, and mice have been and remain the primary wild rodent carriers of the disease in the homeland of the plague. Burrowing hares can also become infected and transmit the disease (James and Harwood 1969). As long as infected wild rodents, hares, and human beings avoided each other, the plague did not become a threat to human populations. Plague infections have occurred sporadically among small nomadic groups, hunters, trappers, traders, and other travelers penetrating wild rodent country and coming into contact with infected fleas.

By the first century A.D. trade across Central Asia had increased dramatically with the demand for goods between the East and the West. Several expanding trade routes connecting cities throughout Central Asia, northern China, Southeast Asia, Western Asia, the Mediterranean region, and Europe traversed wild rodent country. The black rat following these trade routes out of South Asia picked up the plague bacteria from infected wild rodent fleas. The rats then distributed the disease to cities throughout Central and South Asia.

Infected black rats followed early shipping routes from ports in Western Asia to the Arabian Peninsula, up the Red Sea to Egypt, and into the Mediterranean. The plague began to appear in port cities wherever infected rats appeared. Rufus, a physician from Ephesus who died in A.D. 117, described symptoms of the plague based on observations by two physicians practicing in Alexandria, Egypt, during the early part of the first century A.D. (Cloudsley-Thompson 1976).

The first major plague pandemic reaching Europe began at Pelusium, near the Mediterranean port of Said in Egypt in A.D. 531. Pelusium was a major trading hub between the East and West, where overland caravans traded goods to be loaded onto Mediterranean ships. By A.D. 542 infected rats aboard Egyptian grain ships carried the disease to Constantinople (Hendrickson 1983). The great plague of Justinian, named for the emperor of the eastern Roman empire based in Constantinople, had begun. The physician Procopius described the symptoms of the plague that ravaged the city. The disease spread throughout the Mediterranean region and parts of Europe as far north as Denmark, appearing sporadically in and around major trading centers for two hundred years before subsiding (Gottfried 1983; Hull 1941). As the plague marched eastward along trade routes into Asia, the disease reached trading centers in China by A.D. 610 (McNeill 1976).

The second major plague pandemic moved out of Central Asia across the caravan routes, and accompanied advancing Mongol armies. Plague appeared at the caravan city of Aleppo, now Halab in northern Syria, during the fourteenth century. China experienced widely scattered plague epidemics in 1331, following intrusions by the Mongols. By 1347 the plague was everywhere within China. The Nestorian community near Issyk Kul, a lake not far from Ama Alta in southeastern Kazakhstan, near the Chinese border, suffered a plague epidemic in 1338. The plague traveled along trade routes to trading centers on the west side of the Caspian Sea, and as far as the trading center of Sarai on the lower Volga by 1345 (Gottfield 1983).

In 1346 plague broke out among Mongol soldiers attacking the port town of Caffa (the modern city of Feodosiya) on the southeast coast of the Crimea in the Black Sea region. Genoese traders had established a colony there around 1266. The Mongol khan Yanibeg had placed the town under siege in 1343. The plague epidemic drove the Mongols away from the siege, but not before infected rats following the Mongol army invaded both the town and ships anchored off shore. The Genoese sailed off with the rats aboard, taking the infection with them (Herlihy 1997; McNeill 1976).

The Genoese ships carried plague-infected rats to Constantinople, Cairo, and their home port at Genoa by 1347, and to Messina in Sicily by 1348. The disease quickly spread to all of the major cities of Italy, and by 1349 ships had carried rats and plague to England, eastern Ireland, and all the major port cities of Europe. By 1352 the rats and plague had reached Moscow (Herlihy 1997). The bubonic form prevailed during the summer months, while the more deadly pneumonic form dominated during the winter months as people crowded together in their homes, passing the infection around by way of the aerosol route (Burnet and White 1972).

The black rat thrived on human commerce. Expansion of trade routes throughout the Old World worsened the second plague pandemic. Demand from the West for Asian goods such as silk, porcelain, and spices increased dramatically during the Middle Ages. Various local Asian peoples controlled the overland trade routes connecting Asia with Mediterranean ports, while the Arabs primarily commanded the sea routes from Asia. Asian goods delivered to Mediterranean and Black Sea ports were traded for such items as furs, flax, copper, and iron from northern Europe, as well as wine and olives from southern Europe. Italian merchants dominated the Mediterranean and Black

Sea trade, and Italian ships transported more goods and rats to European and Mediterranean ports than any other ships. The intricate web of trade, rats, and plague caused the world's greatest pandemic through repeated introductions of the disease to various trading centers during commercial transactions. The second plague pandemic lasted for four hundred years, as the black rats took over the known Old World.

Plague was not the only disease being traded about. Other deadly diseases, such as smallpox, malaria, and measles, also expanded throughout the Old World with commercial enterprise. Plague alone cannot take the blame for the high death rates caused by the epidemics sweeping through Asia, Europe, and north Africa. Medieval physicians, overwhelmed with the new diseases, often could not differentiate among the various diseases and treat them appropriately. Ignorance killed more people than disease. The lack of knowledge about the causes of the new diseases allowed the infections to run rampant. Poor standards of personal hygiene and public health also promoted the spread of disease. Rats were viewed as nuisances but not as carriers of disease.

The number of deaths from diseases during the Middle Ages throughout the Old World soared. It is estimated that anywhere from one-third to one-half of the populations in Europe, parts of north Africa, and parts of Asia died during the second pandemic. Societies were affected by the loss of workers, specialists, and rulers, forcing political, economic, social, and cultural changes on shrinking populations as people died of disease or fled from local epidemics (Gottfried 1983; Herlihy 1997).

The end of the second plague pandemic coincided with great migrations of the brown rat, moving into territory occupied by the black rat during the eighteenth century. The brown rats displaced the black rats, and wherever the brown rat took over, plague subsided. *Yersinia pestis* had less of a chance of being transferred from fleas infesting brown rats to humans, since the brown rats avoided the kind of close association with humans that black rats favored (Burnet and White 1972).

Yersinia pestis moved from rats to local wild rodents in many parts of the Old World during the pandemic, leaving behind wild reservoirs of the infection after the plague pandemic itself subsided in the late 1700s. Thus, the stage was set for the third plague pandemic, which began in the late nineteenth century and lingered into the mid-twentieth century, killing an estimated 13 million people worldwide (Hendrickson 1983).

CONCLUDING COMMENTS

Plague is forever. It cannot possibly be eradicated from its many wild animal hosts in various parts of the world. Central Asia, particularly Kazakhstan and extending into Mongolia, remains the primary focus of the disease. Secondary foci of infection among wild rodents have been established in other parts of the world. The wild infection has spread to India, China, Myanmar (Burma), Vietnam, and Indonesia. Wild rodents in north-central Africa, eastern Africa, southern Africa, and Madagascar maintain the infection. Wild rodents in the New World picked up the infection from imported rats. *Yersinia pestis* resides in wild rodents in the western United States, in large areas of the Andes in Peru and Bolivia, and in northeastern Brazil. Sporadic human infection occurs with exposure to infected wild rodents, particularly among hunters, trappers, hikers, animal herders, and campers. Some wild rodents die from the disease, such as the American prairie dog, but fleas left behind in their burrows can infect other animals. Wild rabbits and wild carnivores can also be infected. Cats and dogs coming into contact with infected rodents or their fleas can deliver the infection to their owners. Pneumonic plague has been acquired from pet cats in the United States (Benenson 1995).

Plague epidemics rarely happen today, but outbreaks do occur with social disturbances and natural disasters. When public health measures to prevent the disease do not exist, and rodents acclimated to human houses have contact with infected wild rodents, plague epidemics can return. It only takes a small number of house mice or rats to become infected to give rise to an epidemic.

Reports of thousands of cases of plague during the war in Vietnam between 1962 and 1972 included outbreaks of pneumonic plague. The war and social turmoil allowed the disease to move into disrupted human groups from the wild. The last major pneumonic plague outbreak occurred in 1994 among slum dwellers in the western city of Surat on the Arabian Sea coast, 160 miles north of Bombay, India. The infection spread southward to the neighboring state of Maharashtra (Benenson 1995). More than 200,000 people fled in panic when authorities tried to seal off roads out of the area in attempts to isolate the infection. Public health authorities handed out antibiotics to prevent the disease from spreading, and they stopped trucks from the area to spray them with flea killer. Plague broke out in the eastern coastal city of Calcutta that same year, under similar circumstances (Smith and Reisner 1997).

Antibiotics have been used successfully to treat plague, and a vaccine provides temporary protection. As with some other bacterial infections treated with antibiotics, strains of *Yersinia pestis* have developed resistance to drug treatment. Rats have become more difficult to control since some have become resistant to the poisons used to exterminate them (Henrickson 1983).

India has a large number of poor people living in squalor within its megacities. Rats are revered by the Hindus, who allow them to roam freely, and they often get fed at temples revering the elephant-headed god Ganesha. According to tradition, this god was transported by rats (Hendrickson 1983). Large numbers of rats and rat fleas, and large numbers of people living together under poor, crowded conditions create a time bomb ticking away toward an epidemic of plague. Other megacities with urban shanty towns around the world also present a problem. War-ravaged countries where *Yersinia pestis* remains endemic among wild rodents also have the potential to become plague centers.

The disease could quickly spread to other parts of the world as rats hide in cargo containers aboard ships, or manage to board airplanes. A rat was found foraging in the first-class cabin of an American passenger airplane readying for takeoff to New York from Dallas in 1983 (Hendrickson 1983). An airplane leaving Malaysia's new airport in 1999 had to turn back when a rat was spotted in the first-class cabin. More than three thousand rats were caught at this same airport during the first six months after it opened. The new airport had intruded into an oil palm plantation that harbored rats (*International Herald Tribune*, 1 February 1999), so the rats adapted to the changes forced upon them. What if any of these stowaway rats had carried the plague?

CHAPTER 15

OF LICE AND MEN
Plus Ticks, Mites, and Chiggers

Lice and Men at War

The development of civilization made organized warfare possible. Powerful empires and city-states raised large armies and kept them on the move. The conditions of war often created difficulties in day-to-day living for men on the march. Adequate food supplies, clean water, decent living quarters, and good hygiene often proved difficult to obtain. Cities and towns under siege suffered along with the military, creating breeding grounds for many diseases. By the time that the Persians and Greek city-states went to war, epidemics began to rage along with battlefield conflicts. Similar events happened throughout Asia with war campaigns. Mysterious diseases waxed and waned with military campaigns, often becoming the deciding factor in wars. More men would die from disease than from actual battle wounds.

Plague and smallpox formed the vanguard of diseases that ravaged many military campaigns. We know the role rats played in the plague epidemics, by transmitting the disease to humans through their fleas (see chapter 14). Rats and their fleas also carried another disease harmful to humans, typhus.

Typhus is caused by one of the rickettsiae microbes that naturally infect small blood-sucking insects (see chapter 2). They naturally infected fleas and then rats, and both tolerate the infection without signs of disease. When the rickettsiae infect new types of hosts, disease can follow. Rat fleas, as we know, also bite human beings, thus transmitting the rickettsiae that cause human typhus. The disease cannot spread from one human to another on its own, but with the help of another insect that thrives on humans, typhus can spread quickly in filthy, crowded groups. The human louse can become the carrier of the disease as it feeds on infected humans.

The human louse, as discussed in chapter 3, has been with us throughout human existence, traveling with human beings throughout the world. This tiny ectoparasite started out primarily inhabiting hairs on the head and upper body. But as human groups moved into more temperate regions of the world, they needed to wear layers of clothing throughout the cold months. Lice living on the upper body adjusted to this change by shifting residence to the fibers of clothing when feeding on human blood. When people wore the same clothing for months at a time, the louse population exploded, and so did any agent of disease carried by the lice.

Men and lice at war, particularly during cold winter months, risked becoming victims of their own making. The tiny louse helped decide the outcome of many battles throughout Europe from the Middle Ages to World War I (Zinsser 1935).

Rickettsiae have a long and unique evolutionary history associated with blood-sucking fleas, mites, and ticks, since they evolved from bacteria infecting these insects. Most rickettsiae can be maintained in the natural insect host population independent of the natural animal host. They simply pass the infection from one generation to another through the ovaries of the infected female. Human infections have always been accidental, when humans come between the insect and its natural animal host.

Epidemics of human typhus infection evolved late in human history when the rats took over the world. The establishment of large rodent populations throughout Europe, the Middle East, north Africa, and most of Asia made it possible for the disease to enter human populations on a grand scale along with the plague. Black rats following trade routes coming from West Asia carried not only the plague pathogen, but also typhus infection to other parts of the world (Cloudsley-Thompson 1976).

Repeated exposure of human populations to infection by rat fleas led to a new source of microbe interaction through the human louse. Human victims of rat flea—transmitted typhus managed to infect their own body lice, and the exchange of infection between humans and infected human lice favored strains of rickettsiae responsible for epidemic typhus among humans. Crowding louse-infested people into poor housing or encampments that attracted rodents, particularly during cold winter months with inadequate nutrition and poor hygiene, created conditions ripe for the development of human typhus (T-W-Fiennes 1978b; Zinsser 1963).

Wild Flea-borne Typhus

Human typhus infection was an accident waiting to happen. For centuries human encounters with rodent fleas infected with rickettsiae had been sporadic. Infection occurred only when humans intruded into areas where the infection reigned among local rodents or other small mammals capable of carrying infected ectoparasites. People today can become infected whenever they come into contact with wild infections. This type of typhus has been called murine, endemic, or flea-borne typhus. Wild forms of this disease occur worldwide, predominantly in tropical and subtropical regions (Walker and Dumler 1997). Outbreaks occur when farmers burn fields or brush, flushing wild rodents out of their natural reserves and into contact with local people. Zinsser (1963) reported an outbreak among oil palm workers in one area of Malaysia years ago brought on by contact with the infected fleas of tree rats.

Domestic rodents that come into contact with wild rodents and their fleas can become infected and transmit the rickettsiae to their own fleas. The oriental rat flea, *Xenopsylla cheopis*, the primary insect vector responsible for transmitting the plague bacteria to humans, also transmits most of the wild typhus infections to humans wherever people and infected rodents live together (Snyder 1959). Unlike the plague, typhus infection does not kill rats. Seven other species of rodent fleas, along with rat lice and mites, can also serve as vectors for the infection. The house mouse provides the main reservoir for typhus in north Africa and China. Animals such as the skunk, bandicoot, dog, rabbit, opossum, and cat can also become infected (Azad 1988; Horsfall 1962). The cat flea in California has been known to acquire the infection from opossums and in turn infect cat owners (Benenson 1995).

The rickettsiae responsible for wild typhus, *Rickettsiae typhi* (formerly known as *Rickettsiae mooseri*), operate as natural parasites of insect ectoparasites that feed on wild rodents. Both insect and animal hosts have developed tolerance to the typhi, and do not suffer from the infection. Rat fleas consume typhi with a blood meal from an infected rodent, and in turn the infected rat flea delivers the rickettsiae to another host when it feeds. The female oriental rat flea, *Xenopsylla cheopis*, can also transmit the infection through her ovaries to offspring, maintaining the infection within this flea population (Azad 1988).

The microbes enter the epithelial cells lining the flea's midgut where they multiply and pass out of the flea's body during defecation while it feeds. The flea's bite produces irritation, and the host reacts with scratching that forces the deposited infected feces into the wound or abraded skin, helping the rickettsiae with their invasion. Humans infected by rat fleas develop typhus as the immune system reacts to the invading foreigner (Benenson 1995).

The rickettsiae microbes can survive and remain infective for months in rodent feces (Horsfall 1962). When the feces dry out, they can easily be carried with disturbed dust particles into the air. Thus, sporadic infection can occur with inhalation of contaminated dust particles. Sometimes the microbes may gain access to the human host through the eyes as they are rubbed with contaminated hands (Benenson 1995; Cloudsley-Thompson 1976; Walker and Dumler 1997). Most human infections with wild typhus occur where large domestic rat populations have picked up the microbes from wild rodents, particularly around port cities and coastal areas (Azad 1988).

Human rickettsial infections primarily function as diseases of small blood vessels. Once the microbes gain access to the bloodstream of the human host, they target endothelial cells lining small arteries and veins. Tiny blood vessels in the skin, lungs, brain, and gastrointestinal tract become the major attractions. The outer membrane of rickettsial microbes is coated with a slime layer that permits attachment to and entry into targeted cells (Walker and Dumler 1997) where *Rickettsiae typhi* replicate within the cytoplasm (Horsfall 1962). Infected epithelial cells swell with multiplying microbes, and the swelling blocks blood flow within the affected blood vessel. Eventually the infected cells rupture, and rickettsiae spill out to find other endothelial cells to infect, leaving the damaged cells to die. Dead cells add to the congestion within the blood vessel. The host immune-inflammatory cells take action to destroy the invaders and repair the damage, thus adding to the disease process while trying to overcome it.

Symptoms begin to appear after about twelve days of incubation within the host (Benenson 1995). The disease caused by flea-transmitted wild typhus generally appears in a mild form with high fever, headache, and skin rash. This lasts from nine to fifteen days and is followed by prompt recovery. The onset can be gradual or sudden, with loss of appetite, general muscle aches, runny nose, and cough. The rash covers mostly the chest, abdomen, arms, and legs. The eyes become bloodshot and lymph glands become tender. About 1–2 percent of infected individuals will develop severe illness and die from the disease (Snyder 1959).

Human (Louse-borne) Typhus

Strains of rickettsiae that have adapted to humans and their lice are known as *Prowazeki typhi*, often called epidemic typhus. Over time the prominent typhi strains in flea-transmitted infection slowly converted to Prowazeki strains transmitted by the human louse (Woodard 1988). The Prowazeki strains adapted more readily to the human louse and to people than the wild typhi strains when conditions favored maintaining the infection repeatedly within human populations. The Prowazeki strains can also be transferred back to rat fleas and rats (Azad 1988; Zinsser 1963).

Infected lice, including rat lice, react differently than infected fleas to the microbes. While the rickettsiae do not harm their natural insect host—the infected flea—infected lice generally die from the infection. The microbes damage their gut epithelial cells, killing the louse within eight to twelve days. Adult human lice normally live up to thirty days. Also, infected female lice, unlike female fleas, cannot pass the infection through the ovaries to their offspring (Horsfall 1962; James and Harwood 1969).

Most typhus epidemics occur in temperate areas where humans and their lice endure cold winters together under poor, crowded conditions. Epidemics once raged on board ancient ships, as well as among ravaging armies. Outbreaks also commonly occurred in jails and mental institutions (Zinsser 1963).

Human body lice will leave their host for a new host when people crowd together and share louse-infested clothing, when their host's body temperature rises to high levels, or if the host dies. Heavy lice infestation mixed with skin bacteria can produce intense discomfort in the human host when the lice bite, often leading to skin irritations followed by scratching. In time the chronically infested individual will become desensitized to the irritations produced by lice bites as the skin becomes hardened and deeply pigmented (James and Harwood 1969).

Infected lice transmit typhus rickettsiae in the same manner as the infected flea, through feces deposited while feeding, or when they get crushed and expel the microbes along with gut contents. The rickettsiae enter the human host the same way they do with flea bites, through the bite site or abraded skin. And like flea feces, dried louse feces can retain viable microbes for months, and ride dust particles through the air. Aerosol infection rarely happens, but dirty contaminated fingers can introduce the infection through the eyes (Horsfall 1962; James and Harwood 1969).

Most epidemics of louse-borne typhus have appeared in temperate regions, peaking in late winter and early spring. Human beings become the reservoir for the disease instead of rats, and the human louse becomes the vector instead of the rat flea.

Typhus epidemics are manmade. Maintenance of the disease within human populations depends on human behavior patterns. Social disorder feeds this disease that thrives on poverty, crowding, poor hygiene, and plenty of human lice. The only way to break the disease cycle is to get rid of the human lice by enforcing public health and personal hygiene measures.

Human typhus infection resembles the wild form of the disease but generally takes a more severe form. The fatality rate ranges from less than 10 percent to as high as 60 percent, depending on the type of Prowazeki strain and the condition of the affected population. Poor nutrition and poverty compromise host immune systems and increase the chances of dying from typhus. In general, children suffer less severe disease than adults (Snyder 1959).

During the ten- to fourteen-day incubation period of the infection, the rickettsiae spread throughout the bloodstream, damaging small blood vessels to the skin, brain, gastrointestinal tract, lungs, heart, and liver (Walker and Dumler 1997). Sudden fever, chills, severe headache with muscle aches, particularly in the back and legs, and bloodshot eyes mark the onset of the disease. The body temperature may reach 105°F and remain there throughout the course of the disease, generally lasting about two weeks. The frontal headache is intense, not letting up night or day. Vomiting, constipation, loss of appetite, insomnia, and dry tongue frequently occur. When the lungs are affected there may be a slight cough and patchy pneumonia (Benenson 1995; Murray 1975; Snyder 1959).

The hallmark of the disease is the appearance of a raised red rash that comes up between the fourth and sixth day after symptoms appear. The rash begins on the trunk, covering the whole body except for the face, palms of the hands, and soles of the feet. When the rash first appears, the lesions fade with pressure, varying from pink to bright red in color, and measuring 2–4 mm (less than one-quarter inch) in diameter. The skin lesions darken as the illness pro-gresses, no longer fading under pressure, and they last until the fever breaks. The rash may be less prominent and disappear in two or three days, or it may not be present at all in mild cases, especially in children. Bleeding under the skin at the site of the rash lesions appears in severe cases. The face often becomes dusky or flushed, and sometimes appears swollen (Benenson 1995; Murray 1975; Snyder 1959).

Lesions affecting blood vessels to the brain can lead to stupor, delirium, hallucinations, light sensitivity, and excitability. Deafness and ringing in the ears are common complaints. Renal deficiency with decreased urination com-monly occurs. Severe cases may suffer gangrene of the toes, fingertips, ear lobes, nose, and genitals when infected blood vessels to these areas become blocked by the disease. Severe renal failure and vascular collapse usually lead to death between the ninth and eighteenth day. Otherwise recovery begins when the temperature drops, and full recovery may take two to three months. The rash does not leave any scars (Benenson 1995; Murray 1975; Snyder 1959).

Brill-Zinsser Disease

Nathan Brill described cases of typhus-like illness among Jewish immigrants from Poland and Russia to New York City in 1898. For the next thirty years, other physicians in major eastern cities reported similar sporadic cases. They were puzzled by the disease because it had no association with human lice or flea bites. Hans Zinsser followed over five hundred cases in New York and Boston in 1934, and he discovered the disease to be reactivated typhus. The victims, mostly immigrants from Eastern Europe, had previously suffered the disease many years before as children in their native countries (Murray 1975). Typhus epidemics had raged in Eastern Europe in the late nineteenth and early twentieth centuries, especially during World War I and the Russian revolution (Zinsser 1963).

The Prowazeki strains of rickettsiae have successfully adapted to humans. The microbe's ability to survive undetected by the host immune system long after symptoms of the disease disappear proves this success.

Individuals recovering from lice-borne typhus can become silent carri-ers for years. The disease can be reactivated when the carrier comes under stress with a weakened immune system, allowing the infection to take over again. Reactivated disease is generally mild, lasting seven to eleven days with fever, headache, and rash. Sometimes no rash appears, and the temperature curve can be uneven. Very few people die from reactivated typhus. The most serious problem with reactivated disease arises in the potential for spreading the infection among "lousy" populations. Individuals with reactivated typhus can be contagious to human lice, and when the lice become infected they can spread the disease to other people (Murray 1975; Snyder 1959).

History of Typhus

The early history of typhus proves difficult to trace among the many ancient epidemics caused by various diseases. Most likely the wild form of the disease existed long before the epidemic form became known. Outbreaks of wild typhus along with plague probably occurred in ancient port cities and trading centers inhabited by flea-infested rats. Human commerce promoted typhus along with plague, as rats transported both diseases around the world.

The history of human typhus in Asia remains unclear, but rats from Asia apparently carried wild typhus along with plague to the Mediterranean basin. From here the disease spread throughout Europe, where typhus eventually became recognized as a separate disease during the Middle Ages.

The first major plague pandemic lasted for two hundred years, reaching Europe by the sixth century. Wild typhus outbreaks most likely accompanied the plague pandemic. Similar outbreaks may have occurred as plague traveled eastward into China at the same time.

Zinsser (1963) described an early report of disease symptoms with a spotted fever suggesting a wild typhus outbreak at the monastery of La Cava near Salerno, Spain, in 1083. From 1095 to 1270 the crusaders suffered from various diseases on their quests for Jerusalem, including wild typhus. More crusaders died from diseases than from battle (Walker 1988).

The second major plague pandemic, which began in the fourteenth century and lasted for four hundred years (see chapter 14), succeeded largely because human living conditions during this time period in Europe were often abysmal. These conditions allowed wild typhus to evolve into human typhus, as the infection jumped from rat fleas to human lice. Cramped housing for the poor attracted rats, people rarely bathed or changed clothes, and much of the European population were "lousy" people (Cloudsley-Thompson 1976). Similar conditions in Asia may also have prompted the evolution of other strains of human typhus there (Zinsser 1963).

Records of longstanding typhus epidemics in the Balkans suggest that the disease was established there very early, probably carried by Turkish armies from Anatolia. The Hungarian army under King Hunyadi claimed victory at the siege of Belgrade against the army of Mohammed II in 1456. The Turkish army had been suffering from a pestilence that soon afflicted the Hungarian army, even killing King Hunyadi himself. In 1542, Joachim, Marburg of Brandenberg, took an army of mostly Germans and Italians to Hungary to push back the Turks, only to have his army struck down by a deadly disease that killed thirty thousand soldiers. Emperor Maximilian II sent a large army into Hungary in 1566 to push back Suleiman's Turkish army; his own army was soon decimated by diseases, forcing him to make an unfavorable peace with the Turks. For over a hundred years survivors from the battlefields of Hungary carried disease back to their home populations. Perhaps it is not just coincidence that human typhus epidemics have flourished in Hungary, the Balkans, Poland, and Russia up into the twentieth century (Zinsser 1963).

The Spaniards recorded an epidemic of human typhus at Granada in 1489–90. The severe spotted fever killed a large portion of the Spanish army of Ferdinand and Isabella during battle with the Moors. Spanish physicians called the disease *tabardillo*. Seventeen thousand Spanish soldiers died from the disease, compared to only three thousand killed in battle. The Spaniards believed the disease had been brought from Cyprus by mercenary soldiers. Most likely the disease had traveled to Cyprus with Turkish soldiers from Anatolia. Typhus spread throughout the Iberian Peninsula, spilling over into France and Italy during the sixteenth century. The Spaniards carried the disease to New Spain, and a deadly epidemic referred to as *tabardete* struck Mexico City in 1576. Similar epidemics had occurred in Tlascala and Cholula in 1545 (Walker 1988; Zinsser 1963).

Typhus continued to spread during the sixteenth and seventeenth centuries throughout Europe. Wars promoted typhus to the status of a major cause of sickness and death among fighting soldiers and fleeing peasants. Typhus had become a disease of war and revolution, and Europe fostered many wars and revolutions over the centuries. Typhus ravaged prisoners of war, sailors crowded on board ships, and soldiers crowded into cramped quarters. And surviving troops took the disease home with them.

Medieval Europeans tolerated human lice. Both rich and poor accepted lice as a normal part of life. One story shows well how ignorance of the disease contributed to its spread. Jails served as hotbeds for typhus, which was often referred to as "jail fever"; the jails literally crawled with lice. When the opportunity arose, infected lice freed themselves from prison. One such occasion happened in England when a prisoner named Rowland Jencks appeared in chains from his jail cell before a crowded court at Oxford in 1577. He was accused of speaking evil of the government, profaning God's word, abusing ministers, and staying away from church. His lice took advantage of the crowded courtroom, and soon after the trial, more than five hundred individuals who had attended the hearing, including all the judges from Oxford's faculty, died from the disease. Mr. Jencks survived, minus his ears that had been cut off as punishment for his evil deeds (T-W-Fiennes 1978b).

By the beginning of the eighteenth century, typhus had become well established throughout Europe. The most severe epidemics occurred during the French Revolution and Napoleon's campaigns. Napoleon's army suffered more from disease, particularly typhus, than from battle in his march to conquer Russia. Typhus raged among the armies engaged in the Crimean War in 1854–56. Reports of typhus epidemics came from north Africa, Persia, China, and North and South America during the nineteenth century (Cloudsley-Thompson 1976; Zinsser 1963).

By the mid-nineteenth century typhus epidemics began to fade as lice populations shrank wherever improved standards of living and better hygiene took over. The cause of the disease remained unknown until 1909 when Charles Nicolle discovered that the human louse transmitted the disease. When World War I broke out in 1914, typhus epidemics began their sweep through the Balkans and along the eastern front. The Serbian army suffered 150,000 deaths from typhus by 1915. Thirty thousand Austrian prisoners of war died from the disease in Serbian prison camps, along with 126 doctors. Typhus on the western front was kept to a minimum by controlling human lice infestations. Civil war and famine in Russia from 1917 to 1925 created the right conditions for yet another typhus epidemic that claimed the lives of 3 million people (Cloudsley-Thompson 1976; T-W-Fiennes 1978b; Walker 1988).

In 1916 da Rocha Lima finally discovered the causative agent of human typhus. But not until 1931 was the wild typhi form separated from the human form along with its natural hosts (Murray 1975).

DDT helped keep typhus to a minimum during World War II. Most outbreaks stayed confined to small segments of the German army on the eastern front at the beginning of the war, and in parts of north Africa. The worst outbreaks of typhus took place in the German concentration camps.

Outbreaks also occurred in Japan and Korea in 1945–46 (Cloudsley-Thompson 1976). Since then, outbreaks of human typhus have been isolated in those areas around the world wherever social unrest and "lousy" populations collide.

Trench Fever

Human lice also carry another rickettsial infection referred to as trench fever, so named because it was first identified among soldiers fighting in the trench war of World War I. The disease had become endemic in Poland. Allied and German troops reported about 1 million cases in Western Europe. The infection was also recognized among soldiers fighting in World War II, with eighty thousand cases reported. This disease is caused by a different genus of rickettsiae, *Bartonella quintana*. Human beings appear to be the only vertebrate hosts, and both lice and humans serve as carriers. The infection probably exists wherever human lice prevail, and silent infections go unreported. Other endemic areas have been reported in parts of Russia, Mexico, South America, and Africa (Benenson 1995; Cloudsley-Thompson 1976; Horsfall 1962; Ley 1975; Weiss 1988). These data suggest that this rickettsial infection has been with humans far longer than typhus, and that humans reached a mutual tolerance level with the microbes. Disease symptoms probably do not appear until the host immune system becomes compromised by malnutrition and the stresses of war.

The quintana rickettsiae responsible for the infection do not enter host endothelial cells as their typhus cousins do. These microbes remain outside the host cells in the louse intestine and are excreted with feces on the skin of the human host, where they can be rubbed into the bite site or abraded skin. Quintana rickettsiae, like all the other rickettsial infections, infect tiny blood vessels in the human host. Although the microbes remain outside the endothelial cells lining the blood vessels, they can cause inflammation of the blood vessels when the host immune system responds to them (Ley 1975).

When the infection does cause disease, symptoms appear in about two to four weeks after introduction into the host. The disease generally remains mild and not fatal. Symptoms include recurring fever, headache, light sensitivity, severe weakness, and back and shin pains. About 70 percent of cases experience a transient rash. The first attack lasts about twenty-four to forty-eight hours, often followed by recurring bouts every five days before finally abating. The infection has also been called "five-day" or "quintana fever," "shin bone fever," and "Volhynian fever" (Benenson 1995; James and Harwood 1969; Ley 1975).

Ticks, Mites, Chiggers, and Spotted Fevers

Various rickettsiae naturally infect ticks, mites, and chiggers. Transfer of these microbes to human beings produces a group of diseases referred to as spotted fevers. They are characterized by a rash and fever, similar to typhus infection. All of these spotted fevers produce accidental infections in humans, and most of them occur in areas disturbed by human activity where secondary growth of vegetation has been allowed to take over. Thus, humans actually promote tick environments when they rearrange environmental areas, abandon them, and then reclaim them (Sonenshine 1993).

Tick-borne Rickettsioses

Most ticks operate as opportunistic blood-suckers, not loyal to any one animal host. Some species can live for several years, even up to sixteen years or more. Ticks undergo four stages of development, from egg to larva to nymph and finally to adult, completing the cycle in six weeks to three years. Most ticks utilize different animal hosts during various stages of their development, usually starting with very small animals and ending up with much larger ones. The many tick species vary considerably in size, but they rarely exceed 20 mm (less than three-fourths inch) in length when fully engorged with the victim's blood. Most tick bites go unnoticed, and the tick may not be discovered until long after it has engorged itself on the host's blood. Tick saliva contains an anticoagulant to prevent the host's blood from clotting, thus forming a pool of blood from which the tick feeds rapidly (James and Harwood 1969).

Most female ticks drop off the host once they have gorged themselves, in order to deposit their eggs on the ground. The eggs are coated with a waxy secretion that protects them from the environment. They need moisture to survive and hatch after eighty days, and the young larvae generally climb up grasses or other low vegetation to grab hold of passing or grazing animals. Most ticks drop off their animal hosts to molt, finding a new host during the next stage of life (James and Harwood 1969). Dogs commonly transport infected ticks from wild animals to their human owners.

One group of rickettsiae infecting ticks have little or no effect on their wild animal hosts but do threaten humans. These rickettsiae, like those that

parasitize fleas, maintain the infection within their own population by transmitting the microbes through the ovaries to their young. Sporadic, accidental tick-borne rickettsial infections occur worldwide, and produce similar
spotted fevers. Rickettsii strains produce Rocky Mountain spotted fever
throughout the Americas. Closely related sibirica strains cause north Asian
tick typhus in Russia, Central Asia, Mongolia, and northern China. Japonica
strains cause oriental spotted fever in Japan. Conorii strains serve as agents
for what is commonly known as "boutonneuse fever" in the Mediterranean
basin, Africa, and Western Asia. Australis strains produce Queensland tick
typhus in eastern Australia. All these diseases have local names wherever
they occur (Sonenshine 1993; Walker and Dumler 1997).

Tick-carried rickettsiae, similar to flea-transmitted rickettsiae, thrive
within the cytoplasm of the host endothelial cells that line tiny blood vessels. Some also infect muscle cells of the blood vessel walls and the heart.
Unlike typhus-causing rickettsiae, this group of rickettsiae generally does
not kill the infected host cell with rapidly developing offspring. Tick-carried
rickettsiae produce fewer offspring, and they generally leave the cell without killing it. However, as their numbers increase within infected host cells,
they often become trapped in the connecting network of tiny canals that
course through the cell (Sonenshine 1993).

Tick-borne rickettsial infections vary in severity according to the
microbe species and strain, and to the responding host immune system.
Some strains are quite deadly, such as the rickettsii strain found in the
Bitterroot Valley of Montana, where fatality rates reach 90 percent or more,
while most rickettsii strains reach fatality rates of around 20 percent. Some
rickettsii carried by ticks do not infect humans at all (McDade and
Newhouse 1986; Sonenshine 1993).

The best known rickettsii infection is Rocky Mountain spotted fever,
so called because the disease was first noted in the Rocky Mountains of the
western United States. Actually more cases occur today in the eastern and
southeastern regions of the United States than in the West, and it has been
found all over the Americas. Rocky Mountain spotted fever has become the
most severe rickettsial infection in this group of tick-borne pathogens
(McDade and Newhouse 1986).

Major symptoms of Rocky Mountain spotted fever resemble typhus,
with sudden onset of high fever, severe frontal headache, muscle and joint
pains, and rash in most cases. Incubation time is shorter, three to twelve

days, and there may be abdominal pain, vomiting, sometimes diarrhea, cough, ringing in the ears, light sensitivity, and dizziness. The smooth muscles of the blood vessels and heart are injured, and internal bleeding occurs into adjacent organs. The rash usually appears between the second and sixth day, beginning on hands, forearms, feet, and ankles, spreading to the trunk, neck, and face. The rash lesions in severe cases coalesce to form large areas of bleeding under the skin. Gangrene can develop when blood vessels become blocked. Delirium, coma, vascular collapse, and death can happen with this disease. Otherwise, recovery can be slow, leaving some individuals deaf, vision-impaired, or suffering from neurological disorders such as partial paralysis or defective muscle coordination (Sonenshine 1993).

The conorii rickettsial infections, commonly known as "boutonneuse fever," "Mediterranean fever," "Kenya tick typhus," "South African tick bite fever," and "Indian tick fever," among other local names, are closely related to rickettsii, but they usually produce milder disease. The conorii, unlike the rickettsii, do not attack the smooth muscles lining blood vessels, so the patient's vital organs do not suffer from internal bleeding. Almost all cases have a distinctive small ulcer with a brown or black center at the tick bite site. Symptoms resemble rickettsii infections, but the rash rarely appears on the abdomen. Almost all infected individuals recover from the conorii infections. However, an unusually virulent strain attacked a newly established Jewish settlement in the Negev Desert in Israel, causing several deaths, during the late twentieth century (Sonenshine 1993).

Sibirica rickettsial infections range widely throughout Siberia and Central Asia, commonly known as "North Asian tick typhus," while Japonica strains occur in Japan. Symptoms include sudden onset with fever, chills, and muscle and joint aches. The fever gradually increases before becoming intermittent. The rash begins during the first week on the hands and feet, gradually spreading over the trunk. Some individuals may develop a small ulcer with brown crust at the tick bite site. The disease remains generally mild and is followed by rapid recovery. It rarely causes death (Sonenshine 1993).

Australis rickettsiae infection, known as "Queensland tick typhus," the Australian version of tick-borne rickettsial infection, resembles sibirica and conorii rickettsial infections. The disease stays relatively mild. The rash can be more variable, from raised red to large pink lesions (Sonenshine 1993).

Another tick-transmitted rickettsial infection called "Q-fever" or "Balkan grippe," can be found worldwide. This disease first became recognized among workers in a meatpacking plant in Brisbane, Australia, in 1935 (Weiss 1988). The rickettsiae responsible for this infection belong to another genus, and the microbes have been labeled *Coxiella burnetii*. These microbes reproduce within the infected cell's lysosome, a minute structure within the cytoplasm that breaks down large molecules to be used as fuel for the cell. Potent enzymes within the lysosome normally kill microbes that invade this structure, but burnetii rickettsiae manage to survive the deadly lysosome enzymes. They are very hardy outside the host, able to survive dry conditions, unlike the other rickettsiae, and they can survive for years in soil, dust, dried tick feces, dried or frozen infected animal tissues, and even in water. The infection becomes airborne with dust particles, and is inhaled by the exposed host (Horsfall 1962; Sonenshine 1993).

Symptoms of Q-fever develop after about twenty days of incubation with sudden fever, chills, sweats, sore throat, diarrhea, light sensitivity, severe frontal headache, and muscle aches. The fever lasts from six to fourteen days with wide fluctuations. Pneumonia, fatigue, and enlarged liver frequently appear. Unlike the other rickettsial infections, there is generally no rash, but sometimes a rash can appear on the trunk and shoulders. This disease can persist for months or years, affecting tissues of the heart. Few people die from the disease, less than 1 percent of those infected (Sonenshine 1993).

Unlike the other tick-borne rickettsial infections, Q-fever can become epidemic, particularly among people who work with animals or animal products. Domestic animals acquire the infection from ticks that infest wild animals and migratory birds, but they rarely display symptoms. Most humans acquire infection by breathing in contaminated dust particles where infected animals are kept. The disease can also be acquired by handling infected placental tissues, body fluids, animal feces, or contaminated straw or wool. The wind can carry contaminated dust particles for half a mile or more from the source of the infection (Benenson 1995; Sonenshine 1993). An outbreak of Q-fever in northern Kazakhstan in 1954 followed the reclamation of steppe land for domestic use, exposing workers to infected ticks from the local wild rodent population (Horsfall 1962).

Mite- and Chigger-borne Rickettsioses

Almost all mites are so tiny that they can barely be seen by the unaided eye. Some mites act as ectoparasites to animals, birds, and humans, producing a variety of skin irritations, including mange and scabies. They tend to feed on host tissue debris other than blood. The life cycle of these tiny insects varies from eight days to less than four weeks, and passes through five developmental stages (James and Harwood 1969). Like fleas and ticks, mites can be infected with rickettsia and maintain the infection within their ranks by passing it through their ovaries to their offspring. Natural animal hosts of these tiny ectoparasites do not suffer ill effects from the infection.

The tiny house mouse mite will attack humans and transmit *Akari rickettsiae*, causing rickettsialpox disease (James and Harwood 1969). This disease generally stays mild and resembles chickenpox. The disease appears about one week after the initial mite bite, a pimple-like lesion with a dark center. Symptoms last about one week, with fever, chills, sweats, headache, light sensitivity, muscle aches, backache, and a rash. The rash develops into blister-like lesions with red borders, drying and forming dark crusts that fall off without leaving scars (Benenson 1995; T-W-Fiennes 1978b). The disease was first described in New York tenement housing in 1946, and since then it has been identified in other cities in the United States and in the Ukraine. The disease probably goes undetected in many parts of the world (Walker and Dumler 1997; Weiss 1988).

Asian redbug mites live as free insects, feeding upon insect eggs and vegetation, except during the larval stage. About twelve days after the eggs of these mites hatch on the ground, the tiny larvae must find an animal host in order to complete their life cycle. The larva attaches to the host's skin and injects a secretion from the salivary glands to dissolve the surrounding tissue, creating intense irritation to the area. The liquified tissue debris feeds the developing mite larva, allowing it to develop into an adult mite. The irritating larva is commonly known as a chigger, and during its stay on the animal host the rickettsial infection it carries is transmitted to the host. Human beings who intervene between the chigger infected with *Tsutsugamushi rickettsia* and natural field mouse and rat hosts develop a disease commonly known as "scrub typhus." In some areas ground birds play the natural host role (Ley 1975; Zinsser 1963).

Several scattered strains of the chigger-borne tsutsugamushi rickettsial infection inhabit many parts of Southeast Asia, covering a rough triangle from Pakistan to northern Japan and down through the New Hebrides Islands to the north coast of Australia. Outbreaks occur wherever human beings invade the natural habitat of the mites and their natural rodent hosts. Infested areas often remain quite small, sometimes only covering a few square feet. Such areas have been referred to as "typhus islands." Scrub overgrowth forms a common habitat, particularly near the edge of forests and rivers (Horsfall 1962; Ley 1975).

The disease was first recognized in Japan in 1893, and the causative microbe was identified in 1918 (Weiss 1988). Epidemics of the disease do occur, particularly among military personnel and among workers reclaiming scrub areas infested with mites and rodents (Benenson 1995; Ley 1975). The disease goes by many local names, including "ezo fever," "Japanese river fever," "tropical typhus," "rural typhus," and "tsutsugamushi disease." Four major syndromes of the disease most likely relate to different variants of the tsutsugamushi rickettsiae, with mortality rates varying from 5 percent to 40 percent, depending on the variant (Horsfall 1962).

Like other rickettsial infections, tsutsugamushi microbes infect the endothelial cells lining small blood vessels, leading to inflammation of these blood vessels, particularly in the skin, and often involving small blood vessels of the lungs and heart. The disease begins with a punched-out ulcer with blackened scab over the infected chigger bite, followed by symptoms within one to three weeks. Headache, fever, chills, backache, swollen lymph glands, reddened eyes, and enlarged spleen are the early symptoms, followed within a week by a rash that spreads over the trunk, arms, and legs. The rash may last only a few hours or a week. Inflamed lungs, delirium, stupor, deafness, muscle spasms, other symptoms of encephalitis, and heart failure usually occur during the second week of illness, followed by either death or recovery (Ley 1975).

CONCLUDING COMMENTS

Typhus became a major human disease from the sixth century into the early twentieth century. Human behavior and human lice created epidemic human typhus at a time in our history when people accommodated and tolerated lice infestations. The disease went from a sporadic accidental infection derived from rat fleas to human infection transmitted by human lice.

Typhus thrived on war and followed "lousy" armies throughout the Old World, often killing more fighting men than did battle wounds. Typhus first journeyed throughout the world along with plague, rats, and fleas through the avenues of human commerce. War and poverty mixed with "lousy" populations provided opportunities for typhus to jump from rat fleas to human lice and become a major human disease capable of disrupting battles and political outcomes.

Epidemics of human typhus rarely appear among modern nations today, but this does not lessen the importance of this disease. Human typhus still exists wherever infected human lice or rat fleas interact with people. The disease exists in regions of Mexico, Central America, South America, central and east Africa, and numerous regions throughout Asia. Outbreaks can occur whenever social systems and human hygiene collapse, particularly during war and revolution. Megacities with overwhelming numbers of people living in poverty can also be affected. Silent human carriers of typhus can introduce typhus to "lousy" populations when the individual's disease reactivates. Wild typhus reservoirs can never be eradicated, keeping the door open for future outbreaks of typhus (Benenson 1995: Horsfall 1962; Walker 1988).

Tick- and mite-borne rickettsial infections have never posed a global threat to human populations, because outbreaks occur only in isolated areas. Although these rickettsial infections have become accidental diseases of humans, they can cause havoc in expanding urban and rural populations who intrude into previously wild infested areas.

Most of the rickettsial infections have been caused by human disturbance of local natural environments. Displacement of natural flora and fauna, followed by abandonment of the land to secondary growth, provide ideal habitats for wild rodents, ticks, and mites, the primary natural reservoirs of these rickettsiae.

CHAPTER 16

MARCHING TO A NEW WORLD ORDER

European Expansion and the Industrial Revolution

With the dawn of civilization, human history began to change at an ever increasing rate as the forces of greed and power dominated the development of human societies. Throughout the world, the quest for more material wealth and control over others prevailed as the leading forces in human evolution. Trade routes became the life lines of empires.

Expansion of the Roman empire from the first century B.C. to the sixth century A.D. throughout the Mediterranean, Anatolia, north Africa, and Western Europe set the stage for large-scale epidemics. Increased trade links to all parts of Asia brought new diseases to trading centers throughout the empire. Epidemics of new infections, such as bubonic plague and smallpox, waxed and waned in and around major ports and cities. However, the imported diseases could not establish permanent residency as endemic sources of infection in the new environments. Social and cultural conditions had to change before the new diseases could remain full time.

Medieval Prologue

The medieval centuries witnessed large-scale turmoil and chaos throughout the world. The march of civilization had reached a peak of intense rivalry among various peoples.

The Mongol invasions erupting from Central Asia marked the thirteenth century. The Mongols pushed westward into Eastern Europe, eastward into China and Korea, and southwestward into Western Asia, disrupting many different societies and fostering the spread of disease, particularly bubonic plague.

While most of medieval Europe remained stifled in its own inertia, China's civilization managed to survive the Mongol invasions and centuries of turmoil and outbreaks of diseases, to become the Old World's greatest civilization. When the Mongols disrupted their overland trade routes, the Chinese turned to the sea, expanding trade routes to Southeast Asia, India, and the Persian Gulf. Southeast Asia became a major crossroads for trade as various local kingdoms jockeyed for power. Medieval India also suffered Mongol invasions, and endured power struggles among three major kingdoms.

Turkish peoples from Central Asia, having adopted the Muslim faith, moved steadily into Western Asia, setting up a series of local kingdoms. The Muslim Turkish intrusion into the Middle East sparked the Christian Crusades. By the fifteenth century, Muslim Turks controlled Anatolia and parts of the Levant, while local kingdoms dominated Africa, many of them thriving on wealthy trade routes with the Muslims to the north and to the east.

Countless conflicts for domination swept medieval Europe, accompanied by plagues, pestilence, famine, and social corruption following the Mongol invasions. Europe became a major crossroads of repeated epidemic diseases fed by trade routes from the east and from north Africa.

By the fourteenth century, epidemic diseases that had once haunted the Roman empire put down roots and became endemic to most of Europe. These included plague, typhus, smallpox, malaria, syphilis, leprosy, measles, diphtheria, influenza, and tuberculosis. Descriptions of "plague" and pestilence by medieval historians and physicians often referred to any one or a combination of these diseases, not just bubonic plague.

Western Europe sank into an abyss of turmoil as the introduced diseases became entrenched as local diseases, with great losses in population amid social unrest. Years of war between England and France, and frequent famines added to the miseries of the afflicted populations and promoted the spread of disease.

Meanwhile, more stable and less populated Eastern Europe garnered wealth and power during the fourteenth century. Many German and Flemish peasants fled to Eastern Europe to escape the ravages of war, famine, and disease and to work the lands of Slavic princes. Other German migrants pushed into the Baltic, where they gained control of the north-to-south trade, united under the Hanseatic League. To the south, Italian states continued to maintain tight control over their trade routes from east to west, while Spain got caught up in its own dynastic wars.

Rampaging diseases, bouts of famine, and wars became signs of the times throughout the Old World, from Western Europe to East Asia. Disheveled populations forced political and economic changes in many parts of Europe and Asia as large numbers of people died and large numbers of survivors migrated to other areas.

By the sixteenth century major power shifts were taking place around the world. The Muslim Ottoman Turks built their vast empire based in Anatolia (modern Turkey). The Safavid Muslims dominated Persia (modern Iran), Muslim Mughals ruled northern India, and Muslim Berbers controlled trade routes in north Africa, while large and powerful city-states continued to flourish throughout Africa. Russia expanded its boundaries to the east and west following a long disruption by the Mongol invasions that had split it apart.

Following the stabilizing rule of the Ming dynasty established in 1368, China's population increased dramatically to become the largest populated empire in the world. Political stability allowed the population to recover as infant survival rates increased, despite downswings from major epidemics in several population centers.

By inventing firearms (using gunpowder previously developed by the Chinese) during the early part of the sixteenth century, the French changed how wars were fought, setting the stage for modern warfare. From that beginning, men continued to develop even greater weapons of destruction for killing each other.

By the sixteenth century populations exhausted by cyclic epidemics began to recover as the epidemics eased with socioeconomic stability and the lessening of famines. The population in Europe recovered to the levels attained at the beginning of the Middle Ages as a result of social and economic stability. Growth continued at a rapid pace despite the continuing threat of epidemics.

The Great Paradigm Shift

The greatest paradigm shift in human history began with the European Renaissance. Fourteenth-century Italy gave rise to this transition from medieval to modern Europe with the revival of intellectual thought, invention, and creativity based on the recovery of classical works lost during Europe's Dark Ages. Europeans gradually freed themselves from harsh socioreligious controls to rediscover the greatness of the past preserved by the eastern empires. The Protestant Reformation and revolt against the oppression of the Catholic Church paved the way to intellectual freedom. European societies also gained greater literary freedoms with the invention of the first European printing press in the mid-fifteenth century. By the late sixteenth century, Western Europe was well on its way to a cultural revolution that would affect the entire world.

The old manor system of lord and serfs unraveled in many parts of Western Europe and Britain (Gottfried 1983). Disease, war, and famine had wiped out major portions of the work force as well as many of the elite. Surviving workers abandoned their lands to better themselves elsewhere. Many of the rural people migrated into towns and demanded wages for their work. Revolts against established authorities provoked political changes, and with political changes came economic change.

Shortages of farm labor spawned newer and better farming methods, and shortages of tradesmen and laborers brought innovations in technology. With increased wealth and wage earnings, the demand for luxury goods increased, fueling the growing market economies. Trade increased, and European economic power shifted from Eastern Europe and the Italian coast to the west. The Ottomans continued to maintain control of the Middle East, while East Asia insulated itself from the rest of the world.

European expansion began with Spanish and Portuguese explorations for new sea trade routes to Asia. Spanish discovery of the New World by the end of the sixteenth century brought drastic changes in the global balance of power, with intense rivalries among European nations.

The process of globalization of people, plants, and animals had been set in motion. The New World received domestic animals, plants, and people from the Old World, while many New World plants reached the Old World. Old World socioreligious institutions swept the globe along with colonization and global trade.

Diseases that had once ravaged Europe, Asia, and north Africa were quickly introduced to the populations of the Americas, Pacific Islands, Australia, New Zealand, and South Africa, with similar disastrous results (McNeill 1980). These diseases quickly decimated Native American and

South Pacific populations just as they had decimated European populations when first introduced from Asia. Old World diseases reduced most Native American tribes to mere remnants of their former populations, and some tribal entities did not survive the onslaught. However, America's native populations did not decrease from diseases alone. Wars, famine, and population dislocation aided and abetted the new epidemics.

Trade based on agriculture, ironworking, cattle, gold, and slavery fueled powerful African city-states. The slave trade extended to both Arab and African traders across the Sahara. The capture and selling of people were big business for many west African kingdoms long before the first Europeans, the Portuguese, arrived along the coast.

The demand for cheap labor by Europeans lead to a boom in the African slave business. Finding the interior of west Africa controlled by ruling chieftains, the Europeans were confined to enclaves along the coast. Local African slave traders would bring their human merchandise for sale to the newcomers, just as they traded slaves with Arabs to the north. Iberia became the first European stop for African slave shipments, but the slave trade rapidly shifted to the New World. The demand for new sources of labor had grown in the colonies as the numbers of captive native peoples used for slave labor dramatically dropped off with the introduction of Old World diseases. In the course of four hundred years, over 10 million African slaves from all over west Africa, and as far south as Angola, with some from east Africa and Madagascar, moved through the trade routes.

African slaves brought their diseases, particularly malaria, with them to other parts of the world. British convicts sent to Australia paved the way for Old World diseases to wipe out many of the aboriginal populations. Migrants and indentured servants helped spread diseases far and wide throughout the world. The process of germ globalization had begun.

The Great Leap Forward

The industrial revolution that took place in Great Britain fueled European expansion. Shortages of energy sources sparked this change, as Britain ran out of wood and turned to coal during the sixteenth century. Wind- and water-powered mills provided only about one-fourth of the energy needed for developing industry. Britain had abundant stores of coal, as well as iron, tin, and copper. The Britons also developed more efficient farming methods, and utilized their massive river system and harbors for the transport of food stuffs, raw materials, and goods throughout the land. Progress could take place because of social changes that evolved from the labor shortages during the Middle Ages, and the Renaissance that opened people's minds to scientific thought and innovation. Social changes led to changes in governance, allowing science and commerce to take root and grow.

Coal became the major force for change, combined with the invention of the steam engine at the end of the eighteenth century. Steam engines powered by coal spawned technological inventions that brought about great advances in all kinds of industry, from textile mills, breweries, flour mills, and paper mills, to iron works. Mechanical production of many goods increased greatly for domestic use and foreign trade, and Britain quickly became the leading exporter of manufactured goods (Cipolla 1978; Deane 1996; Hughes 1970).

The best example of dramatic change in production took place in the textile industry. Textile production went from a scattered cottage industry dependent on hand tools to a centralized factory system powered by large-scale machinery. This raised production at lower costs, and textiles became a major British export (Peterson 1973).

Large numbers of people began to move, attracted by wage work in towns and cities, and by opportunities in the newly opened colonies. Towns and cities grew at a rapid pace. Industrialization altered the British social structure and way of life, with a growing middle class and a working poor class, while most of the wealth remained in the hands of the elite.

The innovations developed in Britain spread to other parts of Europe and North America. Progress was rapid. The invention of the first locomotive in 1814 led to the first railway system in Britain, and British iron-built steamships soon followed. Other nations quickly followed Britain's example.

By the end of the nineteenth century rural, agrarian Europe had been transformed into a predominantly urban society. Commerce and wage work ruled the land. The world population increased dramatically, along with the economic boom powered by the industrial revolution, as birth rates soared ahead of death rates.

Growing cities could not keep up with the rapid influx of newcomers, and this led to problems associated with crowding into poor housing, pollution of air and water, improper sewage disposal, poor working conditions, lack of safety standards, poor nutrition, and pooling of diseases. These factors increased the death rate and lowered the infant survival rate in crowded cities, while in rural areas older people lived longer, and infant survival rates rose. However, steady migrations from rural areas sustained population growth in the cities (Davis 1972).

Factory work shaped the daily lives of the working poor. They generally worked from dawn to dusk without concern for their safety or health. Children were pressed into the labor force at ages as young as four, particularly in the textile factories and coal mines (Heilbroner 1975).

Sewage waste and effluent from factories often were dumped into the same rivers that supplied drinking water, or were allowed to seep into underground water wells. By 1830 all large manufacturing centers in Britain experienced polluted water supplies. The working poor crowded into small row houses, usually sharing a common water source and outside privies. Cleanliness and sanitation were inadequate. The privies often overflowed and contaminated adjacent shallow wells that supplied drinking water (Cartwright and Biddiss 2000).

Such overcrowded slums became hotbeds of disease, particularly respiratory and intestinal diseases. Alcoholism and poor nutrition contributed to the onslaught of infectious diseases. Tuberculosis and syphilis afflicted rich and poor alike, but the poor suffered the most. Polluted air, poor living conditions, overcrowding, and overwork contributed to high infection rates of the poor (Dubos 1952). Mortality from tuberculosis alone reached very high levels among these people (Cartwright and Biddiss 2000).

The patterns of work-related diseases and injuries differed from those in agrarian areas. The first reported incident of "factory fever" near Manchester in 1784 resulted from malnutrition, combined with fatigue, polluted air, and poor working conditions. This diagnosis soon fit other factory workers throughout the industrial districts, and many died from "factory fever" (Peterson 1973). Coal miners were prone to develop lung diseases; dye workers became susceptible to bladder cancer; chimney sweeps developed cancer of the scrotum (Higginson 1980); hatters developed a neurological disease known as "mad hatter" disease, caused by the chemicals used to smooth hats; and perfume workers developed liver damage (T-W-Fiennes 1978a).

The mid-nineteenth century brought new scientific insights into the health problems associated with the industrialization of cities. Mandated public sanitation measures helped to clean up the cities. Living standards were greatly improved by cleaning up polluted waters and food sources, improving housing, and implementing control of sewage discharges. Eventually wage earners received protection with better working conditions and improved safety measures, and child labor in factories and mines was outlawed. City health improved, but death rates still remained higher than in rural areas (Davis 1972) as epidemic diseases and air pollution continued to take their toll.

Thus, human beings had embarked on a course of great technological change that empowered them to reshape their world with unprecedented control over nature. These technological innovations born of human creativity eventually produced the modern world with its modern mix of diseases.

Once past the rampaging epidemics that had done so much to decimate Old and New World populations, the global population began to spiral out of control with colonization and missionization. Global population had grown from around 300 million in A.D. 1 to about 800 million by 1750 (Coale 1974), despite the onslaught of various diseases. This illustrates the remarkable ability of human immune systems to adapt to ever-changing challenges by pathogens. Despite great losses of human numbers from epidemic diseases over generations, the survivors developed enough tolerance and resistance for human populations to increase in numbers. By 1900 the world's population had doubled (Cipolla 1978) to around 1.6 billion.

As the Old World diseases went global and mixed with new ones, particularly respiratory viruses, patterns of disease began to change throughout the world. Diseases once confined to specific regions moved from their homelands to become established in far distant lands.

CONCLUDING COMMENTS

Civilization arose out of the development of agriculture, and significantly changed disease patterns with the development of trade routes that also acted as conduits for pathogens. Many diseases acquired from domestic animals and insect pests became well-established human diseases.

The troubled medieval period brought major shifting of disease patterns with varying types of infectious diseases. Sporadic epidemics that once haunted the empires of Rome and East Asia became endemic diseases in medieval Europe, Asia, and north Africa. Repeated famines and wars leading to social disruption facilitated the process, and many populations became greatly reduced in numbers, particularly in Western Europe.

By the end of the Middle Ages epidemic diseases began to wax and wane through cyclic appearances in a state of fluctuating equilibrium, depending on social upheavals, food shortages, and lax living standards.

The industrial revolution and European expansion opened the door for the global expansion of Old World diseases. Rapid immigration, together with the high densities of populations in cities and towns lacking the infrastructure for public health, created hotbeds for disease. Crowded housing, polluted air and water, and harsh working conditions provided ideal circumstances for the mixing and spread of infections. These conditions, plus increasing trade routes with various people moving about the globe, allowed many diseases, once confined to the Old World, to spread to all other parts of the world.

Scientific reasoning brought new understanding of many infectious diseases, and caused measures to be put in place by the nineteenth century to keep them from spreading as much as possible. This worked in some places most of the time, but it failed where preventive measures were not put in place. Plus, social disruptions, such as wars or economic downturns, frequently undermined measures taken to prevent the spread of diseases. The battle between humans and pathogenic microbes never ceases.

The microbial pot began to be stirred more rapidly, mixing pathogens from different parts of the world. Populations in the New World, never before exposed to Old World diseases, were ravaged by the new infections. As New World populations decreased, populations in the Old World increased dramatically. Migrations to the New World eased the pressure of European population growth, and European migrants rapidly displaced weakened native populations.

Overall, the world population increased dramatically during the industrial revolution, and with the population explosion, epidemics grew in proportion to the burgeoning populations. Diseases once confined to specific regions or animals went global. A new world order of human diseases was in the making.

CHAPTER 17

EASY ROUTE TO
FAME AND GRIPE

Cholera, the Salmonella Gang, and
Other Prominent Gut Bugs

The early stages of globalization facilitated the spread of various diseases throughout the world. No longer confined to specific regions, many diseases found new havens as they traveled far and wide on board ships that increased in spread and range. They began to appear as if out of nowhere, in places where they had never been before. Progress marched forward, and many geographically localized endemic diseases began to evolve into global pandemic diseases.

European industrialization made possible globalization, and led to the development of new commercial centers throughout the world. Their rapid growth attracted large numbers of people who hoped to benefit from wage work and opportunities to improve their lives. The newly mechanized industries required greater numbers of workers for increasing production. Industrialized towns and cities grew rapidly throughout the world with little regard to basic infrastructure, such as housing and drinking water, sewage and waste disposal.

People often dump factory wastes and raw sewage into rivers and streams, polluting the very sources of water used for drinking. Wells dug to obtain safe drinking water do not always escape pollution. Shallow wells placed near overused public latrines are in line for sewage runoff. The urban poor working classes proved to be the most vulnerable to unsafe drinking water, since they were often crowded into clusters of poor housing units dependent on a single latrine and a single water source (Cartwright and Biddiss 2000).

Contaminated drinking water can serve up unsuspected deadly cocktails loaded with water-borne infectious diseases. Diarrhea, sometimes mild, sometimes deadly, commonly follows.

Humans have always been susceptible to water-borne diseases. The development of agriculture, followed by the process of civilization, created greater opportunities for intestinal (enteric) pathogens to attack. Epidemics often waxed and waned, depending on the type of infectious agent and source. Whenever drinking water became contaminated with human or animal waste, opportunities arose for water-borne agents of disease. Also, undercooked or raw foods contaminated by polluted water or feces carried the risk of infection. The most notorious disease arising from contaminated waters made its formal global debut in the early nineteenth century—cholera. Before industrialization and European expansion, cholera had been a disease of the flood-prone Ganges delta region known as Bengal on the Indian subcontinent (modern-day Bangladesh).

The Story of Cholera

Cholera is caused by bacteria belonging to the genus Vibrio that inhabit estuaries, marshes, and coastal waters. Vibrios require salty waters for growth. They move about by way of a hair-like tail known as a flagellum. Over thirty species exist, but only about ten of them can accidentally infect humans. Cholera has become the most widespread and best known of the pathogenic vibrios, having more than eighty variants (Sakazaki 1992).

Cholera does not naturally infect humans, but instead operates as an accidental infection caused by opportunistic bacteria with pathogenic potential (McNicol and Doetsch 1983). Unlike many other infectious agents of the gut that depend on passage from one host to another by way of fecal contaminated water, vibrios can survive independently when they return to their natural environment. They don't need to invade a human or animal host to survive, but they can adapt to the gut microenvironment of a host when accidentally ingested. Once they escape from a host, they can either return to nature or pass through another host by way of fecal contaminated waters (Colwell and Spira 1992).

"Stick-to-itiveness" is a way of life for vibrios. The bacteria attach to the surface area of a source likely to bring them into contact with minute food particles. They prefer to attach to chitin, the major substance forming the outer shells of crustaceans, particularly the chitin of tiny copepods found in plankton. Vibrios may actually play a role in the life cycle of these tiny creatures by promoting the release of their eggs from the egg sac through their ability to disrupt proteins. Vibrios also attach to the chitin-lined hind gut of the blue crab and other large crustaceans. Vibrios can stick to the roots of water plants, and even to trickling filters used to treat raw sewage (Colwell and Spira 1992).

The evidence points strongly to the Ganges delta as the origin of the pathogenic vibrio that causes cholera; scattered outbreaks of the disease and seasonal epidemics have occurred there for centuries. Cholera remains endemic to that region to this day, and the delta estuaries provide homes to numerous varieties of nonpathogenic vibrios.

We now know that eating undercooked or raw fish and shellfish from vibrio-contaminated waters can be a major source of cholera infection. Large plankton blooms follow the monsoons in the delta area, promoting explosive growth of vibrios. Fish and shellfish become contaminated and pass the infection to humans who eat them raw or undercooked (Colwell and Spira 1992). Passage from the human gut with diarrhea allows the infective vibrios to return to their natural environment or to infect other people through fecal-contaminated drinking water.

Although vibrios require salty water for growth, they can survive near the surface of fresh water if they can find something to attach to with available salt-sparing nutrients. Vibrios can alter their shape and enter a state of dormancy when environmental conditions do not favor growth, and they can survive for years in this state (Colwell and Spira 1992). Artificial ponds have been used for centuries as sources of potable water in the flat rural areas of the Ganges delta. The ponds become flooded and filled during the seasonal monsoons (Cockburn 1963). As the dry season takes over, algae and water plants thriving within the stagnant waters offer a safe haven for vibrios introduced into them either by contaminated flood waters or by leaking sewage from nearby latrines. Infection follows with the drinking of contaminated water or by ingestion of raw fruits and vegetables washed with contaminated water, as well as by consumption of contaminated raw or undercooked fish and shellfish.

Vibrios can survive for several days in contaminated moist foods. They have to remain in a wet environment in order to survive, being susceptible to drying. High temperatures lasting over ten minutes will kill them, and they have poor tolerance for low-acid environments (Sakazaki 1992).

Most vibrios quickly die following ingestion, as they pass into the stomach where gastric acids attack them. However, food particles ingested along with the vibrios buffer the overpowering acidic attack against them, enabling some of them to pass through the stomach without harm (Glass and Black 1992). Some vibrios have developed adaptive strategies to survive and thrive in the human gut, while most other vibrios have not.

The human gut supports a wide variety of host-friendly bacteria and viruses that thrive on sloughed dead cells and debris, keeping the local ecology on an even keel. Their presence and actions keep the surface immune cells that have dispersed among the mucous cells and subsurface of the intestinal lining active and alert with an arsenal of immunoglobins and other immune agents. This makes it difficult for a foreign microbe to move in, unless the immune responses are down, or the intruder can devise a way to get past them.

Pathogenic vibrios have managed to acquire gene sequences (plasmids) that enable them to produce enterotoxins (poisons) to help them fend off competing intestinal bacteria and thwart immune responses as they attach to the mucosal cells lining the small intestine. Anchored to the mucosa, they alter the local ecology to reconstruct their natural salty environment. Similar plasmids have been found in *Escherichia coli* bacteria, normal residents of the human gut. *E. coli* may have picked up the gene sequences from human DNA debris coming from tissue sloughs in the intestine. Transfer of the genetic material from *E. coli* to pathogenic vibrios could have occurred either in the human gut or in sewage-contaminated waters (McNicol and Doetsch 1983).

The enterotoxins released by pathogenic vibrios help them alter the exchange of sodium and chloride ions across the mucosal barrier of the small intestine. This dramatically increases the salinity and fluid levels in the gut to resemble their natural aquatic environment. Nutrients for the body are absorbed in the small intestine, and this part of the gut oversees fluid exchanges from the stomach and internal pancreas, liver, and biliary tree, as well as its own secretions. Up to 11 liters of fluid is exchanged here in twenty-four hours. A much smaller fluid volume reaches the large intestine, where most of it gets absorbed through the colon wall. Pathogenic vibrios severely disrupt this balance, as they hold the fluid within the gut and cause large volumes to pass through the intestine with watery diarrhea (Finkelstein 1992; Holmgren 1992). This leads to severe dehydration of the host.

The hallmark of cholera is sudden onset of painless, profuse watery diarrhea described as "rice water" stools with a characteristic "fishy" odor. Sometimes the diarrhea is accompanied by vomiting of clear fluid. Symptoms usually appear two to three days following ingestion of the vibrios, but sometimes symptoms can appear within a few hours or as long as five days later. Host reactions to the vibrios contribute to the diarrhea as war rages between intestinal surface immunoglobins and the invaders, along with increased mucosal secretions and gut motility. Individuals with type O blood appear to be genetically more susceptible to cholera than other blood groups (Benenson 1995; Rabbani and Greenough III 1992).

Diarrhea can range from mild to severe, depending on the type or strain of pathogenic vibrios and the quickness and efficiency of the intestinal immune cells. Many infections result in mild to moderate diarrhea with excretion of infectious vibrios for up to two weeks. Infants and young children suffer the most with severe diarrhea. Prolonged diarrhea can dehydrate them within hours, with death close behind. Cholera can be severe for many adults as well as for the young when dehydration takes over. Dehydration is the killer with severe diarrhea, and up to 70 percent of cholera victims die from it (Rabbani and Greenough III 1992).

Symptoms of severe dehydration start with thirst and loose skin turgor (tension), followed by hypovolemic (low fluid volume) shock when the victim loses more than 10 percent of body fluid weight and the circulatory system collapses. The extremities cool down, fingers appear shriveled, eyes become sunken, the tip of the tongue and the lips turn blue, the mouth becomes dry, muscles ache, and the victim gasps for breath. Hypoglycemia (low blood sugar) often becomes a complication of cholera, especially in children, as altered absorption of nutrients in the gut interferes with nourishment during the course of the disease (Rabbani and Greenough III 1992).

Simple fluid and electrolyte replacement therapy, along with feedings of rice or grains, has reduced the death rate in recent years to less than 1 percent. The complex carbohydrates in these foods quickly break down into simple sugars and amino acids for absorption through the gut to offset nutritional deficits and low blood sugar levels in young victims. Cereals also help push needed electrolytes and water through the intestinal barrier and into the circulatory system. Recovery due to ample fluid and electrolyte replacement can take four to six days as the diarrhea gradually decreases, and acquired immunity to the disease prevents further attacks (Mahalanabis et al. 1992).

Interaction between vibrios in nature and human beings in the Ganges delta most likely began with the earliest farming villages in this region. This interaction ultimately led to vibrio adaptation to the human gut to produce endemic cholera.

Cholera did not catch the world's attention until the British moved into the Indian subcontinent during the late eighteenth century. The British established Calcutta on the western edge of the delta as a large commercial center that attracted large numbers of rural poor in search of wage work. The new arrivals settled into sprawling slums with poor drinking water and sanitation, ripe conditions for cholera.

The British expanded their control over the new colony by building railroads across the country so that they could move large numbers of troops, commercial goods, and people throughout the region. Shipping fleets increased to carry goods and raw materials from British India throughout the world. The reforms in transportation over land and sea enabled cholera to spread quickly beyond its native habitat.

British Calcutta became a major hub of cholera (McNeill 1977). Crowds of Hindu pilgrims coming to the lower Ganges often carried cholera back to their homes, and advancing railroad networks helped them spread cholera from the growing city more quickly to other areas. Pilgrims from far away could make the trip to the Ganges and return home in record time. Infected army recruits traveling by rail also carried the disease to distant parts of the Indian subcontinent, and ships with contaminated bilge waters and infected deck hands carried it by sea to distant lands.

By 1817 the first cholera pandemic originating from the Ganges delta entered the world stage. Rumors of a new and terrible disease in British India soon reached England. By 1821 ships carried it westward through the Arabian Sea and Persian Gulf region, with thousands dying from the disease. Camel caravans carried it overland across Syria and into southern Russia in 1822. At the same time it spread to the west, it traveled eastward by ship into Southeast Asia, including Indonesia, the Philippines and vast areas of China, finally reaching Japan by 1820 (Longmate 1966).

Another global round of cholera—the second pandemic—emerged from the Ganges delta in 1826, following the same westward and eastward paths as it had before. Cholera quickly established a focus within the

Muslim pilgrimages to Mecca in the Middle East, as it had for the Hindu pilgrimages to the Ganges in India. Cholera would remain a scourge for Muslim pilgrims to Mecca until 1910, when recognition of how to handle the disease among the pilgrims slowed it down (McNeill 1980).

Military troops and commerce again played key roles in the dispersal of this disease. Russian troops fighting in Persia and Turkey, as well as boats traveling up the Volga and Don Rivers brought cholera into Russia, reaching Moscow by 1830. Russian troop movements into the Baltics, large attendance at trading fairs, and travel by boats and ships quickly spread cholera throughout Europe.

Fear of the devastating new disease provoked desperate quarantine attempts to isolate it. The Russians posted soldiers around quarantined villages with orders to shoot anyone leaving them. Borders were closed and ships underwent quarantine as the fear of cholera spread. The working poor suffered from the disease the most, and they rioted out of fear of being deliberately victimized with poisons spread by the ruling classes or by foreigners (Longmate 1966; McNeill 1980; Morris 1976).

Fearful of the new disease that had not yet touched their shores, the British issued quarantine regulations against all incoming ships during the summer of 1831. Over seven hundred ships loaded with flax and hemp from the Baltic port of Riga, along with over three thousand other ships, were subject to a series of quarantine stations along the northeast coast of Britain where they remained confined for fourteen days. However, by the following summer, cholera broke through the quarantine and hit the commercial center of Sunderland on the northeast coast of England (Morris 1976). Perhaps the quarantine of so many ships along this coast guaranteed the dispersal of cholera vibrios from the ships' bilge waters into the local bays and estuaries, thereby contaminating fish and shellfish that were harvested and eaten by the local population. The quarantine to prevent cholera turned into a guarantee of the disease.

The disease quickly spread to London and throughout the British Isles. It was in London that John Snow proclaimed his water-borne theory of cholera in 1853. He postulated that the disease had been carried through the excreta of its victims into sewage-contaminated water sources. He based this on his observations that districts suffering from cholera utilized one particular water company that drew its water from the sewage-contaminated Thames River. He proved this in 1854 with his investigation of the Broad Street pump in the cholera-stricken Soho district. Local privies had leaked sewage into the well, and when he persuaded local authorities to remove the pump handle, the disease faded away. Despite this evidence, Snow could not convince his colleagues that cholera was a water-borne disease. Not until long after his death did his preventive measures gain favor (Morris 1976).

This round of cholera did not spare Australia, with the disease reaching the west coast in 1832. Cholera also crossed the Atlantic for the first time that year, arriving in North American port cities. The city of Quebec was struck first, then Montreal, followed by New York and Philadelphia; the disease steadily spread along the east coast and reached the gulf coast port cities by 1834. Cuba and port towns of Mesoamerica also contracted the disease. By 1836 it disappeared from North America, only to return in 1848 for a longer stay, reaching the West Coast by 1850 (Barua 1992).

The third cholera pandemic began in 1852 with renewed vigor wherever it had prevailed before, and it spread into South America and all over the continent of Africa. The fourth pandemic came in 1863, causing about thirty thousand deaths among ninety thousand Muslim pilgrims to Mecca in 1865. Cholera caused one of the worst epidemics in European history in 1866, killing around ninety thousand people in Russia alone (Barua 1992).

By this time, cholera began to be recognized for what it was, and public health measures to defeat the spread of the water-borne disease began to be imposed in parts of Europe and North America. When the fifth pandemic struck the world in 1881, these measures paid off, sparing those cities that had prepared for it. However, cholera continued to have its way wherever public health measures were not taken and knowledge of vibrio behavior was lacking. Thus, the disease ravaged parts of Europe, Russia, the Middle East, north Africa, all parts of Asia, and South America (Barua 1992).

The sixth pandemic, lasting from 1899 to 1923, struck the same areas that had suffered from the earlier pandemics. Cholera finally left North America in 1911, and it left Europe in 1925. A large outbreak in Egypt in 1947 left over twenty thousand dead (Barua 1992). By the 1950s fluid replacement therapy began to drastically reduce the number of deaths from cholera (Mahalanabis et al. 1992).

The seventh pandemic began in 1961 with an outbreak in Sulawesi, Indonesia. This was the first pandemic caused by a new cholera strain named El Tor. This strain differs from the classic form that originated in the Ganges delta by having less of the genetic code for producing enterotoxin. It has only one copy of the toxin genes, while the classic type contains two copies of the toxin gene (Holmgren 1992). El Tor was first noticed in 1937 as a mild, cholera-like disease occurring in Indonesia (Barua 1992). El Tor generally produces only a few bouts of diarrhea without significant fluid deficit and most often with few or no other symptoms (Rabbani and Greenough III 1992; Sack 1992).

El Tor appears to be hardier than the classic strain. It can withstand greater environmental variations in water salinity, particularly in flood-prone areas. El Tor strains have replaced the classic strains everywhere in the world since the 1970s except in the Ganges delta where the classic type persists alongside El Tor (Siddique et al. 1991).

El Tor spread to West Asia, Africa, Europe, and the Philippines by the 1970s. Imported cases sporadically appeared in countries with safe water, con-trolled sanitation, and public health surveillance. Consequently, El Tor settled into endemic vibrios, inhabiting coastal areas of countries all over the world. Almost half the shellfish along the coast of Portugal harbored El Tor vibrios during the 1970s, and outbreaks have occurred all over the world wherever El Tor vibrios resided. This includes the gulf coast of North America and Queensland, Australia. Undercooked or raw contaminated seafood, especially shellfish, became the chief transmitters for the disease (Barua 1992), along with inadequately treated drinking water, and contaminated water used for irrigation and for washing fruits, vegetables, and other foods.

Ship bilge waters have been primarily responsible for the seeding of cholera vibrios in coastal areas throughout the world. The most recent major outbreak occurred on the coast of Lima, Peru, in 1991. Undercooked and raw shellfish and fish contaminated by vibrios left by bilge waters started the epi-demic. Poor sanitation and water treatment then helped spread the disease throughout the coastal cities, and northward (Lederberg et al. 1992).

A new strain of cholera, called 0139, broke out in India and Bangladesh in 1992, and spread to other parts of Asia. Cholera struck Rwandan refugees in Zaire (now the Democratic Republic of Congo) in 1992 and occurred in Albania that same year (Benenson 1995). Cholera is determined to remain a global player.

The Salmonella Gang

This group of microbes constitutes one of the most commonly occurring bac-teria throughout the world. Approximately two thousand variations exist in association with various life forms, from insects, reptiles, birds, and wild and domestic animals to humans. While many salmonellae have adapted to a specific host, many more exist in nature without a specified host. Water serves as the primary medium for transporting these microbes, as they move from one host to another via the oral-fecal route. They can survive for long periods of time in water and soil, and they can stay alive for a while under freezing conditions (Morgan 1952). Foods contaminated by infected host feces provide a common mode of transmission. Salmonella infection does not always cause disease, since many of these microbes have become quite successful passive gut residents in their hosts (Rowe and Gross 1984; Rubin and Weinstein 1977).

Like so many microbes, salmonellae are opportunists, always on the alert for ways to adapt to new surroundings. Most strains that occur as natural infections of animals, and some nonspecific host strains, can infect humans. These types of infections generally come under the guise of "food poisoning," and they usually require high doses of ingested salmonellae to produce disease.

As with many other gut-invading microbes, the ability of salmonellae to bind to cells lining the gut determines their ability to cause harm. Salmonellae target the specialized antigen transporting membrane cells (M cells) scattered among the mucous cells and overlying lymphatic tissue, particularly in areas rich in lymph nodules, called peyer's patches. The M cells constantly sample intestinal contents for potential foreign antigens, and transport them from the gut lumen to the underlying lymph cells, where macrophages destroy the foreign material.

Salmonellae attach to the M cells and subvert them for their own use. Some accidental salmonellae infections in humans stay confined to the M cells on the surface of the gut with just local immune reactions. More virulent salmonellae can pass through the gut wall by way of M cell transport, provoking underlying macrophages to attack them. Many of these bacteria manage to survive and multiply within the macrophage vacuoles (Raupach et al. 1999; Rubin and Weinstein 1977). The infected macrophages then become subject to destruction by the immune system in order to destroy their unwanted parasites. Usually the battle is confined to the local tissues, but some highly virulent strains manage to escape the onslaught and get past the local tissue response, seeding out to other areas of the body (Sereny 1977).

The antigen arrangement on the bacteria cell surface determines how quickly the host immune system will recognize them. Some bacteria have ways of covering up their surface antigens to shield themselves from initial attack. Salmonellae with easily recognizable antigens provoke immediate host immune responses as they attach to M cells. Some salmonellae sneak in under cover and are able to delay the immune response until after they have invaded underlying lymph tissue. Most salmonellae not adapted to a specific host that invade the human gut provoke immediate local immune reactions. This generally limits the disease to acute inflammation of the gut lining (gastroenteritis) with immediate immune response, lasting only twelve to forty-eight hours after ingestion (Rubin and Weinstein 1977).

Various salmonellae adapted to different animal hosts that accidentally infect humans cause similar symptoms of gastroenteritis. This includes nausea and vomiting, subsiding in a few hours, followed quickly by abdominal cramps and diarrhea. Diarrhea can last three to four days, and then disappear rapidly. Sometimes diarrhea can be severe and persist for two to three weeks, and the abdominal pain can mimic appendicitis symptoms (Rubin and Weinstein 1977).

Typhoid Fever

Some of the salmonellae transformed themselves into strict human pathogens sometime in the distant past. This may have coincided with the origins of agriculture and animal husbandry, when humans mixed the raising of crops and animals with water-management schemes. Repeated human exposure to certain salmonellae strains excreted by animals into water used for irrigation and drinking may have enabled the bacteria to jump species and adapt to the human gut.

Salmonellae strictly adapted to the human gut cause typhoid fever and related paratyphoid diseases. They have developed effective means for evading initial surface immune responses while they multiply within M cells. Then they invade subsurface macrophages in large numbers, provoking a general immune system alarm affecting the whole body. As immune responses attack and break down the bacteria, the battered foreigners release endotoxin damaging to the mucous membranes of the intestinal wall. This induces fever and provokes the immune system into action to counteract the toxin (Rubin and Weinstein 1977). Paratyphoid fever is less common and produces milder symptoms and lower fatality (1 percent) than typhoid fever (10 percent) (Benenson 1995).

Human typhoid fever spreads by the oral-fecal route with human fecal-contaminated food or water. Contaminated water provides the major source of transmission. Shellfish from sewage-contaminated waters, especially oysters, can be a source of infection. Raw fruits and vegetables fertilized by human excreta and eaten raw can also lead to infection (Benenson 1995).

Industrialization brought large epidemics of typhoid fever, caused by wholesale production of contaminated milk products and other food products, as well as contaminated water. Industrialization also allowed the disease to quickly spread throughout the world (Rubin and Weinstein 1977).

Infection can be mild with little effect on the intestinal tract when the host immune response quickly contains the infection (Benenson 1995). Some individuals become chronic carriers of the bacteria without showing any symptoms of the disease. Infected food handlers excreting contaminated stools who don't adequately wash their hands often transmit the disease to others. The most famous chronic carrier of the disease cooked for several families in and around New York City in the early part of the twentieth century. Mary Mallon became known as "Typhoid Mary" when it was discovered that she had been responsible for several outbreaks (Wukovits 1990).

Salmonella typhi, when ingested, invade the M cells where they multiply in the first four to five days of the infection before passing below the surface of the intestine into the lymphatic tissue. The initial infection usually involves only a small area of the bowel. If the bacteria cannot be confined to the subsurface lymph cells by the immune system, they can spread through the mesenteric lymphatics that drain the gut and can reach the circulatory system to invade other organs of the host. The liver, spleen, bone marrow, gallbladder, and bile become common targets. Infected bile can dump the bacteria back into the intestinal lumen to start the cycle all over again. Paratyphoid species follow similar tactics (Rubin and Weinstein 1977).

The interplay between the host immune system and the bacteria determines the course of the disease. Local competing flora within the host's intestine can contribute to the demise of these foreign bacteria. When host immune responses limit the infection to the intestine, the affected portion of the bowel swells and becomes inflamed. The immune cells try to seal off the focal area of infection with granulomatous tissue that often ulcerates as tissue dies and sloughs off, sometimes leading to hemorrhage or perforation of the intestine. Otherwise the ulcerated areas heal with eradication of the invaders (Rubin and Weinstein 1977).

Genetics plays a role in the host's immune response. Individuals who suffer from congenital anemias, such as sickle cell anemia, are highly susceptible to systemic invasion by *Salmonella typhi*, resulting in severe chronic forms of the disease with recurring outbreaks. Other diseases suffered by the host can affect the course of this infection. Individuals with chronic schistosomiasis often have chronic mild or asymptomatic typhoid fever (Rubin and Weinstein 1977).

Symptoms of typhoid fever usually begin to appear from one to three weeks following the microbes' arrival in the gut as the systemic immune response reacts to the invaded lymph tissue. Sometimes it takes only a few days or it may take as long as sixty days before symptoms appear. Reaction to the bacteria and its toxin affects the whole body, and symptoms can vary from one individual to another. Typical early symptoms include severe headache, weakness, general aches and pains, sometimes cough or nosebleed, and constipation more often than diarrhea. Body temperature gradually rises within a few days, and rose-colored spots usually appear on the abdomen, sometimes extending to the back and chest, and appearing in successive crops for several days. The lower abdomen becomes tender, and the spleen enlarges. Transient hair loss and bronchitis commonly occur. Bacteria shed through the bowel, and about 25 percent of victims also excrete bacteria in their urine. Infected pregnant women in the early stages of pregnancy will often abort, and premature labor can be triggered in later stages (Benenson 1995; Rubin and Weinstein 1977).

Recovery is gradual, taking three to four weeks. A small percentage of victims retain *Salmonella typhi* in their gallbladders to become chronic carriers of the disease. Various organs of the body can be damaged in some way from the infection, leaving recovering individuals with a variety of impairments. Some individuals harboring hardy bacterial strains can suffer relapse of the disease, sometimes months or years later. Their immune systems cannot end the infection. They can only contain the bacteria by sealing them off in granulomas, until an upset in the host triggers their release. The granulomas containing the bacteria commonly form in bones and joints, particularly the spine, ribs, and long bones, not unlike the granulomas of tuberculosis. *S. typhi* granulomas often form in the bones and joints of young children and infants (Rubin and Weinstein 1977).

With modernization of the industrialized world, typhoid fever and its cousins have become a rarity wherever modern standards for treatment of drinking water and waste disposal have drastically reduced the human fecal/oral contamination cycle. Those parts of the world without these modernized controls continue to harbor the disease.

Salmonella Postscript

While the human-adapted salmonellae infections of typhoid fever and paratyphoid fever no longer pose a threat to modern nations, infections from animal salmonellae have become a growing threat to modern life. We may have broken the human cycle of infection, but we have managed to increase the animal cycle of infection along with increasing access of animal infections to humans.

Modern methods of farming and food processing on a mass scale have allowed greater numbers of salmonellae to infect domestic animals and to enter the human food chain. Concentrating large numbers of animals and poultry into small areas has increased the exchange of salmonellae strains among them, allowing for selection and exchange of genetic material for greater virulence. Once rare strains are now becoming common (Rowe and Gross 1984).

The practice of recycling animal waste, particularly poultry droppings and bone meal, for animal feed has guaranteed wholesale inoculation of animals and poultry with salmonellae capable of infecting humans. One particular type of salmonella that affects fish off the coast of Peru accidentally became introduced into European poultry in the 1960s. The fish were processed into fishmeal and added to poultry feed. The salmonellae survived the process and quickly adapted to life in the intestines of chickens, ultimately infecting humans (Mims 1980).

The constant recycling of salmonellae strains through their animal hosts has turned them into steady asymptomatic carriers of more virulent strains. Salmonellae infections have grown so common that susceptible young animals routinely receive antibiotics to prevent them from succumbing to the disease. This has just added fuel to the fire as animal strains of salmonellae have taken on antibiotic resistance factors and continue to evolve into more potent bacteria. Salmonella in poultry has become so successful that it now passes into eggs, making them a source for human infection. Raw and undercooked eggs and meats, even frozen meats thawed at room temperature, can harbor salmonella.

Commercial food-processing plants and abattoirs producing large amounts of animal products can be silent hubs of salmonellae distribution into the human food chain. The bacteria can survive and grow in foodstuffs at warm temperatures without altering their taste or appearance. Meat products such as sausage and luncheon meats, egg products such as frozen egg whites and dried egg powders, dairy products such as dried milk, and other foods containing animal ingredients can be affected (Morgan 1952; Rubin and Weinstein 1977).

Other Prominent Gut Bugs

While viruses, protozoa, and some bacteria can attack the human gut, only two other bacteria of global prominence will be discussed here.

Shigellosis

Four groups of shigella bacteria with many variants have successfully adapted to the human gut. They prefer to inhabit the colon, or large intestine, and sometimes the lower end of the small intestine. With the help of acquired plasmids, shigellae press themselves into the M cells and break into their cytoplasm, where they grow rapidly and escape into surrounding epithelial tissue. Strains of shigellae that have not been able to acquire the necessary plasmid remain harmless, unable to force their way into the intestinal tissues. Those strains with the plasmid that can break through the intestinal barrier trigger the immune system with an acute inflammatory reaction as they attack epithelial tissues. Unlike salmonella, shigella bacteria do not survive macrophage ingestion, making it easier for the local immune response to contain the infection (Hale and Keren 1992; Raupach et al. 1999; Sansonetti 1992).

The mildest and most common forms of shigella belong to the *S. sonnei* group that produce short-term diarrhea. The *S. flexneri* and *S. boydii* groups cause more severe disease, while the *S. dysenteriae* group causes the most serious disease with fatality rates of 20 percent (Benenson 1995; Goodwin 1984). *Shigella dysenteriae* and some *Shigella flexneri* strains excrete a toxin (exotoxin) into surrounding tissue. This toxin inhibits protein synthesis in the epithelial cells and destroys tiny blood vessels (capillaries) feeding into them. Hemorrhages can follow, along with ulceration of the colon wall, with the possibility of bacteria escaping into the bloodstream (O'Brien et al. 1992).

Usually the disease remains confined to the colon. Genetically susceptible individuals who cannot keep the bacteria confined to the colon can develop Reiter's syndrome in the joints. This develops when the bacteria escape into the bloodstream and lodge in the joints, triggering inflammatory responses from the immune system (Benenson 1995).

Quick immune response mixed with milder strains of shigella often goes unrecognized by the host. Diarrhea, sometimes watery and with severe forms containing mucous and blood, is the major symptom. The extent of damage to the colon by shigella determines the type of diarrhea.

Symptoms generally appear within one to three days from the time of ingestion, sometimes within twelve hours or as long as one week with *S. dysenteriae*. Milder forms can last four to seven days, while severe forms can last several weeks, depending on host immunity status. Onset is usually abrupt with abdominal cramps relieved by defecation. Bowel spasms, fever, nausea, and vomiting often follow, along with abdominal tenderness (Benenson 1995; Cuff 1975).

Infected cells gradually die and shed along with the bacteria from the intestinal wall as healing progresses. Abscesses can form in severe cases, leaving raw areas—that is, ulcers. With limited ulceration of the colon, healing occurs without scarring. Healing following severe ulceration can lead to scarring and possible constriction or narrowing of the space within the intestine. Chronic colitis can also develop from severe shigella infection (Cuff 1975).

The shigellae have existed for centuries all around the globe. *Shigella dysenteriae* has often been confused with amoebic dysentery, since they produce similar symptoms, but shigella is more widespread and much more common than the amoebic form (Goodwin 1984). Poor sanitation and water standards, coupled with overcrowding, lead to endemic infections of the disease. Infection can be rampant wherever people crowd together in confined spaces under poorly controlled conditions: military camps, refugee camps, prisons, orphanages, and day care centers.

Feces containing shigella spread the disease through sewage-contaminated drinking water and food. The bacteria can survive for days in contaminated foods. They can be transmitted from contaminated hands and fingernails following defecation, and sometimes flies pick them up and deposit them on food. The bacteria can survive for several weeks in cool, humid areas with little direct sunlight (Goodwin 1984).

Wherever proper measures have been taken for drinking water and sewage disposal, the milder shigellae strains have replaced the strains producing more severe forms of disease. Outbreaks of the more severe forms of the disease continue to plague the world wherever conditions favor easy fecal-oral transmission. So-called "traveler's diarrhea" is often produced by a hardy strain of shigella acquired in an underdeveloped area of the globe (Goodwin 1984).

Escherichia coli

This group of bacteria normally resides in mammalian and human colons, where they help maintain a healthy intestinal environment. Their complex and readily changeable antigen patterns keep the local immune cells alert with constant stimulation that promotes immunoglobin production. This keeps the gut defenses ready to quickly respond to invading microbes. There are numerous strains of *Escherichia coli*, and all of them can borrow a variety of genetic information contained in plasmids from other bacteria. This gives them tremendous range of variability that allows them to adapt to changing environmental conditions.

The human and animal gut resembles a very popular swap meet with all kinds of microbes wandering in and out, checking over the merchandise to see if they can find anything to use to their advantage. They pick their way through pieces of discarded "junk" genetic material and debris until they find something that fits their particular needs. *Escherichia coli* are major shoppers, selecting various bits of genetic information with a variety of uses that come in handy when they need to make changes as their intestinal environment changes.

The greatest environmental challenge to bacterial survival has been the recent overuse of synthetic antibiotics. These antibiotics threaten the resident gut bugs, forcing them to quickly evolve or perish as a species. Strains of *E. coli* have managed to grab plasmids that allow them to resist destruction by synthetic antibiotics, and in the process they transform themselves from host-friendly bacteria into bad guys.

Consequently, renegade *E. coli* have entered the realm of intestinal pathogens, following the same easy fecal-oral route used by other gut bugs to find new victims. Six major categories of pathogenic strains have been identified in recent years, based on the different ways they have altered their behavior and affect the host intestine (Benenson 1995). Some have taken on salmonella-like characteristics, while others have adopted shigella-like characteristics (Novgorodskaya and Polotsky 1977).

These new pathogenic strains are particularly dangerous to the very young. The first recognized pathogenic group of *E. coli* in the mid-twentieth century attacked babies throughout North America and Europe. Most babies in modern countries during this time period were bottle-fed. The major factors leading to the success of this group of salmonella-like strains known as *Enteropathogenic Escherichia coli (EPEC)* may be the widespread use of artificial milk formulas in place of natural mother's milk, and the response of the bacteria to synthetic antibiotics. Newborns enter the world with sterile guts and begin to acquire their natural friendly intestinal bacteria shortly after birth. What the newborn ingests as food determines the developing composition of intestinal bacteria, causing a difference between breast-fed infants and those fed artificial formula. Bacteria such as *E. coli* do not gain prominence in the breast-fed infant gut until the introduction of other foods, while they takehold in the bottle-fed infant gut from the beginning (Dubos 1980). Thus, the formula-fed infant became more vulnerable to *EPEC*.

Outbreaks of *EPEC* have decreased in industrial countries as the spread of the disease has been contained through better controls over transmission of the bacteria, and as more mothers choose to nurse their infants. Infants fed artificial formula in developing countries around the world remain at risk of *EPEC* along with another group of pathogenic strains known as the *Enteroaggregative* strains (*EAggEC*). The watery diarrhea resulting from the infections can be severe and deadly. Toddlers in developing countries can be susceptible to yet another group classified as *Diffuse Adherence* strains (*DAEC*) (Benenson 1995).

Cholera-like *Enterotoxigenic* strains (*ETEC*) form one of the major causes of "traveler's diarrhea." They attack the upper portion of the small intestine in a similar manner to cholera, using the same endotoxin-producing plasmids that the vibrios use to increase the fluid content of the gut. The symptoms of escherichia cholera-like strains resemble cholera, but they generally have a weaker and shorter effect on the host gut than do the vibrios (Benenson 1995; Novgorodskaya and Polotsky 1977).

Shigella-like strains of *Escherichia coli* include *Enteroinvasive* strains (*EIEC*) and *Enterohemorrhagic* strains (*EHEC*). They have acquired the same plasmids that shigella use to attack the colon tissues, and produce similar symptoms to shigellosis (Benenson 1995; Sasakawa et al. 1992).

The actions of the *Enterohemorrhagic* strains (*EHEC*) resemble *Shigella dysenteriae* with similar symptoms. It takes only a small number of bacteria to cause infection within three to eight days after ingestion. This group of strains populates the guts of cattle, crossing into human gut territory through meat contaminated with cattle feces, especially ground meat. Outbreaks have occurred in the United States from undercooked hamburgers. Raw milk can also be contaminated with cattle feces, and a recent outbreak of this disease derived from apple juice when the apples became contaminated by cow manure used as fertilizer. The bacteria can also be transmitted from infected human feces through drinking contaminated water and even from swimming in contaminated waters (Benenson 1995; Sasakawa et al. 1992).

CONCLUDING COMMENTS

The quest for safe drinking water and food has always been a concern for humans. This remains a difficult task today in many parts of the world that lack controls over water purity and food handling. Sewage and water problems that existed during the early period of industrialization in the West linger among populations in underdeveloped countries. Cholera, typhoid fever, and dysentery caused by shigella remain serious threats to many of the underdeveloped countries of the world. Modern nations rarely have exposure to these more serious forms of intestinal infections, but they do retain the mild forms of them.

Rapid transit of people and foods from underdeveloped areas to various other parts of the world provide opportunities for mixing of the many types and strains of gut bugs, synthetic antibiotics, and environments. This has speeded up the ongoing evolution of gut bacteria and host immunity with successes and failures on both sides throughout the world.

The battle continues. The indiscriminate use of synthetic antibiotics throughout the world has signaled a revolution among all kinds of pathogenic bacteria, particularly the various gut bugs fighting for survival against these new weapons. Different types of bacteria have turned to each other for help, sharing plasmids capable of resisting synthetic antibiotics. This has also made them more powerful against their hosts' immune fighters. Foreign intervention into the host immune defensive line with synthetic antibiotics acts like a special strike force with rapid assault on the enemy, but at the same time interferes with the hosts' natural defense responses, particularly within the gut. How quickly the natural host immune response can recover from this artificial intervention and take over more effectively will determine the outcome of the war.

Underdeveloped countries may be hotbeds of disease dissemination, but developed countries unknowingly contribute to evolutionary changes in pathogens. Most notable are the silent changes taking place in intestinal bacteria. Modern food processing brings a mixed blessing: in general, it has provided us with safe foods on a grand scale, but at the same time it has enabled any bacterial contamination within the system to spread rapidly. Cattle feed-lots and crowded pig and poultry pens become major sources of bacterial exchanges of genetic material useful for antibiotic resistance and increased virulence. Beef contaminated with new strains of virulent *Escherichia coli*, and new strains of salmonella from poultry, have already passed through the food-processing system to infect people. Many coastal shell-fishing areas have turned into breeding grounds for vibrios, and some of our own resident gut bugs have turned against us in order to survive the synthetic antibody onslaught.

Our war on bacteria with synthetic antibiotics has backfired in many instances, speeding up the evolutionary cycle of many different kinds of microbes. How then do we stop this vicious cycle?

CHAPTER 18

TRANSOCEANIC
HITCHHIKERS

Yellow Fever and
Its Dengue Cousin

Y ellow fever and dengue fever belong to a large group of viruses called arboviruses carried by blood-sucking mosquitoes, ticks, sandflies, and biting midges capable of infecting vertebrates. Over five hundred of these arboviruses, representing several groups of different but closely related viruses, have been recognized around the world (Lederberg et al. 1992). Every part of the globe has its own set of insect vectors and arboviruses interacting with local fauna. Many of them infect primarily lower vertebrates and migratory birds without causing any harm to their natural hosts (Ray 1984).

Human beings become accidental hosts to some of the arboviruses whenever they intrude into insect vector territory and disrupt the normal animal host–vector cycle of infection. Over a hundred arboviruses have spilled over into human populations. Most of these viruses produce few, if any, ill effects in human hosts. Some, like yellow fever and dengue fever, can generate acute infections with varying degrees of illness, depending on the type of virus and the host's immune reaction. Symptoms can range from influenza-like illness with or without joint pains, to more severe illnesses, such as encephalitis, and hemorrhagic disease (Benenson 1995).

Most of the arboviruses causing severe disease have been restricted to remote areas of the world and have had negligible impact on major human populations. However, as transoceanic commerce has expanded, some of these viruses have managed to break out of their geographical isolation to find new habitats and vector-host cycles to their liking. Outbreaks of disease from some of these arbovirus infections have had major impacts on human settlements and commerce wherever they have been introduced.

Yellow Fever

The mosquito-transmitted arbovirus that causes yellow fever escaped from confinement in the jungles of west Africa with expansion of the slave trade in the seventeenth century. Along with malaria, slave ships carried this disease to the New World where it quickly established itself in a reign of terror over European immigrants and native peoples alike. The disease became known as "Yellow Jack" during its early history. The nickname derived from the requirement of ships carrying the infection to hoist a yellow flag when they approached ports (McNeill 1976).

Unlike malaria infection, yellow fever was not carried to the New World by the African slaves themselves. The infection lasts only a short time and would not have survived the long sea voyages in the blood of the slaves. The only way the virus could have been shipped out of its homeland was through vector mosquitoes traveling as stowaways on board the slave ships, laying their eggs in the ships' water casks, and attacking crewmen and human cargo alike (McNeill 1976).

The mosquitoes would have found it difficult to survive without some form of nectar or other plant juice feedings. Without these feedings, the adults could only have survived for a few days, not long enough for females to produce the next generation of eggs (Nasci and Miller 1996). The ships' crews must have provided some form of plant juice or sugar-laden feedings for its winged stowaways. Once they landed in the Caribbean, the mosquitoes quickly adapted to the tropical climate, so similar to their native habitat.

The mosquito responsible for spreading yellow fever outside of west Africa proved to be *Aedes aegypti*. This particular mosquito evolved a close relationship with humans as they settled down to farm and build settlements. The mosquitoes primarily became attracted to the water containers people made, finding them ideal for egg laying. As day feeders, the females in their search for blood meals also grew attracted to the lactic acid oxidation products in human sweat. Their most active times coincide with human activities in the early morning and late afternoon, and they hunt their prey between 50 cm (2 inches) and 1 m (about 3 feet) above the ground (Ribeiro 1996).

Wild *Aedes* females choose natural small containers of clean water, such as rot holes in trees or leaf axils of plants, in which to lay their eggs. They avoid water with dirt or sand bottoms. Each female lays about seventy eggs around the damp zone just above the water's edge, and the eggs hatch in installments over time. Several females may lay hundreds of eggs in the same container, forming a large mass of eggs above the water line. The eggs can go dormant for months if the container loses water, as long as there is some remaining dampness (Gillett 1971).

The virus does not harm the mosquito, and infected female mosquitoes pass the virus through the gametes to the eggs, thus maintaining the infection within the mosquito population without introduction from animal or human hosts (Benenson 1995). When infected mosquito eggs must wait out dry spells, the virus also goes dormant and waits with the unborn mosquito to come back to life when adequate moisture returns.

The yellow fever virus has coexisted with nocturnal wild *Aedes africanus* mosquitoes in the canopies of tropical west African forests for millennia. Monkeys, especially colobus and red-tailed guenon monkeys, living in the treetops of these forests serve as primary hosts without any ill effects from the blood-sucking female mosquitoes. Woodcutters felling trees in the forest inadvertently bring down hungry canopy mosquitoes along with the trees and serve as transient blood meals. The woodcutters carry the infection back to their villages where the local resident *Aedes* mosquitoes pick it up from them. Also, as farmers have moved closer to the tropical forests, the red-tailed guenon monkeys descend from their lofty habitat to raid village crops. This has allowed the local mosquitoes, particularly the *Aedes simpsoni* mosquitoes living among favored plant crops near villages, to sample the monkeys' infected blood and transmit it to the local folk (Cooper and MacCallum 1984). These mosquitoes like to lay their eggs in the water-containing axils of the plants (Stanley 1980). This process of transferring the yellow fever virus from the canopies to human settlements continues to this day, and the disease has become a common, mild childhood disease in west Africa (Burnet and White 1972).

Aedes aegypti established itself as the primary mosquito acclimated to villages and towns (Stanley 1980), picking up the yellow fever virus from infected people and transmitting it to other humans, thus breaking the infectious cycle between monkeys and mosquitoes of the tropical forests. When *Aedes aegypti* landed in the tropical New World, the virus managed to reach indigenous *Haemagogus* mosquitoes inhabiting the high canopies of tropical rain forests (Stanley 1980). When monkeys would come down from the treetops to raid village crops, the imported *Aedes* mosquitoes bit them and infected them with the virus, which they then carried back to their own treetop mosquito population. The natural infectious cycle between canopy mosquitoes and monkeys occurring in west Africa became duplicated in the tropical forests of Central and South America.

However, the virus has proved to be just as deadly to many of the New World monkey hosts as it can be to human hosts. Infected howler monkeys, squirrel monkeys, and owl monkeys can die from the disease, but infected woolly monkeys and capuchin monkeys show no symptoms of the disease (Nasci and Miller 1996).

American woodcutters experience similar attacks by treetop mosquitoes with felled trees as their west African counterparts, picking up the new virus from the mosquitoes. The men take the virus back to their villages where it is acquired by *Aedes aegypti* with the potential to repeat the human-to-human cycle. Infected monkeys raiding village gardens can also carry the virus to rural villages.

The Spaniards opened up new horizons for yellow fever when they started the transatlantic slave trade in 1501, buying slaves from Guinea traders for export to the New World. The first yellow fever epidemic documented in the New World occurred in the Caribbean in 1648, almost a century and a half later. *Aedes aegypti* and the yellow fever virus became established in their new outposts throughout tropical areas of the New World by the early part of the eighteenth century.

Infected mosquitoes traveled from the Caribbean islands to major port cities of eastern North America along shipping lines to cause outbreaks of the new disease in those cities. However, seasonal cooling in the northern temperate zones limited yellow fever outbreaks to the warm seasons. The tropical mosquito vectors died when temperatures dropped below 60°F (Garrett 1994). The disease had to be reintroduced during warm months for further outbreaks. Similar outbreaks also occurred in port cities of Spain, Portugal, and south Wales (Stanley 1980).

Epidemics of yellow fever played havoc with the history of the New World. Admiral Vernon set out from Southhampton, England, in 1741 with 27,000 men to conquer Mexico and Peru, only to fail in his efforts when yellow fever killed all but 7,000 of his troops. Napoleon's brother-in-law, General Charles Leclerc, encountered a similar problem when he tried to put down a rebellion in Santo Domingo in 1802, only to be defeated by yellow fever when 29,000 of his 33,000 soldiers died from the disease. The following year Napoleon offered to sell the Louisiana territory to the United States—coincidence? (Gillett 1971; McNeill 1976).

Outbreaks of yellow fever haunted the New World up until the early twentieth century. How people contracted the disease remained a mystery until 1881 when Carlos Finlay in Cuba discovered the role of the *Aedes aegypti* mosquito. At this time the French were trying to build a canal through the Isthmus of Panama, only to be defeated by mosquitoes carrying yellow fever and malaria (McNeill 1976).

The U.S. Army set up a yellow fever commission in Cuba led by Walter Reed. In 1900–1901 the commission proved that a virus carried by the mosquitoes caused yellow fever. Armed with this knowledge, the Americans took over building the Panama Canal from the French in 1904, and successfully completed it in 1914 by enforcing strict control over local mosquito populations. Lacking mosquito control methods elsewhere, outbreaks of yellow fever continued to flare up in various parts of South America. Rio de Janeiro suffered a major epidemic in 1928–29 in which almost 60 percent of those afflicted died (Sawyer 1951). A succession of campaigns were conducted to wipe out *Aedes aegypti* culminating in the use of DDT following World War II. This and the use of vaccines drastically reduced the mosquito population in the Americas, finally resulting in the eradication of yellow fever epidemics in the Western Hemisphere (McNeill 1976).

The Yellow Fever Viral
Impact on the Human Host

The yellow fever virus belongs to a group of RNA viruses known as flaviviruses. The virus protein core encloses itself in a lipoprotein envelope with projecting short spikes that help it attach to target cells. These spikes also set off the host immune intruder alarm that calls for various immune responses to neutralize the enemy virus. This response works somewhat in favor of the virus, drawing its favorite target cells, the macrophages that act to engulf foreign material. The confrontation allows the virus to attach and enter its target cell, where it sheds its alarming spiked envelope and quietly invades the network of microcanals coursing through the nucleus and cytoplasm of the macrophage to replicate undisturbed (Monath 1995).

Initial viral replication takes place within the infected macrophages inside the lymph nodes, and when the viral population increases, it spills out into the circulating blood system in search of new territory. The major attractions for the circulating virus become the resident macrophages of the liver, known as kupffer cells. Kupffer cells attach to the lining of the minute blood vessels interlaced among the liver cells, the hepatocytes. Kupffer cells act to remove circulating debris and foreign material, as well as aged and damaged red blood cells. Damage to the kupffer cells by the virus extends to neighboring liver cells that degenerate into translucent hyaline "councilman bodies," typical of yellow fever infection. Damaged cells appear scattered among healthy cells throughout the liver. The many metabolic activities of the hepatocytes (Downs 1975; Monath 1995) become disrupted, including the conversion of the yellow pigment in bile, known as bilirubin, to its greenish counterpart, biliverdin. This conversion is necessary for the excretion of bilirubin by way of bile through the small intestine. Otherwise the unaltered form builds up and circulates in the blood, leading to yellow jaundice as it collects in the skin, whites of the eyes, mucous membranes, and body fluids. Hence the name "yellow fever."

Trouble occurs in other organs, especially the tubules of the kidneys. Since the hepatic cells also produce clotting factors, disruption of clotting time can lead to internal bleeding, particularly within the gastrointestinal tract. The brain may suffer microscopic hemorrhages, and heart muscle may deteriorate with fatty degeneration (Ray 1984; Sydenstricker 1951).

The disease produced by the yellow fever virus can range from mild to severe, depending on the immune response of the host. Most attacks prove to be mild, with few if any symptoms, particularly among children living in endemic areas. They may have only a short period of fever and headache (Downs 1975).

Three to six days after the virus has invaded the lymphatics, symptoms abruptly appear, often with chilling, as the virus floods the circulating bloodstream. Severe headache, fever, backache, leg pains, and exhaustion appear and last about three days. The face becomes flushed, eyes become sensitive to light, and the tip of the tongue turns bright red. Nausea and vomiting with tenderness and discomfort affect the stomach, along with constipation (Downs 1975).

This initial phase of the disease often precedes a brief remission before the next phase of the illness takes over by the fourth day as liver damage begins to take its toll. While the headache and backache diminish, yellow jaundice gradually appears, and the face turns pale, sometimes with a bluish tinge. Depression and sometimes mental confusion occur, along with the feeling of exhaustion. Signs of internal bleeding from the gastrointestinal tract appear with vomit containing clear fluid with specks of old brown blood. Minute hemorrhages in the form of swollen and bleeding gums and nosebleed occur, small purplish pinpoint spots on the skin, known as petechiae, appear, and the pulse rate drops. Recovery can begin by the seventh or eighth day, and convalescence takes place rapidly with lasting immunity. Hiccups, copious vomiting, black stools, and inability to produce urine usually signal death from the disease. Fatality rates can range from 10 percent to 85 percent (Downs 1975; Sydenstricker 1951).

Yellow Fever Epilogue

No major urban epidemic of yellow fever in the Western Hemisphere has occurred since 1942 (Benenson 1995), indicating that campaigns to eradicate the primary mosquito vector, combined with mass vaccinations against the disease, have proved effective. Sporadic rural outbreaks of yellow fever among men working in the tropical forests of Central and South America have continued to occur from infected wild canopy mosquitoes. Compulsory vaccinations in west Africa brought urban epidemics to a halt there for a while, until the disruption of vaccination programs. Outbreaks began to reappear in eastern Nigeria in the early 1950s, and they have continued with increasing frequency. Hundreds of thousands of people became infected in Nigeria between 1987 and 1991 (Monath 1991, 1995).

Aedes aegypti was reintroduced during the 1970s and 1980s into Central and South America, and the southern United States, placing residents in these areas at risk for renewed urban yellow fever epidemics. *Aedes aegypti* has reached east Africa and northern Australia with a similar threat. Thirty thousand people died from the virus in southwest Ethiopia during the 1960s (Monath 1991, 1995).

Dengue Fever

The yellow fever virus apparently never reached eastward into Asia when it expanded out from its west African homeland (Nasci and Miller 1996). This is curious since *Aedes* mosquitoes capable of carrying the virus exist in eastern Asia. Perhaps competition from its closely related cousin, another flavivirus causing dengue fever, prevented the yellow fever virus from moving into Asia. Also, far less demand for slaves from west Africa limited slave trade (and the spread of the yellow fever virus) to Asia, while great demand for slaves from the Americas fueled the slave trade with west Africa.

The dengue fever virus appears to be transmitted through a natural wild mosquito and monkey cycle, similar to the cycle for the yellow fever virus, among wild mosquitoes living in the canopies of tropical forests in Asia. *Aedes niveus* mosquitoes inhabiting the canopies of Malaysian tropical forests provide the best example of this cycle, infecting not only monkeys, but also slow lorises, squirrels, and civets (Sabin 1959). And like the yellow fever virus, dengue fever viruses appear to be maintained independently within the mosquito population by passage through eggs to the young (Stanley 1980).

Evidence suggests that the Asian *Aedes albopictus* mosquito, commonly known as the tiger mosquito because of its black and white stripes, most likely became the bridge for dengue fever viral infection between canopy mosquitoes, tree-dwelling animals, and humans. Wild albopictus mosquitoes thrive in rural tropical areas, breeding primarily in tree holes, and taking blood meals from various mammals within their territory. When human settlements intruded into their territory, some variants of these mosquitoes adapted their egg-laying habits to manmade water containers, bamboo stumps, and coconut husk litter. This brought them into close contact with humans, but unlike aegypti, which prefers human blood, albopictus turns to human blood as a secondary choice (Benenson 1995; Hawley 1991).

Tiger mosquitoes thrive throughout tropical areas of rural Southeast Asia and India. Some variants of this species have been able to move northward into the temperate zones of Korea and Japan by adapting their life cycle to cooler temperatures. Eggs laid in the fall can withstand cold winters to hatch in the spring, unlike their tropical relatives' eggs, which cannot survive the cold (Hawley 1991).

The dengue fever virus appears to be centuries old in Southeast Asia, sporadically attacking humans via their mosquito vectors whenever people intruded into infected mosquito territory. At least four distinct strains of the virus have developed in different areas of Southeast Asia, originally separated by geographic barriers (Stanley 1980).

Merchant ships from the West brought *Aedes aegypti* mosquitoes to Asian port cities during the eighteenth century, where they picked up the virus. Aegypti became the ideal urban vector for dengue fever virus in place of the more rural tiger mosquito. *Aedes aegypti*, a seasoned ship traveler, also carried the virus to different parts of the globe over the next two centuries.

Epidemics of dengue fever transmitted by *Aedes aegypti* first appeared in Egypt and Java in 1779. The American city of Philadelphia recorded an outbreak in 1780. This new disease became known as "joint fever" or "breakbone fever" for the intense pain produced in the back and major joints (Sydenstricker 1951; Sabin 1959). Outbreaks followed in Cadiz, Seville, Granada, and Lima. Epidemics during the nineteenth century affected hundreds of thousands of people in India and the Americas, quickly spreading to west Africa, northern Australia, and some of the Pacific Islands (Stanley 1980). The virus was able to establish itself in new indigenous mosquito-monkey cycles in Polynesia and west Africa (Benenson 1995).

Primary Infection of Dengue Fever

The term *dengue fever* for this infection did not come into use until 1869 when the Royal College of Surgeons in London designated it as the proper term. *Aedes aegypti* mosquitoes first became implicated as the vector for the disease in 1906, but the virus itself was not identified until 1944. The role of *Aedes albopictus* as the original mosquito vector for humans became known in 1931 (Monath 1995; Sabin 1959).

Primary infection with dengue fever rarely kills, with less than one death out of ten thousand infections (Sydenstricker 1951). Children tend to have a mild form of the disease or show no symptoms at all, and the disease has been known as a common childhood infection in its homeland of Southeast Asia.

It takes newly infected mosquitoes at least nine days for enough of the virus to be produced within their midguts for infiltration of the saliva to infect human hosts with their bite. Unlike yellow fever virus, this virus does not target the liver. Dengue fever virus hunts for roving macrophages—monocytes, in small blood vessels—invading them as they try to squelch the invaders. This triggers a cascade of events with killer T cells alerted to destroy the infected white blood cells. The release of cytokines by the T cells and other released mediating substances during the battle have an adverse affect on the tiny blood vessels of the battlefield. They swell and leak fluid out into neighboring tissues (Monath 1995; Ray 1984). The symptoms of primary dengue fever stem from the immune reaction of the host.

Three to five days after the host receives the virus, symptoms appear abruptly: severe headache, particularly focused behind the eyes; severe pains in the back, knees, hips, and other joints; and aching muscles. Joint pain grows so intense that the victim can hardly move. Extreme weakness, loss of appetite, constipation, nausea, and vomiting follow, with body temperature rising to 104°F or higher within a few hours. Eyes turn red, the face becomes flushed, and a fleeting pale pink rash covers the knees, ankles, and elbows as lymph nodes swell (Benenson 1995; Johnson 1975; Sydenstricker 1951).

Often the fever drops temporarily about the fourth day with profuse sweating, sometimes with bleeding from the nose or gums and with diarrhea. After about twenty-four hours, the fever climbs even higher than before. The pulse slows, and a raised reddish rash appears over the trunk, spreading outward and lasting about three days before becoming itchy and finally fading away. Very small pinpoint skin hemorrhages may appear on the last day of the illness, usually on the feet and legs, occasionally in the armpits, wrists, hands, and mouth. They fade in one to three days, leaving behind a transitory brownish discoloration. Symptoms can last up to seven days or just three days, depending on the virus strain and the host immune system response. Symptoms also vary with each strain. Unlike yellow fever, recovery is slow and may take weeks (Benenson 1995; Johnson 1975a; Sabin 1959; Sydenstricker 1951).

By the 1920s urban epidemics of dengue fever recurred in the Americas, Australia, Greece, and Japan. Over 500,000 people became infected in Queensland, Australia, in 1925–26. Mosquitoes infected nearly 90 percent of the population of Athens during an epidemic in 1928–29. Infection of at least 30 percent of the population of Miami, Florida, occurred in 1934. Nearly half the population of Osaka, Japan, became infected in 1944. The Pacific Islands suffered epidemics of dengue fever during World War II (Benenson 1995; Sabin 1959; Stanley 1980; Sydenstricker 1951).

Mosquito eradication programs following World War II eliminated dengue fever from the Pacific Islands and from the Americas. However, by the 1970s *Aedes aegypti* mosquitoes returned to these areas, bringing back the dengue fever virus with them (Benenson 1995; Stanley 1980).

Dengue Hemorrhagic Fever

During World War II massive troop movements, distribution of war supplies, and flight of war refugees promoted the spread and mixing of different strains of the virus that had been geographically isolated from one another for centuries. The wars in Korea and Vietnam, as well as other social upheavals and civil conflicts raging throughout East Asia, added to the dislocation of the different strains of dengue virus throughout Asia. Rapid air travel has made it even easier for the different strains to be spread throughout the world, just in the past thirty years.

Now multiple strains of the virus have become endemic throughout the tropical regions of Asia, the Pacific Islands, and Queensland, Australia. All four major strains of the virus have become endemic to west Africa, and recently on the east coast of Africa and its offshore islands. Jeddah and Saudi Arabia have also reported more than one strain of the virus. All four major strains arrived in the Caribbean by 1977, with two or more of the strains extending into Central and South America. More than one strain was identified in Texas during the 1980s (Benenson 1995).

Outbreaks of dengue fever in Manila and Bangkok in 1954 showed a new side to this disease that had only been seen sporadically before: in Queensland, Australia (1897), South Africa (1927), Greece (1928), and Taiwan (1931) (Monath 1995). The usually mild dengue fever of children suddenly turned into a dangerous illness. Singapore was struck by this new form of dengue fever in 1960, and this attack was followed by outbreaks in Malaysia, South Vietnam, Indonesia, India, and Oceania, wherever *Aedes aegypti* had become well established in urban settings. Most of the victims were children under the age of eight (Johnson 1975b).

Apparently this serious malady strikes individuals who have had a previous mild infection with one viral strain followed by infection with a different viral strain. Infection from a single strain provides immunity to that particular strain but not against other strains. Instead of cross-immunity from one strain to another, the victim experiences cross-reaction. The host immune system overreacts to the familiarity of the virus as it replicates quickly within monocytes, triggering a massive immune response that wrecks the small blood vessels of the vascular system. Diffuse leakage from damaged small blood vessels leads to loss of circulating fluid as fluid gets pulled out of circulation and dumped into the tissues and body cavities. Blood clotting factors become disrupted, leading to internal focal bleeding in most organs. When blood vessels leak severely, the circulatory system collapses into volemic (low fluid volume) shock, followed by death (Monath 1995; Ray 1984; Rothman and Ennis 2000).

Initial symptoms resemble the early phase of primary dengue fever infection, with abrupt onset, fever, nausea, and vomiting. Sometimes there can be a dry cough with congested throat. By the second or third day, small pinpoint hemorrhages appear on the face and/or arms and legs, followed by larger hemorrhages or bruises under the skin. Hemorrhages into major organs can also occur. Sudden severe pain and tenderness in the abdomen signals gastrointestinal bleeding and a severe turn for the worse. By the third or fourth day this leads to vomiting of large amounts of old blood, which looks like coffee grounds. This lasts from twelve to twenty-four hours, followed by a fall in temperature and blood pressure, rapid weak pulse, pale face, and profuse sweating, while the arms and legs turn mottled purple or brown and cool to the touch. Restlessness and apprehension signal the onset of shock as the circulatory system collapses before the sixth day of the illness. Fatality rates can reach 50 percent (Benenson 1995; Johnson 1975b).

The mixing of two or more of the dengue fever viruses with *Aedes aegypti* mosquitoes has produced urban outbreaks of dengue hemorrhagic fever among children throughout Southeast Asia, the Philippines, South Pacific Islands, the Caribbean, and South America since the 1980s (Benenson 1995). The 1981 outbreak of dengue hemorrhagic fever in Cuba followed interaction with Vietnam for professional training and reconstruction projects. Apparently the exchange brought a second strain of the dengue fever virus to Cuba to cause havoc among Cuban children who already had been sensitized to another strain of the virus (Garrett 1994).

CONCLUDING COMMENTS

Dengue fever and yellow fever share the same urban mosquito vector, the globe-trotting *Aedes aegypti*. Yellow fever came out of west Africa, while dengue fever came from Southeast Asia. The two would never have overlapped if not for global commerce. Where yellow fever reigned from the seventeenth century through the early twentieth century as the most prevalent arbovirus, dengue fever has since assumed that role in the world, and dengue hemorrhagic fever has emerged as a new disease (Lederberg et al. 1992).

The natural vector for dengue fever, *Aedes albopictus*, has recently managed to reach outside its Asian homeland, thanks to modern commerce.

This black and white mosquito, known as the tiger mosquito, immigrated from Japan to Houston, Texas, in 1985 aboard a freighter loaded with used tires for the retread industry. The mosquitoes had been using the water accumulated in the old tires for breeding. The immigrant Japanese variant of *Aedes albopictus* tolerates temperate weather, and its eggs are capable of withstanding cold winters. Soon after its arrival in the United States, it promptly headed northward by way of truck transport of the imported tires, reaching the Great Lakes area in less than fifteen years (Hawley 1996; Rothman and Ennis 2000). We know that some of the immigrant mosquitoes carried the virus with them (Lederberg et al. 1992).

The biggest problem with the introduction of *Aedes albopictus* to North America lies not so much in the threat of dengue fever, as in the catholic tastes of the mosquito, permitting it to acquire native arboviruses from feeding on birds and animals. They more likely will be able to transmit native arboviruses to people than local mosquitoes, with their habit of hanging around people's houses. Arboviruses sporadically introduced to humans may have opportunity to become epidemic threats if this mosquito interferes with the natural mosquito–animal host cycle (Lederberg et al. 1992).

While in the past the most dangerous arboviruses have been restricted to remote areas around the globe, the possibility of outbreaks increases with rampant human population growth into rural areas throughout the world. Air travel opens up the potential for them to leave their native lands. Chikungunya, a viral infection similar to dengue fever and transmitted by *Aedes aegypti*, has already migrated from Africa into Southeast Asia and the Philippines. West Nile virus, carried by wild birds native to parts of Africa, recently moved into other parts of Africa, the Middle East, southwest Asia, and southern Europe (Johnson 1975c). This same virus showed up on the East Coast of North America in 1999, and, having been picked up by local mosquitoes and migratory birds, it has moved across the United States.

The future mix of rapid travel, growing populations seeking out more land, and the globe-trotting domestic Aedes mosquitoes throughout the world most likely will change the geographic patterns of many arboviruses. One country's local arbovirus may well be another country's unwelcome and dangerous immigrant.

CHAPTER 19

FOOD FOR THOUGHT

The Mystery Diseases

Y ou are what you eat—or, more correctly, your body builds on what you feed it. We all need the same basic ingredients from our diets for adequate human functioning and health. This includes sufficient amounts of protein, certain fats, carbohydrates, vitamins, minerals, and fiber. Disease and poor nutrition often operate synergistically. The immune system, like the rest of the body, cannot function effectively when adequate amounts of required nutrients are lacking in the diet. Outbreaks of disease often shadow times of famine.

Carbohydrates provide the chief sources of energy for the body. Plant foods, such as fruits, vegetables, legumes, seeds, nuts, and whole-grain cereals, contain carbohydrates. Plant foods also provide fiber needed for healthy functioning of the gut. Protein consists of amino acids that the body uses primarily for a variety of building materials. The body can manufacture many of the amino acids it needs, but at least eight of them have to come from outside the body, and must be consumed at the same time in proper proportions before the body can use them. Animal meats contain all the essential amino acids, while most plant food sources lack one or more of the necessary ones. When the diet lacks meat, the needed amino acids can be gained from plant foods only by mixing different ones that contain complementary types of amino acids.

Different kinds of fats come from animal and plant sources. They break down into various fatty acids used by the body tissues, and they also act as back-up energy sources for the body. Vitamins and minerals come from a variety of plant and animal sources. Vitamins help make enzymes work. Enzymes act as the catalysts for reactions essential for metabolism, growth, and development. All cells of the body need minerals, and they play various roles in certain body functions.

Whenever certain nutrients are missing from the diet or are in short supply for a long time, bodily functions requiring those nutrients become dysfunctional. When one aspect of bodily functioning is disturbed, the whole body suffers, since the human body forms an integrated system. Amazingly, the human body can take a lot of punishment and nutritional neglect for some time before it displays evidence of system breakdown. This allowed our ancestors to weather seasonal changes in food resources. Human beings can usually survive hard times when our food supplies fall short of meeting all our nutritional needs over the short haul, but if deprivation lasts too long, we suffer the consequences. Those people who have greater needs for any missing nutrients suffer the most, while those individuals who can survive on minimal amounts of missing nutrients survive much better.

Human evolutionary history has been checkered with periods of optimum food supplies and poor or negligible food supplies, related to cultural and/or ecological upheavals. Wide swings in nutrition may have contributed to shorter lifespans and poor infant survival rates in many societies, acting as a brake on population growth. Wherever adequate nutrition lasts for more than one generation, lifespans lengthen and infant survival rates increase, allowing for population growth.

Food Choices and Availability

Over twenty thousand varieties of edible plant foods exist around the world (Pfeiffer 1975). They provide a rich diversity of plant food sources for human consumption. Environmental and geographical barriers throughout most of human evolution have limited the availability and types of plant foods, as well as animal foods, in the different regions of the world. However, each ecological region used by humans usually could produce enough diversity of food sources to meet basic nutritional needs for people from early times onward.

As early human beings spread over the globe, evolutionary adaptations to local food resources took place. The human body has the evolutionary capacity to adjust to diverse environments and diets. Evolutionary adjustments in basic nutritional needs have ranged from low marginal subsistence to highly dependent subsistence levels with regard to certain nutrients found in local food sources. Where certain required nutrients fell short, humans adjusted by subsisting on marginal levels of those nutrients. People living in regions containing overabundant supplies of certain nutrients eventually developed a need for greater amounts of those nutrients than did their counterparts in other regions. This may explain why so much variation in individual requirements for various nutrients developed. Long-term evolutionary interaction with specific regional food sources may also help explain why today many people exhibit sensitivity or allergic reactions to certain foods that would have been foreign to their early ancestors (Pfeiffer 1975).

Our earliest human ancestors survived as omnivorous opportunists searching for both plant and animal foods. Plant foods, more accessible than animal foods, formed the bulk of their diet. They most likely moved about from one seasonal food source area to another, as diverse plant foods became available, such as seeds, nuts, fruits, tubers, and vegetables. Small animals, as well as occasional large animals, could be taken when opportunity allowed. The hunting and gathering Bushmen of the Kalahari Desert in southern Africa exemplify how our earliest ancestors must have lived off the land. Bushmen diets generally provide all the nutrients that they need from a variety of seasonal plants that make up the bulk of their food, with occasional meat and fat from hunted animal sources. The small, slim bodies and slow maturation of the Bushmen reflect evolutionary adaptation to seasonal fluctuations of food sources in their environment, allowing them to survive during occasional shortages of food (McElroy and Townsend 1989).

Where food resources proved inadequate, our ancestors most likely moved on to other areas in their quest for the nutrients their bodies needed. Some, such as people around the North Sea, discovered fishing and shellfish gathering as valuable food resources. Some avid hunters, such as the Inuit (Eskimo), adapted to cold-weather areas and adjusted to diets high in animal meat and fat, with few plant foods available. Wherever our ancestors went, they exploited available food resources to meet their nutritional needs.

Environment determines what food sources will be available, but human beings decide what qualifies as food. What one culture considers food, another may not. For example, people in the United States do not consider dogs as food, but dogs constitute a choice food item in many parts of Asia. Corn (maize) may be a food item in the Americas, but it serves only as animal food in some countries. Southwestern Pueblo native peoples do not recognize fish to be appropriate food, while most people in the United States consume fish readily.

Sometimes societies place restrictions of certain foods on all their members, or on particular members or age groups. Most Christians eat pork, while Muslims and Jews do not. Some Christian sects do not eat meat, while most do. Many African societies do not allow weanling children to eat protein foods until they reach a certain age. Pregnant women in many societies around the world are often prohibited from eating certain foods deemed harmful to their unborn fetus.

The Mystery Diseases: For Lack of Certain Nutrients

The agricultural revolution, followed by civilization, brought cultural and dietary changes to most people around the globe. The first farmers had the best of both food worlds, a domestic staple plant supply mixed with gathered wild plant and animal foods for a diverse and nutritious diet. Domesticated animals eventually supplanted wild animal foods in many parts of the Old World. Eventually, overreliance on specific domesticated staple plant foods at the expense of food diversity often led to chronic and sometimes severe nutritional deficiencies. Diets restricted to domesticated staple plant foods may provide ample calories for energy and population growth, but they often lack certain nutrients needed for good health and longevity.

Ecological upsets, such as drought and floods, have often led to famine and severe nutritional deficits, while wars and sociocultural changes usually played havoc with both diets and available food resources. Nature and culture have always interacted to affect availability and choice in human food resources.

Culture dictates not only what constitutes food, but also how to prepare food. Processing can affect the quality of food, altering either the nutrient content or the bioavailability of the nutrients. Some processing methods can alter the chemical nature of nutrients in negative as well as positive ways. Food processing can either bind nutrients so that they cannot readily be absorbed through the small intestine and used by the body, or can break down bonds that would otherwise keep nutrients from being absorbed. Overcooking can also destroy nutrients such as water-soluble B complex vitamins and vitamin C.

Mysterious diseases, often unexplained, appeared throughout the world at various times, sometimes associated with certain diets or with specific social groups. Some were thought to be infectious diseases, poisoned foods, or genetic disorders. By the nineteenth century obvious associations with specific dietary deficiencies became known for some of the mystery diseases, but not until the 1920s and 1930s could we correlate specific nutrient deficiencies with the various dietary disorders.

Beriberi

Sometimes food processing leaches out nutrients from plant foods. The remaining food substance often consists of empty calories—carbohydrates without companion vitamins. Energy can be extracted from these empty calories, but the enzyme systems involved lack the necessary vitamins naturally found with the carbohydrate food. To make the systems function properly on these empty calories, the necessary vitamins have to be taken from other sources. If the diet is missing alternative sources of the missing vitamins, nutritional deficiency disease develops.

Records of the use of polished white rice as a staple food first appeared during the third century B.C. in China (Wood 1979), and from there it spread to other parts of Asia. The rice gets milled and washed until all the water-soluble vitamins leach out, in order to reach the pure whiteness preferred over the dull brown color of natural whole-grain rice. Wheat flour similarly became transformed from a vitamin-rich food source to a vitamin-empty white flour during the early twentieth century in Western countries.

Chinese physicians noticed the appearance of a new disease following the introduction of polished rice, and by the seventh century A.D. this disease had been well defined by characteristic symptoms. The disease became known as beriberi, endemic among rice eaters in the south of China, but nonexistent among wheat and millet eaters in northern parts of China. This mysterious disease also became well known among the Japanese as *kakke*, especially prominent among upper-class people who disdained any form of rice not highly polished (Guggenheim 1981; Pfeiffer 1975).

The disease commonly occurred throughout Southeast Asia wherever polished rice served as the staple food with little else in the diet. Groups of men forced to live and work together in various enterprises from mining to shipping, inmates in crowded insane asylums and prisons, as well as men in military camps often suffered from this mysterious disease (Guggenheim 1981).

The industrialization process in Southeast Asia during the late nineteenth century compounded the problems with polished rice. Steam-powered mills took over the processing, producing large quantities of rice quickly and cheaply, and efficiently removing all nutrients from the grain. Often this highly processed, cheap rice represented the only food source for poor and confined individuals. The disease became more rampant, especially among the Japanese (Guggenheim 1981).

Studies in Malaysia by Braddon at the beginning of the twentieth century confirmed earlier suspicions that dietary dependence on polished rice caused the disease. Braddon described how Malays using crude pounding methods and little washing to process their rice lost very little of the vitamin content. Tamil immigrants from southeast India soaked their rice in the hulls in a process known as parboiling, and then dried it in the sun before cooking. This process helped retain some of the vitamins in the grain. Chinese immigrants working in remote tin mines ate imported polished rice provided by their employers. This rice proved to be empty of vitamins, and the disease known as beriberi commonly occurred among them (Guggenheim 1981; Wood 1979).

Rice cooked without polishing contains all of the B vitamin complex. Parboiled rice loses most of its B vitamins, but retains thiamine (B1), niacin, and some riboflavin from the B complex. Polished rice loses all of the B vitamins except for a trace amount of folic acid (Kirschmann 1975). The Japanese and other Southeast Asians further compounded the loss of thiamine with their polished rice by eating it with raw fish that contains the enzyme thiamase. Fish have to be cooked to inactivate this enzyme, otherwise it destroys whatever thiamine may be present in the diet (Pfeiffer 1975).

The total loss of thiamine from polished rice with little if any other source for the vitamin available in the diet leads to the deficiency disease beriberi. Thiamine combines with pyruvic acid to help produce quick energy from the carbohydrates in rice and other plant foods for all cells in the body. Cells in the nervous system depend the most on this form of energy, and they usually become the first cells to suffer from thiamine deficiency (Scrimshaw 1975).

Symptoms of beriberi can vary from mild to severe, depending on how long the deficiency lasts. Mild symptoms often appear with temporary depletion of thiamine from the diet, but they disappear when the vitamin is restored to the diet. Mild symptoms are often vague, with loss of appetite, constipation, fatigue, insomnia, headaches, poor concentration, faulty memory, and irritability. If the deficiency remains uncorrected, other symptoms, such as numbness, tingling and burning sensation in the hands and feet, tender calves in the lower legs, and vague abdominal pains, follow. Muscle cramps, especially at night, become frequent (Pfeiffer 1975; Scrimshaw 1975).

If the deficiency continues for too long, more severe symptoms develop with mental disturbances, severe weight loss, plugged hair follicles, weak and sore muscles, paralysis of the legs and sometimes the arms, and enlarged heart. Death can occur with congestive heart failure associated with fluid retention in the legs, abdomen, and lungs. "Wet" beriberi refers to thiamine deficiency disease accompanied by this fluid retention (Pfeiffer 1975; Scrimshaw 1975). "Dry" beriberi refers to the deficiency disease dominated by neurological symptoms causing disability that culminates in death. Sensation disappears in hands and feet, and motor nerve function disappears, resulting in the inability to control movements. Confusion followed by coma in the final stages precedes death (Pfeiffer 1975; Scrimshaw 1975).

Nursing mothers severely deficient in thiamine pass the deficiency to their infants. The babies become restless and pale. They vomit, refuse to suckle, and cannot sleep. Eventually they have difficulty breathing, turn blue, and die. Infants with less deficient nursing mothers develop symptoms resembling adult beriberi (Scrimshaw 1975).

Today, throughout the modern world, most food processors fortify grains with synthetic vitamins to replace the natural vitamins lost in the processing. This has drastically reduced the overall global incidence of beriberi. However, sporadic cases of beriberi can still be found among poor people in times of famine who have nothing to eat other than polished rice without vitamin fortification.

Pellagra

Having been ravaged by infectious diseases for centuries, eighteenth-century Europe was struck by a new and mysterious disease. The Spanish physician Gaspar Casal first noted the disease in 1730 among poor rural peasants in Asturia, northern Spain. He called it *mal de la rosa* because of the red skin associated with it. Casal related the disease to their poor diet, consisting primarily of bread or gruel made from imported corn (maize). The disease, later to be known as pellagra, also occurred among poor peasants subsisting on corn in northern Italy, southern France, Austria, Romania, and the Balkans. By the nineteenth century the disease had appeared among the poor in Egypt. The disease also appeared in parts of India and southern Africa among poor peasants subsisting primarily on millet. The mysterious disease among corn eaters in

Europe persisted until the beginning of the twentieth century, then disappeared when agrarian reforms improved people's diets (Guggenheim 1981; Roe 1973).

Corn had been introduced to Europe from the New World in the early part of the sixteenth century. At first, some Europeans planted it in herbal gardens as a curiosity, but by the eighteenth century peasants planted it for use as a highly productive food crop. The new grain was used as a substitute for other grains in the diets of poor peasants (Guggenheim 1981; Roe 1973).

The same mysterious disease made its appearance among imprisoned federal troops at Andersonville, Georgia, during the American Civil War in 1864. The disease also haunted poor sharecroppers in the South, particularly blacks, from the Civil War until the early twentieth century. Like the corn eaters of Europe, they ate mainly cornmeal mush or bread with little else (Roe 1973; Wood 1979).

In 1914 pellagra officially became recognized as a nutritional disorder. In 1935 the missing nutrient responsible for the disease was found to be niacin (B3), one of the vitamins from the B complex. This knowledge brought an end to the disease in the southern United States following World War II (Guggenheim 1981; Roe 1973).

The highest quantities of niacin occur in animal protein foods and tuna fish, followed by sunflower seeds, whole wheat flour, halibut, brewer's yeast, peas, and peanuts (Gerras 1977). Small amounts may be present in other plant foods, such as corn. Animal protein and some plant proteins also provide the body with the amino acid tryptophan, which can be converted into small amounts of niacin. Most of the other B vitamins will not be present when niacin deficiency occurs, and their absence contributes to the various symptoms of pellagra (Roe 1973).

Corn lacks the amino acid tryptophan, and although corn contains small amounts of niacin, the vitamin cannot be released from its biochemical bonds with ordinary cooking. When the diet lacks other sources of niacin, long-term corn eaters become niacin deficient. People totally dependent on millet can also develop niacin deficiency even though millet contains some tryptophan that could be converted to niacin. Millet may contain an amino acid imbalance when too much of the amino acid leucine interferes with the conversion of niacin from tryptophan (Roe 1973).

Niacin comes in two forms, and both can serve to form a coenzyme vital for the integrity of the cells in all of the tissues of the body. Consequently, deficiency of this vitamin disturbs cell maintenance and cell division to form new cells. Tissues with the highest cellular turnover rate, the skin and lining of the gastrointestinal tract, become the first to feel the effects of niacin deficiency (Roe 1973). Cell turnover slows, and the vulnerable tissues become prone to irritation and breakdown.

Many poor and elderly people subsisting on low levels of niacin with protein-poor diets develop mild (subclinical) pellagra. They exhibit poor appetite, dull headache, dizziness, weakness (especially in the legs), irritability, depression, sleeplessness, mental fatigue, digestive disturbances, and sore tongue. Some develop a skin rash resembling prickly heat, followed by dry, scaly skin with fine wrinkles and coarse texture (Gerras 1977; Scrimshaw 1975; Spies 1951). Symptoms of pellagra often appear seasonally, showing up in the spring when food supplies fall short, and then disappearing with more plentiful and diverse foods until the following spring (Roe 1973).

Pellagra unfolds progressively. Symptoms increase with prolonged niacin deficiency. Digestive disorders, dermatitis, and dementia often are cited as the classical "three Ds" of severe forms of this disease. The tongue, mouth, and throat become very sore and swollen with burning sensations aggravated by hot or acid foods. The abdomen distends and hurts, usually accompanied by watery diarrhea and severe weight loss. Areas of the skin exposed to sunlight turn red, resembling sunburn. Other easily irritated parts of the skin, such as elbows, knees, groin, feet, areas under breasts, and underarms, also turn red. Reddened areas peel and turn reddish-brown with a distinct border to adjacent normal skin. The affected skin thickens while turning rough and scaly. Prolonged niacin deficiency wreaks havoc on the nervous system. Burning sensations of the hands, feet, and other body parts, with altered tendon reflexes, lead to altered muscle coordination, numbness, or paralysis. Psychotic symptoms include periods of manic depression, apprehension, hallucinations, confusion, delirium, and disorientation. Many victims of pellagra over the years have ended up in asylums for the insane. Death occurs in 50 percent of severe cases, generally from heart failure (Roe 1973; Scrimshaw 1975; Spies 1951).

Could this new disease, pellagra, actually have been an old disease of the New World where corn originated? Early Spanish conquerors did not mention any signs of the disease among the people of the Americas. Archaeological records show that prehistoric Native Americans domesticated corn and used it as a major food source for centuries before European invasion. Analysis of early Native American diets reveals that corn provided only a portion of a very diversified diet, often consisting of beans, squash, and other plant foods along with animal protein. This diversity alone would have prevented niacin deficiency.

What if the prehistoric farmers of the Americas faced periodic food shortages and famines similar to those of their European counterparts, forcing them to depend on corn for survival? Pellagra would still have been a rarity because of the way they processed their corn from prehistory up to this day, as seen in Mexico. Native Americans soak corn kernels with wood ash (alkali) in earthenware jars to loosen the outer layers. This makes it easier to grind the corn into a paste for cooking round, flat griddle cakes known as tortillas. The alkali treatment releases niacin from its biochemical bonds, making it available as a nutrient in the diet (McElroy and Townsend 1989; Roe 1973). Unfortunately, when corn gained export to Europe, the method for processing it did not go with it. Otherwise, outbreaks of pellagra probably would not have occurred in Europe.

Scurvy

Scurvy arises from a deficiency of ascorbic acid, commonly known as vitamin C. Most animals produce their own vitamin C from glucose by way of glucuronic acid, and they never suffer from a deficiency of the vitamin. Their livers produce whatever amounts are needed, and it gets distributed throughout their tissues (Scrimshaw 1975).

Humans and great apes are among the few animals that cannot make their own vitamin C. They lack the liver enzyme, 1-gluconulactone oxidase, necessary to synthesize the vitamin (Pfeiffer 1975). This evolutionary quirk made humans and great apes dependent on food sources for the vitamin. Perhaps their common primordial ancestors could find far more of the vitamin in food than needed, making it unnecessary to synthesize it in their bodies.

A wide variety of biochemical reactions in the body require vitamin C. The immune macrophages use large amounts of the vitamin to fight off foreign invaders. Among its many other duties, vitamin C helps detoxify harmful toxins introduced into the body, and it acts as an antioxidant to disarm free radicals that can damage tissues. It is vital for the formation of collagen—the protein substance used to build connective tissues in skin, ligaments, and bones, and in healing wounds. Vitamin C activates folic acid from the B vitamin complex so that it can be used to form red blood cells, and it helps iron absorption, protects other vitamins from biochemical damage, and regulates cholesterol (Pfeiffer 1975).

The threat of vitamin C deficiency has haunted human populations throughout history. Many of our early ancestors adapted to surviving on very low levels of the vitamin (Pfeiffer 1975) in order to weather seasonal shortages of fruits and vegetables, the major sources of vitamin C. Where diets fell short of fruits and vegetables, particularly in the far northern climates, the vitamin could be found in raw meat, since it saturates animal tissues, especially livers. Raw liver would have provided high quantities of several other vitamins as well as vitamin C. When our ancestors discovered fire and began cooking their meat, much of the vitamin C would have been lost, since heat destroys it.

Fortunately, serious effects of vitamin C deficiency take at least three months to develop (Carpenter 1986). Symptoms have often appeared in the spring in temperate zones, and at the end of dry seasons in tropical zones, disappearing when fresh fruits and vegetables again become available (Scrimshaw 1975).

Anemia develops when vitamin C is not around to activate folic acid for making new red blood cells and help with the absorption of iron needed for hemoglobin development. Symptoms of fatigue, weakness, and shortness of breath develop. Bones and joints ache from weakened collagen development. Wounds heal slowly, and the immune system grows weak (Carpenter 1986; Scrimshaw 1975).

These symptoms disappear when vitamin C reappears in the diet. Otherwise, more obvious signs of deficiency begin to develop about six or seven weeks later. Damaged collagen formation in the skin leaves it dry and rough. Hair follicles on the buttocks, backside of the calves and thighs, abdomen, and forearms plug up and turn into hard lumps with the hairs breaking off or coiling into the follicles. More severe symptoms develop over a period of several weeks, or much sooner when the afflicted individual becomes stressed. Prolonged vitamin C deficiency weakens the body's ability to react to stress and prompts rapid development of scurvy (Carpenter 1986; Pfeiffer 1975; Scrimshaw 1975).

Severe scurvy weakens the connective tissues throughout the body as collagen is depleted. Tiny blood vessels become so fragile and porous that they leak blood into surrounding tissues to cause pinpoint hemorrhages in the skin. The gum tissues in the mouth swell, turn spongy and purple, and bleed easily. Infection cannot be stopped in the gums, and the teeth quickly decay. The damaged gum tissues, bleeding and infected, produce a foul mouth odor. Bone tissue around tooth sockets recedes, and the teeth loosen and fall out. The bones lose minerals, becoming thin and fragile, particularly the vertebrae of the spine (Jaffe 1972). Wounds do not heal at all. Exhaustion follows any activity. Severe pain and difficult breathing often accompany exertion. Muscles, joints, and bones suffer when subjected to the slightest pressure or trauma. Sudden pain in feet and legs just from walking or marching develops as weakened ligaments cannot support the joints in motion. Feet and lower legs often turn black and blue from hemorrhaging beneath the skin. Similar subsurface bleeding frequently affects the back side of the thighs, as well as any joint or muscle of the body exposed to trauma or pressure. Prolonged severe scurvy usually ends with death caused by heart failure (Carpenter 1986; Pfeiffer 1975; Scrimshaw 1975).

Following several weeks or months of deficiency, severe symptoms of scurvy develop in children and infants (Jaffe 1972). Developing teeth and growing bones of children form poorly and remain thin and porous. Sometimes bleeding occurs in the shaft of long bones where it interfaces with the cartilage-growing end plate, causing the bone ends to dislocate, separate, or become impacted into the shaft, leading to bone deformities (Schrimshaw 1975).

Babies develop severe hemorrhaging beneath the outer covering (the periosteum) of long bones. The periosteum loosens and bellows outward from its bony anchor to create large outward swellings. Movement causes the baby to cry with pain. Usually the lower end of the femur in the thigh, the upper end of the humerus in the upper arm, and both ends of the tibiae in the lower legs receive the greatest damage. The mid-rib ends facing the chest can also be affected when small swellings referred to as "scorbutic rosary" show up (Scrimshaw 1975). Infants with severe scurvy generally die from some infection, since the deficiency affects their immature immune systems (Jaffe 1972).

Infant scurvy usually appears in artificially fed babies lacking any vitamin C source. Human breast milk generally contains sufficient amounts of the vitamin, even when the mother's diet contains little vitamin C (Carpenter 1986). Only when the mother has suffered from complete, prolonged deficiency will her baby suffer.

The earliest description of infantile scurvy appeared in Europe in 1650 (Jaffe 1972). Undoubtedly, instances of infant scurvy showed up unrecognized throughout human history.

When bottle feeding using evaporated cow's milk became popular during the mid-nineteenth century, scurvy cropped up frequently in infants between six and twelve months of age. Epidemics occurred in institutions housing young infants, and the disease became known as "Barlow's disease," after a British physician who determined that vitamin C deficiency caused it. Eventually, infant formula received fortification with the vitamin to prevent this deficiency disease (Carpenter 1986; Scrimshaw 1975).

Sparse evidence exists for scurvy in ancient human bones. Ancient cities under extended siege, populations suffering from prolonged famines, prisoners, and stranded armies with limited supplies of fresh fruits and vegetables would have been at risk for scurvy. Parts of medieval Europe most likely suffered seasonal bouts of mild scurvy, and reports of scurvy appeared among the first crusaders (Guggenheim 1981).

I found evidence of scurvy in a young woman who had lived at Corinth, Greece, under the Frankish occupation during the thirteenth century. She must have been confined for several months and limited to a diet lacking both vegetables and fruits. It is highly unusual for an individual to develop severe scurvy in the Mediterranean region. Her bones appear paper thin, especially the vertebrae in her spine. She showed signs of periosteal hemorrhaging on the bones in her feet, lower legs, and right forearm. Her gums had rotted and her jawbone had shrunk. She had lost several teeth, while the remaining teeth exhibited large caries.

Famine may have led to the presence of the disorder in the bones of a group of ancient Maya adults (Saul 1972, 1973). Prolonged siege of sixteenth-century Antwerp produced evidence of scurvy on some adult bones (Janssens et al. 1993). Scurvy was a scourge among early whalers in Arctic waters, with evidence for it discovered on the bones of seventeenth- to eighteenth-century Dutch whalers buried at Spitsbergen on the island of Zeeusche Uytkyck (Maat 1982). The raw meat diet of native Inuits in the Arctic spared them from the deficiency, while European explorers in the Arctic who spurned the native diet suffered severely from the disorder (Carpenter 1986).

By the end of the fifteenth century Europeans had launched their global explorations. Long ocean journeys with poor food provisions that lacked fruits and vegetables caused ships' crews to experience scurvy after three months at sea. Many crew members died from the deficiency, and sometimes only a few survived to return home. Scurvy remained a serious problem associated with long sea voyages to the end of the eighteenth century, before the diets of sailors improved.

In 1605 an East India Company physician named Lancaster became the first to use lemon juice to prevent scurvy, but most other physicians disregarded his advice. Another physician named Lind published a paper on the use of lemon juice as a preventive in 1757, but only after his death in 1795 did the British navy begin to follow his recommendations. Fresh fruits and vegetables were finally used to bolster sailor's diets at the beginning of the nineteenth century (Guggenheim 1981).

Rickets

Rickets primarily attacks the very young. The disorder appears mostly during the rapid growth period between four months and two years of age. Growing bones and teeth soften because normal mineralization cannot take place. Various skeletal deformities develop, depending on how long and at what age bones did not receive adequate mineralization (Weech 1951). Softened bones also tend to fracture easily.

Skull bones of young infants yield easily to pressure. With rickets the bones become thin, the anterior fontanel (soft spot) closes more slowly than usual, the skull takes on a square shape, and a flat spot develops on the side of the head habitually favored by the baby. Fast growing rib ends enlarge and become rounded, often bending inward, putting pressure on the lungs. Learning to sit up and walk puts pressure on soft bones of the limbs, back, pelvis and rib cage. The lower back becomes twisted under the weight of the upper body, and the pelvic bones flatten. Ends of long bones in the arms and legs enlarge and affect the developing wrists and ankles. Applied pressure bends the long bones into deformity. Bones in the fingers enlarge with excessive build-up of outer bone. Movement becomes painful, so the baby sits for hours, placing more pressure on the weakened skeleton (Weech 1951). Developing teeth show defects and erupt more slowly than usual, often failing to appear in normal sequence (Steinbock 1976).

Normal mineralization of bones and teeth requires adequate absorption and regulation of calcium and phosphorus in the body. Vitamin D deficiency results in poor mineralization. This vitamin is crucial for the absorption of calcium and phosphorus from the intestine and for availability of the minerals in the proper balance for use by bone and dental tissues.

Vitamin D is often called the "sunshine vitamin." The human body can make ample amounts of the vitamin from precursors beneath skin tissue when exposed to sunlight. Small amounts of the vitamin also exist in fish, egg yolk, and liver (Pfeiffer 1975).

Excess vitamin D can be stored in fat tissues for future use. Newborns usually possess enough of the vitamin for their first few months of life, acquired from their mothers before birth and stored in their livers. For this reason, young infants lacking sun exposure or dietary vitamin D generally do not develop signs of deficiency until they reach four to six months of age, when rapid growth takes its toll on the vitamin.

Rickets can develop in children up to fifteen years of age, following several months of deficiency as the youngsters use up their liver stores and lack new sources. Developing bone deformities do not occur as severely in the child as they do in the infant (Steinbock 1976). However, bowlegs and spine and pelvic deformities can be pronounced, and bones tend to fracture easily.

Mature bones of adults can also succumb to prolonged vitamin D deficiency, a condition known as osteomalacia. Bone tissue constantly undergoes remodeling throughout life, as old bone cells are replaced with new ones. This process requires a steady supply of calcium and phosphorus. Without vitamin D to maintain normal mineralization during bone turnover, mature bones will soften, bend, and fracture readily (Steinbock 1976).

Primarily, vitamin D deficiency derives from lack of sunshine for prolonged periods without any available dietary sources. Arctic inhabitants, who lack adequate sunlight throughout the year, can meet their vitamin D needs with a diet of fish and raw liver. During the nineteenth century, cod liver oil provided an effective cure for rickets (Guggenheim 1981).

The earliest known evidence of rickets comes from nine-thousand-year-old human settlements in the Iron Gate (Djerdap) Gorges region of the Danube River, located in a triangular area between Romania, Bulgaria, and Serbia in the Balkans. These people had settled in the bottom of the river's deep gorge, which was densely forested and remained covered in shadow most of the day (Zivanovic 1982). Signs of rickets in the bones of young children from these settlements suggest that the young spent their first years inside the dark settlement and away from sunlight.

Similar environmental absence of sunlight affects pygmy children living in the dark tropical forests of the Congo in Africa. They receive very little exposure to sunlight, and in addition, their dark skin filters out ultraviolet light. These children commonly suffer from rickets (Wood 1979).

References to rickets appear in medical literature dating back to 300 B.C. in China, and some evidence of osteomalacia has been found in a few early Egyptian skeletons (Ortner and Putschar 1981). Soranus of Ephesus on the western coast of Anatolia described infantile rickets in the second century A.D. (Guggenheim 1981). Skeletal evidence for rickets shows up in Neolithic, Iron

Age, and medieval Scandinavia, as well as in medieval towns elsewhere in Europe (Steinbock 1976).

The industrial revolution in Europe and North America offered a mixed blessing. The increased use of coal to power the new industries created high levels of air pollution in crowded cities and towns, filtering out ultraviolet rays from the sun. Poor children who labored most of the day indoors became more vulnerable to vitamin D deficiency than nonworking children. Rickets first manifested itself as a problem among city children in the sixteenth century. By the eighteenth century it was widespread throughout the industrialized urban areas, affecting up to 80 percent of the children. Adult vitamin D deficiency, osteomalacia, also flourished in northern European and North American cities and towns, especially among poor elderly women who stayed indoors most of the time (Guggenheim 1981).

Cultural habits or customs frequently influence the development of vitamin D deficiency. Babies swaddled, kept indoors, and artificially fed can suffer deficiency. Muslim and Hindu women required to cover themselves completely when away from the house, and women shunning full sunlight to keep their skin light, become vulnerable to developing vitamin D deficiency (Wood 1979). Young women who have suffered from the deficiency often have difficulty having their babies because their birth canals narrow and flatten with softening of the pelvic bones.

Following many theories about causation, the true cause of rickets finally became known in the 1920s. Fortification of milk with vitamin D, enforcement of child labor laws, and lowering of the pollution levels in industrialized cities and towns helped to eradicate the deficiency disease from Europe and North America (Guggenheim 1981).

Night Blindness and Xerophthalmia

Night blindness—the inability to see in dim light—marks one of the first symptoms of vitamin A deficiency. The retina requires vitamin A in order to perceive variable intensities of light and color, and it is very sensitive to the loss of this vitamin. Epithelial cells forming the skin and mucous membranes also depend on vitamin A. Without it these cells become abnormal and die quickly. Dead cells pile up on the surface of mucous membranes, preventing mucous secretion (Pfeiffer 1975), and the skin grows dry and roughened.

Continued vitamin A deficiency leads to damage of the mucous membranes lining the eyelids and covering the eyeballs, a condition known as xerophthalmia. The mucous membranes become dry and hard, and the eyes take on a murky appearance. The abnormal mucous membranes develop shiny gray triangular spots known as "bitot's spots," ranging from a few tiny blobs to a frothy white coating overflowing onto the cornea. Loss of vision occurs when the bitot's spots enlarge rapidly, causing the iris to collapse (Scrimshaw 1975). Microbes can easily infect abnormal mucous membranes of the eyes, respiratory system, mouth, gastrointestinal system, and genito-urinary systems with prolonged vitamin A deficiency.

The human body converts carotene found in fruits and vegetables to vitamin A. The vitamin can also be gained directly from certain animal sources such as fish liver oil, fish, animal liver, and egg yolks (Pfeiffer 1975). The body stores surpluses of vitamin A and its precursor, primarily in the liver, for later use. Thus, signs of deficiency take several months to develop.

Assyrian medical texts around twenty-seven hundred years ago described eye disorders that match vitamin A deficiency night blindness and xerophthalmia. Although the cause of these visual disturbances was unknown until the 1920s, the use of raw liver rich in vitamin A to treat eye disorders goes back centuries. The ancient Egyptians used raw liver directly applied to the eyes. Ancient Greek and Roman medical texts mention the eating of raw liver mixed with honey to treat eye disorders. Chinese physicians prescribed similar treatment thirteen hundred years ago. Visual disturbances caused by vitamin A deficiency plagued armies and populations suffering from crop failures and famine throughout the centuries. Vitamin A deficiency frequently caused blindness among whole groups of people suffering from poverty and poor diets (Guggenheim 1981).

Blindness or near blindness from vitamin A deficiency remains a problem in many poor countries of the world today (Pfeiffer 1975), and it is the leading cause of blindness in Bangladesh, India, and Indonesia (McElroy and Townsend 1985).

Endemic Goiter

The thyroid gland at the base of the neck stores iodine and uses it to form thyroxine, a hormone that regulates metabolic actions. When iodine intake becomes low or nonexistent, the pituitary gland senses it and stimulates the thyroid gland to use more and more of its stores of iodine to make thyroxine. This overactivity enlarges the thyroid gland, producing a simple goiter. Quite often this does not cause harm unless the iodine deficiency becomes prolonged to the point where no thyroxine gets produced, resulting in disturbed metabolic actions. Even then the disturbances usually produce only mild symptoms that include chronic fatigue, salt and water retention, some muscle weakness, menstrual disturbances, and lowered resistance to infection (DeGroot 1975; Sodeman 1956).

Physiological stresses, such as puberty, pregnancy, and infectious disease, can trigger the development of goiter in individuals who have limited sources of iodine. The first signs of goiter often appear during puberty, and the thyroid gland gradually enlarges with age. The nodular goiter can become so enlarged that it looks like a huge collar around the neck. This can interfere with swallowing, and cause difficulty in breathing with exertion (Barr 1951). Grossly enlarged goiters can be so common in some parts of the world that they are considered a normal part of life. Most adults with endemic goiter have adapted to the disorder and can function within the normal parameters of their society (DeGroot 1975).

Most people obtain iodine from salt or drinking water. Seafood and kelp also supply iodine. Most mountainous areas of the world and many areas that were covered in the last glaciation lack iodine in both soil and water. Such areas include the European Alps, the Pyrenees, Papua New Guinea, the Andes of South America, the Himalayas, the Pamir plateau in Central Asia, the Atlas Mountains of north Africa, the Great Lakes basin in North America, the Pacific Northwest, the valley of the upper Mississippi River, the southern part of the Nile River Valley, and the Congo River area (Aufderheide and Rodriguez-Martin 1998; Barr 1951). People living in these areas who depend on local sources of water and salt risk developing iodine deficiency. Quite often, as if by instinct, they will trade for imported salt or seafood containing iodine.

More serious effects occur in the developing fetus of a mother suffering from iodine deficiency in regions where severe endemic goiter occurs. The fetus develops thyroid deficiency causing growth disturbances that can lead to dwarfism and mental retardation. Babies born with severe deficiency often appear deaf-mute and suffer from paralysis (DeGroot 1975). If the deficiency does not become pronounced until after birth, less severe symptoms appear, but physical and mental growth remains stunted. Goiter that develops in late childhood has some effect on growth and mental capacity, but not enough to interfere with normal development (Aufderheide and Rodriguez-Martin 1998).

Endemic goiter has been around for centuries. Chinese medical texts describe it in the third century B.C. Several hundred years later they began prescribing seaweed as a remedy, long before anyone knew that iodine deficiency caused it. Marco Polo described endemic goiter among some of the Central Asians he encountered during his travels to China in the thirteenth century (Guggenheim 1981). Roman historians described the disorder among peoples living in the Alps. Goiter has been identified in the mummified remains of a 100 B.C. Nazca woman from the Ica valley in southern Peru, and in an eighteenth-century man from Sicily (Aufderheide and Rodriguez-Martin 1998).

By the mid-nineteenth century, in certain areas of the world, the cause of goiter came to be linked to some sort of deficiency in drinking water. Iodine was identified as the missing nutrient in the 1920s. Shortly after this discovery iodine routinely began to be added to table salt in many countries to prevent goiter (Guggenheim 1981). However, not all parts of the world have followed this form of prevention, and endemic goiter continues to plague millions of people (Aufderheide and Rodriguez-Martin 1998).

The Land of All You Can Eat

People in modern urbanized societies live very mechanized lives dominated by fixed schedules and routines. Most of us do not grow our own food anymore. Instead, we depend on commercial outlets for our food supplies. Modern diets have changed dramatically from human diets of a century ago and before.

For the first time in human history we now see populations subsisting mostly on highly refined, processed foods. Affordability and advertising propaganda frequently dictate food choices. Most of us purchase the food we eat with little knowledge of where it comes from or how it has been prepared for sale. Food shortages and famine have become unknown in modern societies except among the very poor. People are encouraged to buy more and eat more than they need. Welcome to the land of all you can eat.

The United States forms the epicenter of modern eating. Most people find food available at reasonable prices, and seasonal foods can be purchased throughout the year. There are more meat and plant food choices than our ancestors ever dreamed possible, plus artificial foods unheard of before the twentieth century. The modern food system has evolved over the past hundred years from simple farm products sold at local markets to highly commercialized agribusinesses selling to food outlet chains all over the nation. Food has become a commodity, greatly processed and refined from the fields, dairy barns, and feed lots to the supermarket.

Artificial food products, now common in modern societies, have been fabricated from original food sources. Refinement and processing effectively remove most or all of the original nutrients, producing an artificial end product often referred to as "junk food." It looks good, tastes good, is easy to get, and it takes little or no effort to prepare for eating. Processors usually add ingredients such as salt, sugar, hydrogenated fats, artificial flavorings, and chemical preservatives to encourage people to develop a taste for the item and to buy more. Some additives also prolong "shelf life." Sometimes they add to the product a few synthetic nutrients to replace natural ones removed during processing, but rarely enough to make up for lost ingredients.

Repeated use of chemical fertilizers and continued overuse of agricultural fields have leached minerals, particularly zinc, from the soil that would normally be taken up by plants and ultimately ingested by humans. Many vegetables and fruits get picked and shipped before they completely mature, and hence they lose much of their nutritive value. Most chickens, cattle, and pigs receive artificial feed supplements along with antibiotics and growth hormones that affect both the taste and the nutritive value of the meat. Mass processing and refining of meat and plant products in food factories often further compromises the nutritional status of foods. The end products look nice and appetizing, but often lack the full nutritive value that they should contain.

The typical American diet contains high quantities of refined or hydrogenated fats, refined sugars, salt, animal fats, bleached white flour, and chemical additives. Many key nutrients are limited in supply or missing in many foods. Hydrogenated vegetable fats found in margarine and vegetable shortenings contain trans-fatty acids unusable by the human body. The hydrogenation process of vegetable oils into solids transforms natural fatty acids in the oils to abnormal trans-fatty acids. The unusable synthetic fatty acids build up on blood vessel walls and contribute to the modern epidemic of heart disease among Americans (Finnegan 1993).

There may be plenty to eat, but not everything people eat has nutritive value. People subsisting primarily on highly processed foods often eat more than they need because they are starved for missing nutrients.

While great numbers of people do not have enough nutritious food to eat in many developing parts of the world, overeating of highly processed foods has grown into a serious problem in modern societies. Malnutrition underlies both problems. The overfed often exhibit mild (subclinical) nutritional deficiency diseases, while the underfed commonly have more pronounced deficiency diseases.

Obesity and Diabetes

Obesity has reached epidemic proportions in the United States. The majority of adults and rising numbers of children are overweight and malnourished. They eat too much with poor nutritional intake, and their habits are largely sedentary. Eating without sufficient exercise at any age upsets the caloric/energy burning balance and adds to the build-up of fat. Empty calories from junk foods and sugar-laden drinks, and artificially created trans-fatty acids derived from hydrogenated vegetable oils that the body cannot use, are the main factors leading to obesity.

The most prevalent disease in the United States related to diet and obesity is diabetes type II. Both diabetes type I and II result from the failure of insulin produced by the pancreas to regulate blood sugar and metabolize carbohydrates and fats. Insulin allows glucose from carbohydrates to enter cells of the body to make energy for the cell, and when necessary, it also allows fatty acids to do the same as a backup source of energy. When glucose enters the bloodstream following a meal, the pancreas receives a signal to release insulin into the blood to metabolize it and lower blood sugar. If glucose builds up in the blood, it becomes toxic to the body.

Type I diabetes differs from type II. In type I the pancreas no longer produces insulin to regulate blood sugar and metabolize carbohydrates and fats, while in type II the pancreas continues to produce some insulin but the body's cells have grown resistant to it. Type I diabetes develops when infection destroys the insulin-making cells in the pancreas. Type I diabetes is far less common than type II, occurring in less than 5–10 percent of all diabetics (Chopra 1994). Type II diabetes is associated with diet. Perhaps overeating highly processed sugary foods produces too much glucose at frequent intervals that leads to overload and subsequent resistance by the cells to letting in so much sugar. Or the sensitivity may derive from allergy to refined sugars.

Type II diabetes used to be thought of as a disease of older adults, but since the 1960s the disease has increased dramatically among younger age groups, and since the 1990s it has even been showing up in children as young as eight. This dramatic rise correlates with a similar rise in obesity in both adults and children, along with increasing consumption of junk foods and sugar-laden soft drinks.

Globalization of commercial foods has brought a pandemic of obesity and diabetes type II as people around the globe replace their traditional foods with artificial foods. A good example of this can be seen on the Pacific island of Nauru where diabetes had been virtually unknown until the recent discovery of phosphates there. Mining of this mineral brought wealth to the islanders, and they spent it to upgrade their lives by adopting popular Western ways, including dietary habits. They adopted commercial foods along with a sedentary life style, and diabetes quickly became a common disease (Chopra 1994). A similar rapid rise in obesity and diabetes has happened . among Native Americans who have adapted to a diet of white flour, white sugar, and high-fat foods. By following the same diet, their children are now suffering from the disease along with obesity.

Diabetes is a serious progressive disease if not reversed or treated adequately. Long-term damage to cells throughout the body results when their energy needs become compromised. Such damage can impair the heart, blood vessels, kidneys, eyes, and nerves. Heart attacks or strokes can happen easily, the kidneys can fail, blindness can occur, hearing can be impaired, and nerves can be so damaged that loss of sensation occurs in hands and feet. Loss of sensation can lead to injury with poor healing and infection that can end in gangrene and the need for amputation (Chopra 1994; Quillin 1989).

CONCLUDING COMMENTS

Throughout human history food supplies have waxed and waned under both environmental and cultural constraints. Mysterious diseases appeared whenever food supplies lacked certain nutrients over long periods of time. Scientific knowledge of human nutritional needs in the early twentieth century led to drastic reductions in diet-related mystery diseases around the globe. However, many peoples subsisting on poor diets in underdeveloped areas of the world remain at risk for nutritional deficiency diseases and starvation.

While the poor in many parts of the world worry about enough to eat, people in modern societies worry most about how to lose weight. Both can suffer from malnutrition. The dramatic changes in food production in the past hundred years among modernized nations have led to overconsumption of commercialized foods. Processed foods often contain few nutrients, leading to progressive health problems related to malnutrition and overeating. Diabetes type II and obesity have become byproducts of modern living. While the modern world has a rich supply of diverse foods, it frequently devalues foods through refinement and overprocessing as part of mass production. People in modern societies may live longer with their modern diets, but they often suffer chronic ailments related to subclinical malnutrition.

CHAPTER 20

THE GLOBALIZATION OF INFLUENZA

nfluenza, better known as the "flu," is familiar to most of us. We have grown up with it, and the familiar flu season comes around every year with a new variation of the flu bug. It does not matter whether you had the flu the year before, you can still catch the new flu bug since it differs slightly from the previous year's version. And if you don't catch this year's version of flu, then you might get it years later. Some people try to hedge their bets against catching the flu with a vaccination prepared ahead of time each year and tailored to combat the predicted seasonal variant. Despite annual vaccinations in the United States, between thirty and forty thousand people die from influenza each year. It takes at least six months to prepare vaccine. By the time the vaccine is ready for the flu season, the targeted virus may have changed enough to thwart the vaccine, or another variant may have taken over.

What Is Influenza?

Influenza picked up the nickname "flu" during the early twentieth century. Since then "flu" has become a catchall term for many unidentified and unrelated short-term illnesses. The term has been applied to "stomach flu" and other gastrointestinal disturbances, as well as to many other viral infections of the upper respiratory tract.

Influenza, like cold viruses, attacks the upper respiratory tract—nose, throat and the major airways leading into the lungs. The infection stems from a closely related group of viruses carried through the air from an infected individual on a sneeze or cough, or transmitted by direct contact with infected nasal or oral secretions.

The respiratory illness caused by influenza generally ends within ten days. The virus targets the hair-like cells (ciliated epithelia) lining the upper respiratory tract. These cells act as the first line of defense against invaders entering the airways. The targeted cells are infected and destroyed, leaving intact the underlying basal cell layer. New transitional epithelial cells generate from the basal layer within five days, and new ciliated cells reappear within two weeks following the infection (Kilbourne 1975).

Most influenza infections generally do not threaten life, with less than a 1 percent mortality rate among highly susceptible individuals (Kilbourne 1975). Symptoms of illness can vary from mild to severe, with rapid onset following an incubation period of one to three days. Common symptoms growing out of the immune reaction to the virus infection include fever, throbbing frontal headache, aching muscles, backache, general discomfort, exhaustion, loss of appetite, stuffy runny nose, and sore throat with dry cough. Frequent sweating, dizziness, aching eyes, or light sensitivity can also be present. The fever drops within two to five days, and most of the general symptoms fade, leaving the respiratory symptoms to linger for a few more days. Some adults complain of soreness in the center of the upper chest area from viral irritation of the underlying trachea, and some develop hoarseness. Children usually have more vague symptoms than adults. Some children suffer nausea, vomiting, and diarrhea along with the respiratory symptoms (Benenson 1995; Stuart-Harris 1965).

Complications rarely occur from most types of influenza, but they can pose problems, either directly or indirectly, for highly susceptible individuals, particularly with the introduction of a new strain of the virus. Individuals most likely to suffer from complications have immune systems unable to react adequately to the infection. This includes individuals under high stress, malnourished people, and those with preexisting health problems such as emphysema and heart disease. Pregnant women and heavy smokers have high susceptibility to complications. Influenza infection can pave the way for other microbes to enter areas of the upper respiratory system damaged by the virus and spread into the lungs or occasionally other parts of the body. Sometimes the influenza virus itself can reach into the lower branches of the bronchial airways and attack the lungs. Bronchitis and pneumonia are the most common complications associated with influenza. Existing heart problems can be amplified by the illness, and evidence has been found that the virus may trigger encephalitis (Benenson 1995; Kilbourne 1975, 1987; McCullers et al. 1999; Sugaya et al. 2002).

Pneumonia directly caused by influenza virus can be deadly. Symptoms of severe viral pneumonia usually develop quickly, within twenty hours of the onset of the flu. The fever goes up, bloody sputum is coughed up with difficult breathing, the individual suffers anxiety, and begins to turn blue. Death usually follows within five to ten days (Kilbourne 1975).

The Agents of Infection

Three types of related influenza viruses exist, referred to as types A, B, and C. They operate independently of one another, and infection with one type does not confer resistance to the other types. All three viruses have the same basic RNA genome enclosed and protected by a lipid coat derived from the outer membrane of host cells. They acquire this coat when the newly formed virus buds from the infected cell. Hundreds of spike-like projections of two types of proteins protrude from the lipid membrane. One of these helps the viruses attach to and enter host cells, while the other one lets fledgling viruses out of host cells.

Most of the spikes consist of a protein known as hemagglutinin (H). The tip of each hemagglutinin spike holds the key binding activity that fits into the landing lock, the dimpled receptor site, on the surface of the selected host cell. The remaining protein spikes consist of neuraminidase (N) acting as an enzyme to help newly formed viruses break out of infected host cells (Ruigrok 1998). Both proteins provoke antigenic-antibody reactions from the host immune system, but hemagglutinin holds by far the major attraction, while neuraminidase plays a lesser role.

Influenza viruses cannot gain access to host cells without the hemagglutinin spikes. Even when the hemagglutinin spikes locate and bind to the dimpled receptor sites on the target cell, they cannot get through the "door" of the outer membrane until they split into two parts. The depression formed by the receptor site contains a specific acidic fluid that facilitates this act, allowing the two parts of the hemagglutinin to penetrate the cell membrane and enter the cell, while shedding the protective coat in the process. Within just a few hours, around a hundred newly formed viral offspring line up along the inside perimeter of the infected cell, wrapping themselves in the cell's membrane as they bud outward. The neuraminidase enzyme spikes cut them loose as the host cell dies in the process (Hope-Simpson 1992; Kilbourne 1987).

As with all pathogens, each influenza virus type comprises a population of variant subtypes and variant lineages of subtypes, all jockeying for dominance. Changes in their microenvironment, host type, or the host's immune response can favor one variant subtype or lineage over the others. Influenza viruses also have the capability to alter their identity by changing antigenic proteins within a lineage to evade host immunoglobins that have come to recognize them.

Type A influenza viruses represent the most unstable group, frequently changing hemagglutinin antigenic identity with point mutations to escape the immune response of the host. While other viral proteins exposed to the host immune system can trigger immune reactions, hemagglutinin plays the key role in host immune response. Any change in antigenic identity takes place by genetic drift away from the original antigenic form (Kawaoka and Webster 1988; Stuart-Harris et al. 1985). Drift allows for reinfection of a host, since the immune system does not recognize the "new look" of the same virus that caused a prior infection. Vaccines and natural antibodies for last year's influenza virus may not recognize this year's new look of the same virus.

Influenza viruses hold the added potential for change through the capability of producing hybrid viruses from two different subtypes. The structure of the viral genome allows hybrids to be formed since the RNA consists of divided segments (eight for types A and B, seven for type C), and each segment replicates independently. Segments can be swapped between different subtypes of a virus when both infect the same host cells, thus producing hybrid offspring. This maneuver represents a genetic shift away from the parent types (Stuart-Harris et al. 1985).

The instability of the type A viruses can be attributed to their ability to jump species and on occasion produce hybrids from subtypes infecting different host species. Wild waterfowl, pigs, horses, domestic fowl, and humans represent the major players in a web of interaction between these viruses. Types B and C confine themselves primarily to human populations (Hay 1998), having reached a state of mutual tolerance through their adaptation to human hosts. They generally manage to survive by making the rounds of the new batches of nonimmune young children in large populations. Therefore, they are more stable with little need for antigenic change through time, and we see no evidence for hybridization among subtypes. Only pigs have been found on occasion to be infected with types B and C, transferred to them from humans (Kilbourne 1987). Thus, with few counterparts in other host species, it is difficult to produce a hybrid.

Type C shows a more distant genetic relationship to type A than does type B, and type C has adapted better to humans, producing mild to silent infections. Type C viruses make the rounds of newly susceptible young children each year, while type B viruses tend to target older children. Infection from type B viruses also generally produces mild symptoms. Type A viruses attack susceptible individuals of all age groups, and infection can range from mild to severe.

All three types of influenza viruses have a common ancestor. Type C is the oldest, having infected humans for centuries, followed by type B viruses (Scholtissek 1998). Type A viruses represent a more recent acquisition by human populations.

All known subtypes of type A influenza viruses also appear in wild waterfowl throughout the world, with differences between Old World and New World subtypes. They have operated as natural infections for these birds for millennia, having established a state of mutual tolerance with their water bird hosts.

Infected water birds do not succumb to any illness, and remain free of disease while the viruses infect the surface cells of the birds' intestinal tract where they replicate to be shed in feces for about two to four weeks. The viruses have no need to readily change antigenic proteins since the birds' immune system does not react to the infection. The viruses can survive in feces and in water contaminated by them for up to thirty days. Migratory water birds and shore birds congregating in breeding areas ensure that a significant number of the next generation of birds stay silently infected each year, continuing the cycle of infection (Ito and Kawaoka 1998; Webster and Bean 1998).

Human beings generally have no direct contact with wild waterfowl viruses. Even if they do, only a few virus subtypes can infect humans, and they fail to make the transition from a zoonotic disease to a human disease to be transmitted from humans to other humans. Pigs, horses, and domestic fowl can be infected with the wild bird viruses, and as the viruses modify to fit their new hosts more readily, they become more suitable for fomenting human infections when transmitted from the intermediary animal host to humans. Humans can also pass infection back to the intermediate animal hosts. By the time the wild viruses reach the human population and become established human infections, the modified viruses lose much of their potential for infecting their native bird hosts; human hybrid viruses cannot infect wild waterfowl at all (Ito and Kawaoka 1998).

Domesticated ducks may provide the major link for transmission of wild viruses to domestic animals and poultry. The viruses infect ducks the same way they infect their wild cousins, so that they show no signs of disease but carry the viruses in their feces (Kilbourne 1987). Pigs, horses, chickens, and turkeys pick it up from infected duck droppings contaminating water or feed and develop infection of the upper respiratory system, with symptoms similar to those of humans. The virus is then transmitted by droplets in the air from the infected animal to other animals and humans.

Shifting Subtypes and Drifting New Lineages

Fifteen different types of hemagglutinin (H) and nine different types of neuraminidase (N) protein spikes of type A viruses have been identified in wild waterfowl, and all of them exist in wild ducks (Webster and Bean 1998). They appear in specific combinations that have been labeled by assigned numbers, such as H_1N_1, to delineate each subtype of influenza A virus. Only a few of the subtypes infect humans. Each subtype produces antigenic variants within its lineage (genetic drift) affecting one or both protein spikes without altering its subtype identity. Therefore, more than one variant of subtype H_1N_1 can be circulating within host populations at the same time or at different times. Subtypes of A influenza virus tend to progressively change antigenic appearances in response to animal or human host immune responses in order to survive within their host populations.

When a subtype changes host species, the virus often makes adjustments to the new host by modifying its inner core to adapt to and reproduce more efficiently in the new host's target cells (Scholtissek 1992). Otherwise the change in host species might not allow the virus to reproduce sufficiently for it to be transmitted within the new host population.

Occasionally a hybrid virus (genetic shift) arises from two different subtypes and exhibits a new combination of protein spikes, such as an H_2N_2 subtype versus H_1N_1. The new hybrid subtype may produce only mild infection at first. More serious disease occurs with progressive changes in antigenic identity as the hybrid virus continues to adjust to its host, or when it changes host species. Or the reverse can take place, with the new hybrid virus first producing severe disease before adjusting to its host and tempering its effects to produce mild disease.

Pigs have been known to act as the primary "mixers" for creating hybrid subtypes. They easily get infected by both human and bird subtypes of the same viruses, and when infected by both at the same time, the different subtypes can swap genetic segments to produce a hybrid virus (Scholtissek et al. 1998; Webster 1993). The new hybrid can then be transmitted from pigs to people, where it can modify its inner core and become capable of transmission between humans. The new hybrid virus will also undergo progressive changes in antigenic identity (genetic drift) to offset host immune responses.

Major changes in the antigenic nature of any of the subtypes of A virus can spark outbreaks or epidemics of influenza. When a new subtype or hybrid enters the human population for the first time from an intermediate animal host, it can generate an outbreak or epidemic of influenza that may lead to a global pandemic.

The 1918 Influenza Pandemic

The world's best known and most severe influenza pandemic struck in 1918 toward the end of World War I. With amazing speed, a new influenza virus raced around the world in less than four months (Crosby 1976). Approximately half the global population became infected within a short time, but only half that number suffered illness from the infection. Early estimates of 20 million deaths from the pandemic have been revised upward to 40 million–50 million deaths between 1918 and 1920 (Potter 1998). The death toll constituted less than 3 percent of the total estimated world population at that time (Coale 1974).

Some parts of the world suffered more illness and death than others, with the small Pacific Islands hit the hardest. Western Samoa lost 22 percent of its population to the disease. The infection raced through communities, leaving large numbers of sick and dead within a few weeks, and then it vanished as quickly as it arrived. The outbreaks overwhelmed local medical and funerary services very quickly. Healthy young adults suffered the highest fatalities, unlike other influenza outbreaks, which primarily killed the very young, the elderly, and the chronically ill. Basic community institutions, such as schools, public works, and businesses, often had to shut down for lack of staff well enough to come to work. Local governments discouraged public gatherings and told people to stay home. Yet people rarely panicked, while around the world they pitched in to help the victims and fill in for those taken ill (Crosby 1976). Perhaps most people did not panic because they were familiar with influenza outbreaks, which had happened almost annually since the late 1800s (Hope-Simpson 1992).

The 1918 pandemic is notable for the number of deaths among young adults, as well as the high numbers of patients who experienced a protracted recovery that lasted weeks. Most of the deaths were attributed to pneumonia, either directly from the virus or from a secondary infection from another pathogen. For some reason this particular strain or subtype could descend into the lungs quickly and target lung tissue, causing hemorrhaging in the lungs and death within forty-eight hours (Schoch-Spana 2000).

The first recognized wave of the pandemic appeared in early spring of 1918 in several places across the United States. Simultaneous outbreaks of "grippe" had been reported among workers at the Ford Motor Company in Detroit, Michigan, among prisoners in San Quentin prison in California, and among recruits at military bases in Kansas and South Carolina (Bollet 1987; Crosby 1976; Potter 1998). There may also have been unaccounted sporadic infections by this particular subtype throughout the country during the winter of 1917–18.

Interestingly, Vaughn (1921) reported an influenza epidemic in China at about the same time, suggesting that Chinese migrant laborers may have introduced this new subtype of the disease into North America. The American railroads used Chinese immigrant labor, and we know that the virus traveled along the rails with the movement of military recruits and troops as the United States prepared for the war in Europe. New recruits from various parts of the country showed up at military camps in the Midwest and eastern states that spring, many of them sick with the "grippe," and soon the camps reported influenza outbreaks accompanied by significant numbers of deaths (Crosby 1976).

The first wave of influenza fed by the massive movement of men crossing the country by rail lacked the severity of following waves of infection. Reports of influenza outbreaks poured in from all over North America during the spring of 1918 without much alarm. Most of the deaths related to the disease happened in military camps where young recruits underwent enormous stress training for war.

The 1914–18 war provided a staging ground for globalizing the new influenza virus. Ship traffic between the European powers and their colonies in Africa, India, Southeast Asia, and the Pacific provided avenues for rapid transport of the virus worldwide. The infection received the nickname "Spanish influenza," blaming Spain for the outbreak, but it was U.S. troops entering the war during the spring of 1918 that brought the virus to Europe from North America. The earliest outbreak in Europe occurred in France during the month of April, following the landing of U.S. military forces at a camp near Bordeaux. American soldiers crowded on transport ships suffered severely from the virus, with up to 20 percent of them dying from the disease on the voyage. By May the virus had spread to British and German forces, and throughout Europe, and was well on its way around the world (Bollet 1987; Crosby 1976).

War-weary soldiers suffered more severely from the new virus than did civilians. Some military attack plans had to be postponed for the lack of sufficient numbers of men well enough to carry them out. Army horses also suffered from the virus with respiratory illness similar to the human illness. As the virus spread among fighting men on both sides of the battle during the summer, it progressively changed its antigenic identity, gaining virulence. The virus killed almost as many American soldiers as the war did, as well as unknown numbers of Allied and German soldiers (Crosby 1976).

The more virulent form of the virus led to a second wave of influenza outbreaks around the world, all more deadly than those in the first wave. The second wave of the pandemic reached its peak in the fall of 1918. This time around, civilians suffered as much as the military, with more severe disease and increasing death rates. The largest numbers of influenza-related deaths occurred during this wave (Crosby 1976).

Outbreaks from the second wave subsided with the end of the war in November of 1918. However, the ever-changing virus made yet another round during the winter of 1918–19, and a final appearance in January and February of 1920 before it faded into obscurity (Stuart-Harris et al. 1985).

Influenza outbreaks among farmers in Iowa in the fall of 1918 engendered similar outbreaks among their pigs. The disease spread quickly through pig markets around the country, killing thousands of the animals. The infection passed back and forth both between farmers and their pigs for over a year. Following the waning of the human pandemic, the virus became firmly established in North American pigs. This "swine flu" virus remained in the pig population, infecting market-aged pigs just about every nine months. Over the years the swine virus and North American pigs have developed a state of mutual tolerance, resulting in mild to silent infection from the virus (Crosby 1976; Reid and Taubenberger 1999).

In 1931 the virus infecting pigs was identified as subtype H1N1. Blood studies taken from people born before 1933 who survived the 1918–20 influenza contained immunoglobins to a similar H1N1 virus (Potter 1998). Recent DNA studies of influenza virus fragments in preserved lung tissue samples from two soldiers who died in 1918 from this disease, and frozen lung tissue from an Inuit woman who died during an influenza outbreak in Alaska in 1918, support the identification of the 1918 pandemic as an H1N1 virus. Phylogenetic analysis shows that the virus originated as a hybrid with relationships between human, swine, and bird sources, but more closely related to human and swine variants than to bird variants (Cox and Subbarao 2000; Gibbs et al. 2001; Reid and Taubenberger 1999).

When and where did the mixing take place? Type A subtype H1 viruses are native to wild waterfowl in the Old World (Webster and Bean 1998). Most likely an H1 subtype had passed to domesticated ducks and was transmitted to pigs somewhere in China at the same time that a human subtype infected the pigs. Phylogenetic studies of influenza A viruses support this view. This would have provided the right mix to create a new hybrid virus transmitted to humans, with modifications as it passed from host to host, until it gained a foothold in the human population. By the time it reached North America and moved on to Europe, progressive changes in antigenic behavior had reached a high level of virulence. Infection peaked in the pig population of North America as the more virulent subtype returned in the fall of 1918.

Early History of Influenza

Evidence suggests that wild influenza viruses have to pass through an intermediate host before they enter the human population to become successful human infections. If this is correct, then human beings experienced no risk until they domesticated animals, especially pigs, ducks, and horses, in the Old World. New World populations were spared the disease until the European invasion in the sixteenth century (Patterson 1987). Most likely, C type influenza viruses became the first to be introduced to human beings from domesticated animals, followed by the B type viruses. Both types probably had greater virulence when first introduced into human populations than they do today.

The most likely region for the first human contacts with the viruses had to be Asia, where domestication of both pigs and ducks occurred. One or more viral types could also have passed from wild waterfowl through domesticated horses in Central Asia. Each type and subtypes may have gained access to human populations in separate regions at different times. Outbreaks would have been limited to local areas until large population centers with major trade routes developed to support epidemics and maintain the infection within the larger populations. The viruses then could travel from one major population center to another along trade routes and expand into other parts of the Old World.

Epidemics of influenza most likely happened in the mix of infections striking early Old World civilizations from East Asia to the Mediterranean. As civilization and trade expanded, so did the incidence of influenza.

The first definitive description of influenza appeared in A.D. 1173 in Europe as the disease spread northward from the Mediterranean region. Several recorded outbreaks followed, including simultaneous outbreaks of similar symptoms among horses (Crosby 1976). The world's first recorded pandemic struck in 1580 as the disease fanned out from Asia to Africa, then within six months reached Europe, and ultimately arrived in North America (Patterson 1987; Potter 1998).

The industrial revolution, urbanization, and European expansion promoted influenza as a permanent player on the global stage. Outbreaks of the disease have taken place at frequent intervals in various parts of the world since the sixteenth century, varying in severity, depending on the dominant subtype circulating at the time. Horses may have served as major intermediate hosts for the introduction of new subtypes into human populations, since abundant numbers of horses provided the bulk of transport around the world.

At least six pandemics, possibly nine, punctuated with regional epidemics and local outbreaks, occurred over the four hundred years before the 1918 pandemic. Most, if not all, of the pandemics originated in Central Asia, South Asia, or Southeast Asia, and then moved westward (Kilbourne 1987; Patterson 1987; Potter 1998).

The pandemic of 1898–1901 that preceded the 1918 pandemic produced generally mild infections. An earlier pandemic in 1889–91, more serious with a greater attack rate, appeared in three waves with the number of deaths increasing with each wave. Serological studies of elderly survivors from both these pandemics showed that the 1889–91 pandemic had been caused by an H2N8 subtype, and the 1898–1901 pandemic resulted from an H3N8 subtype, while an H1N1 subtype caused the 1918 pandemic (Potter 1998; Webster 1993).

Post-1918 Influenza

Every year since 1918 influenza outbreaks have occurred around the world. Two new influenza viruses that produced pandemics have also been introduced into the global population since 1918.

The identification in 1931 of the virus causing influenza paved the way for tracking both changes in the existing viruses and the introduction of new viruses into human populations. Outbreaks caused by B type viruses as well as A type viruses have been separately identified. Usually causing mild infections in children and adolescents, the B viruses occasionally cause more serious disease in adults, as noted in three outbreaks in the 1940s, 1959, and 1962. Outbreaks of B type influenza often occur along with outbreaks of A type influenza (Stuart-Harris et al. 1985).

Variants of the type A H1N1 subtype of 1918 continued to cycle with progressive modifications in people and pigs without much competition (Smith and Palse 1989) until a new hybrid virus subtype appeared in 1957. The new virus subtype, H2N2, came out of Yunan province in China in February 1957 and spread mostly by ship traffic around the globe within six months. Two waves of infection with equal severity hit several countries. The very young and old suffered the most severe symptoms. Just under half the world's population became infected with about 30 percent of them suffering illness. Deaths from this pandemic, known as the "Asian influenza," ranked far below the death rate for the 1918 pandemic: no more than 1 million out of 2.5 billion people in the world (Potter 1998). Despite its severity and the large numbers of deaths, only 0.04 percent of the world's total population died, compared to slightly under 3 percent for the 1918–20 pandemic.

The 1957–58 hybrid subtype derived from a combination of human and bird subtypes mixed together in pigs (Potter 1998; Stuart-Harris et al. 1985). The wild virus most likely passed through domestic ducks in close contact with pigs and farmers in Yunan province, and the farmers gave a human virus to the pigs. The pigs in turn gave the farmers the new hybrid virus that readily adapted to human transmission.

Another hybrid subtype entered the global population from southeastern China in July 1968, spreading more slowly than the previous pandemic. It did not hit South America and South Africa until a year later. This subtype, H3N2, known as the "Hong Kong influenza," also resulted from a combination of human and bird subtypes mixed in pigs. This pandemic virus produced a milder illness than did the previous pandemic virus, attacking the very young and old more than any other age groups (Potter 1998; Stuart-Harris et al. 1985).

Outbreaks of a mild influenza in China during May 1977 heralded the global resurgence of another H1N1 subtype within the human population, but one far less virulent than the 1918 variant. The virus, known as the "Russian flu," reached around the globe by June 1978, striking mostly individuals born after 1957. The H1N1 variant proved genetically similar to the modified H1N1 subtype that had been circulating before 1957, suggesting that the variant subtype never disappeared from circulation and resurfaced to infect the young who lacked immunoglobins for it (Potter 1998; Smith and Palse 1989; Stuart-Harris et al. 1985).

Variants of H1N1, along with other subtype variants, survive in pigs all over the world, while variants of H7N7 and H3N8 often infect horses (Stuart-Harris et al. 1985). Horses in northeastern China suffered a severe outbreak from an H3N8 subtype variant in 1989 that killed 20 percent of some herds (Ito 2000). Influenza attacked harbor seals off Cape Cod on the northeast coast of North America in December 1979, with a 20 percent die-off; the seals had contracted subtype H7N7 from shore birds. The same colony was hit again by another influenza subtype, H4N5, in 1982 (Campitelli et al. 2002), followed by infections with H4N6 and H3N3 subtypes in 1991. Stranded whales have also exhibited infection by influenza viruses (Ito 2000). Poultry are especially susceptible to a wide variety of subtypes associated with their wild cousins.

The 1976 Swine Flu Fiasco

Shortly after new army recruits and soldiers returning from the Christmas holidays arrived at Fort Dix, New Jersey, in January 1976, an outbreak of influenza ensued. Most of the illnesses remained mild with only a few hospitalized victims. One sick recruit who refused to answer sick call died from influenza-related pneumonia. Tests showed that he and three others had been infected with an H1N1 swine virus, while all the others had been infected with a variant of the H3N2 virus that had been circulating every year since it was introduced to human populations in 1968 (Neustadt and Fineberg 1978). There had been a few reported cases of human infection by the swine flu since 1974, but the virus had grown so adapted to pigs that it could no longer adjust well enough in the human host to be transmitted from person to person (Ito 2000).

Fearful that the H1N1 subtype of 1918 had begun to resurface within the human population, with the prospect of a similar pandemic, scientists debated the issue and considered what should be done to prevent such a disaster. Some scientists believed this was not the same subtype variant of 1918, while many others feared it could be. This debate was leaked to the media, thus forcing a decision before the debate could be resolved. President Gerald Ford, following recommendations coming out of the debate, announced in March the federal government's intent to immunize the entire population of the United States against the swine flu to prevent a disastrous outbreak expected in the fall of 1976, similar to the 1918 pandemic. Congress appropriated $135 million for the vaccine program (Neustadt and Fineberg 1978).

Vaccine trials in April of that year revealed that it could not be safely used on children without serious side effects. Therefore, individuals under eighteen would not receive the vaccine. Manufacturers of the vaccine delayed production when the insurance companies refused to insure them against lawsuits stemming from side affects of the vaccine. Congress had to pass a bill to cover litigation costs, and President Ford signed the bill in August. Although vaccine production was thus assured, the vaccination program was delayed until the money appropriated for it became available at the start of the federal fiscal year on October first (Neustadt and Fineberg 1978).

Many additional problems with the vaccine program cropped up, and by the time all had been readied, only about half the adults in America agreed to take the shots. Many angry parents refused vaccination when they found out their children could not be vaccinated (Newstadt and Fineberg 1978).

Ten days after the vaccinations began, three elderly individuals with heart conditions died shortly after receiving their shots. The news media jumped on this to create a fear of the vaccine. This prompted President Ford and his family to encourage people to take the shots by televising their own vaccinations. Over 40 million people did receive the vaccine before the program ended in December. The vaccinations stopped when the risk of developing Guillain-Barre syndrome proved to be a dangerous side effect (Neustadt and Fineberg 1978). Guillain-Barre syndrome, a neurological disorder that usually follows infectious disease, leads to progressive muscle weakness that can end in paralysis.

The feared pandemic never arrived, and only one human case of swine flu H1N1 influenza could be confirmed in North America during the flu season of 1976–77 (Neustadt and Fineberg 1978). The modified swine flu variant of H1N1 could not make the right changes to become a human disease. The swine flu vaccination program finally was shelved in March 1977 as the prospects of swine flu for the coming year appeared to be nonexistent and the risks associated with the vaccine seemed too great.

Ironically, the "Russian flu" H1N1 variant did circle the globe during the flu season of 1977–78, unlike its swine flu cousin that remained in the pig population. This shows that the various subtypes can have a wide range of variants coming from different sources, and that not all of them achieve success as human infections.

The 1997 Bird Flu Scare

Fowl plague among chickens first became recognized in Italy in 1878. Its cause remained unknown until 1955, when it was discovered to be an influenza A type virus. Sometimes the disease appeared as a mild infection and at other times it killed all the chickens in a flock. Turkeys and quail also suffered from the disease, while it spared domesticated ducks. As knowledge of the influenza viruses increased, it came to be known that several subtypes infected domesticated poultry, contracted from wild waterfowl either directly or indirectly through domesticated ducks (Stuart-Harris et al. 1985).

Outbreaks of mild chicken influenza H5N2 appeared on Pennsylvania poultry farms in April 1983, and by October the disease turned into a killer with a 100 percent death toll among infected chickens. The same subtype producing mild infection returned in 1985, when it was traced to major poultry markets on the East Coast. This suggested that the poultry markets had been maintaining the potentially deadly virus within the market system. The virus remains harmless until it undergoes a single-point mutation allowing it to invade every part of the chicken's body (Kawaoka and Webster 1988). Similar incidents probably occurred in the past, which would explain the variability of infection in poultry since fowl plague first became known.

Influenza caused by various subtypes has appeared in domestic fowl around the world, but until recently caused little alarm as a potential human disease. This changed with the outbreak of a deadly chicken flu in Hong Kong in 1997. Subtype H5N1 arrived with poultry from mainland China and quickly spread among the poultry markets and farms of Hong Kong. Infected ducks remained free of symptoms, while chickens died from the disease. The virus attacked eighteen humans and killed six of them. Fear of an impending disaster prompted Hong Kong authorities to destroy over 1 million chickens, ducks, and geese to eradicate the disease from the island (Guan et al. 1999; Matrosovich et al. 1999).

Subtype H5N1 had been circulating in the Hong Kong poultry markets together with a variant of another subtype, H9N2. Studies suggest that they may have swapped gene segments to create a more deadly strain of H5N1 (Guan et al. 1999). Although the virus did infect humans and caused severe illness, it appeared to lack the capacity to replicate sufficiently within human host cells to become a human disease (Matrosovich et al. 1999). That situation could readily change in the future.

Six weeks after eradicating domestic poultry from Hong Kong, authorities allowed mainland chickens back into the country following quarantine measures and testing free of the virus. Four years later, in May 2001, another outbreak of deadly chicken flu raised another alarm (*International Herald Tribune*, 19–20 May 2001). Again, eradication of all poultry took place to stop the spread of the virus. Another outbreak in early 2002 led to the destruction of more chickens on three farms (*Arizona Daily Star*, 7 February 2002). By the end of 2003 another deadly strain of H5N1 bird flu from southeastern China had spread throughout Asian poultry markets and farms, along with other, less lethal bird strains. Millions of domestic fowl died or were destroyed to contain the diseases as human deaths from H5N1 infections began to occur in Southeast Asia (WHO Communicable Disease Surveillance and Response report, 15 January 2004).

CONCLUDING COMMENTS

The capricious nature of the influenza viruses has become more evident in recent years with advancing scientific studies of them. World authorities now monitor any virus lineage changes plus movements of the various subtypes. Lineage changes follow relatively uniform patterns of succession, while the appearance of new subtypes remains unpredictable (Cox and Subbarao 2000).

Variants of both H1N1 and H3N2 subtypes continue to circulate among human populations around the globe today, along with B type viruses. A new subtype, H1N2, appeared in mild outbreaks from November 2001 to January 2002 in the Middle East, Britain, and North America (*Weekly Epidemiological Record* 2002). What will happen with this subtype remains to be seen.

The 1997 outbreak of severe H5N1 bird flu in Hong Kong raises the possibility of a deadly pandemic arising from poultry instead of from the traditional intermediate host, the pig. While Southeast Asia's farms and live animal markets have spawned most new subtypes and variants, poultry markets have proved to be major reservoirs for avian viruses with the capability of acting as swap meets for exchange of gene segments among different circulating subtypes (Capitelli et al. 2002). The leap to human beings has already been demonstrated. What remains to be seen is whether or not a particular fowl variant can quickly adjust to human host cells to become a human disease. Another possibility may arise from reassortment when a bird subtype and human subtype mix within a human instead of within an animal intermediate host. This would require a human suffering from one subtype of influenza, such as H3N2 or H1N1, to become infected at the same time with a subtype such as H5N1 contracted from a chicken (Claas et al. 1998).

The rapidly growing global population inhabiting numerous overcrowded cities, plus increasing global air and sea transportation, places the world at risk for severe influenza pandemics in the near future. The rising demand for chicken and pork has increased the numbers of large commercial farms and live animal markets overcrowded with pigs and poultry. With or without the introduction of wild viruses into their ranks, domestic animals are already loaded with various subtypes of influenza viruses capable of changing species and reassorting.

It is not a matter of if, but of when and how a new influenza pandemic develops that will be far more deadly than any previous pandemic. Vaccines may help ward off a pandemic if produced in time. The 1918 pandemic rounded the globe in four months by way of ships. Today that same virus could move by air transport around the world within days. If a modern pandemic were to kill the same proportion of the global population as it did during the 1918 pandemic, that would amount to about 180 million people dead out of a total of 6 billion, all within a short time.

CHAPTER 21

DISEASES OF MODERN CIVILIZATION

The sociocultural revolution triggered by industrialization accelerated during the nineteenth century to evolve into modern civilization during the twentieth century. Those regions around the world that did not industrialize continued to lag behind modernized parts of the world as underdeveloped or developing countries.

The twentieth century marked the end of colonialism, and the world soon divided up into nation-states. Global, regional, and local wars, plus revolutionary attempts to reorganize human societies, disrupted many parts of the world throughout this century. Millions of people were slaughtered, and millions more died from starvation and disease, yet the global population soared to unprecedented heights. Despite the extremely high loss of lives throughout the twentieth century, overall infant survival rates steadily increased, leading to ever increasing numbers of breeding-age humans.

On the Road to Affluence

Great strides in public health during the early twentieth century contributed to a dramatic decrease in contagious diseases among industrialized nations. Clean water and food, sewage treatment, and improved living standards and personal hygiene paved the way for the prevention of many diseases. For example, tuberculosis once haunted the industrialized world, but it receded dramatically when improved public health and hygiene prevented it from spreading.

Dramatic changes in technology brought new challenges to humankind. The invention of electricity, the combustion engine, the telephone, automobile, and airplane played key roles in modernization, leading up to the era of computers and high technology. New energy and power sources, the development of synthetic materials and chemical compounds, speedy communication systems, jet air travel, and the development of modern medicine altered many societies around the world. The so-called "green revolution" during the mid-twentieth century brought chemical alteration of agricultural practices that artificially increased plant yields. The demand for meat foods inspired changes in animal husbandry that altered the way farm animals were fed and raised. Urbanization soon outpaced rural life in many parts of the world, and megacities evolved throughout the world.

Modernization led to changes in human behavior patterns and human interaction with the environment that in turn altered patterns of human disease. For example, major portions of populations around the world smoked cigarettes on a daily basis by the mid-twentieth century, promoting changes in patterns of upper respiratory and lung disease. The dramatic increase in outdoor and indoor air pollution also contributed to changing respiratory disease patterns with skyrocketing numbers of lung disorders and asthma victims during the last quarter of the twentieth century.

So called "diseases of affluence," such as obesity, diabetes, and heart disease, increased dramatically with modernized processed foods and sedentary life styles. Rapid air travel and increasing immigration from poor countries raised the risk of spreading infectious diseases that did not exist in other countries. Increasing use of injectable drugs, both legal and illegal, has became commonplace around the world since the 1970s, contributing to the increase and spread of many blood-borne diseases.

Some infectious agents have taken advantage of modern hospitalization and surgery procedures since the mid-twentieth century to produce *nosocomial infections*—that is, infections acquired in hospitals. Approximately 5 percent of patients in today's modern hospitals in the United States develop nosocomial infections (Lederberg et al. 1992). Hospital-acquired infections claim an estimated sixty thousand deaths in the United States alone (Sharpe and Faden 1998). This does not include thousands of deaths caused by medication side effects and errors.

Nosocomial infection rates are much higher in poor hospitals in underdeveloped countries trying to emulate their modern counterparts, and they often become epicenters for the spread of disease. The routine use of hypodermic needles throughout the twentieth century, routine blood transfusions over the last sixty years, and illegal hypodermic drug use for as many years have opened up new channels for rare infections to spread in human populations.

The twentieth century saw a dramatic shift in the relationship between humans and the microbial world. Modernization has reshuffled the deck of diseases, and—to use a different metaphor—the microbe pot has been stirred faster and faster as humans have reshaped the landscape in their quest for progress. However, the shift has been uneven, leaving a "checkerboard" pattern of diseases throughout the world. While improved living standards among modernizing nations drastically lowered the number and severity of epidemic diseases that haunted previous generations, many of those same epidemic diseases continued to prevail in nonindustrialized parts of the world.

Operation "Clean Sweep"

Modern medical science came to believe that it could wipe out infectious diseases by the mid-twentieth century. Synthetic antibiotics introduced during the 1950s, following the development of penicillin in the 1940s, became the leading arsenal against infectious diseases. Although they only worked against bacterial infections and were ineffective against virus infections, doctors dispensed antibiotics for every suspected infection from the slightest viral cold to major life-threatening diseases. They became the "magic pill" solution, and by the late 1960s medical scientists were predicting the end of the battle with infectious diseases. Antibiotics flooded the world. They could be bought over the counter in many countries, were freely dispensed by prescriptions in other countries, and became common additives to animal feed.

After twenty years of overusing antibiotic drugs, it became apparent that the war with infectious diseases remained far from over. More dangerous "superinfections" developed as targeted pathogens developed resistance to the arsenal of antibiotics thrown at them. Indigenous bacteria also got in on the act. Hit unintentionally by the onslaught of antibiotics, they also changed to resist the drugs and to form new pathogenic strains harmful to their human hosts. Many infectious agents went underground to avoid the antibiotic deluge, waiting for opportunities to reappear when host immunity weakened (Dubos 1980). Many of them have become "sleeper" diseases, chronic forms of disease that continue to puzzle modern medicine.

Modern medical science developed childhood vaccinations to replace early childhood exposure to common infections (Burnet and White 1972) as part of the "clean sweep" approach to knocking out infectious diseases. Before vaccinations to elicit immunity became routine, young children would often deliberately be exposed to contagious individuals in the knowledge that they would suffer far less from the infection at a younger age than when older. Most early childhood infections in healthy individuals generally present mild symptoms or none at all, and infection results in lifelong immunity. However, children fighting malnutrition and other health-related problems will suffer more severe effects when exposed to childhood infections. As the immune system matures with adolescence, infections such as mumps, if not encountered during early childhood, often cause more severe illness than they would if acquired earlier in life.

Vaccinations against targeted infections have been protecting whole populations from common diseases in modernized nations and in many underdeveloped parts of the world for over half a century. However, infections targeted for vaccination continue to circulate throughout the world, attacking those not vaccinated. Smallpox became the exception as massive vaccination campaigns carried out around the globe supposedly wiped out the disease in the 1970s (see chapter 13). We now realize that the virus has been secretly designated as a biological weapon by rogue governments. We also must worry that incomplete vaccination of populations around the globe will encourage targeted microorganisms, such as whooping cough and diphtheria, to change antigenic structures in order to evade the vaccines and evolve into more potent forms.

Many chemical compounds developed for use as insecticides and pesticides designed to destroy disease-carrying insects have backfired. Many targeted vector mosquitoes have developed resistance to DDT and other chemicals dumped on environments around the world. Also, chemical residues left in the environment have become major damaging pollutants of water and soil, poisoning many life forms and hence threatening human lives.

Drugs developed to conquer malaria met with success, but eventually the parasites developed resistance to them. Modern medicine successfully controlled tuberculosis with drugs, but the bacteria soon developed resistant strains even more potent than the old strains. Consequently, new battle lines have been drawn between humans and familiar pathogens.

Vaccines, insecticides, and antibiotics were supposed to wipe out major infectious diseases by the end of the twentieth century. Instead these "cure alls" deflected many infectious diseases into far more dangerous pathogens than before. Fortunately, many people with good health and strong immune systems can rearrange their vast arsenal of immune responses to meet the new enemies. Yet individuals with impaired immune responses from poor health, poor genes, or malnutrition remain vulnerable to old and new forms of infectious diseases.

We have changed disease patterns throughout the world with the uneven spread of modernization and attempts to control various infectious diseases. Successes have often been tempered by unexpected changes in microbe responses to our efforts to control or eradicate specific infectious agents. The following examples illustrate how disease patterns evolved along with changes in human behavior during the twentieth century.

Epidemic Poliomyelitis

The story of poliomyelitis shows how successful public health measures to eradicate infectious diseases can inadvertently contribute to harmful changes in disease patterns.

Poliomyelitis was rarely mentioned until the mid-nineteenth century. The first described epidemic of poliomyelitis occurred in Stockholm, Sweden, in 1890, followed four years later by a similar epidemic in the United States, centered in Vermont. The epidemic returned to Sweden in 1913 on a much larger scale. Epidemics of poliomyelitis, nicknamed "polio" or "infantile paralysis" for the more severe forms of the disease, continued to appear throughout industrialized countries during the first half of the twentieth century (Howe and Wilson 1959).

Epidemic poliomyelitis primarily evolved as a byproduct of modern living, although the infection has been around for a long time. Three major serotypes of the tiny RNA virus have survived as noncombatant residents in the human gut for centuries. Occasionally the virus breaks through the gut into adjacent lymph nodes and the bloodstream of susceptible individuals. This can lead to various expressions of disease, from transient generalized illness to meningitis or paralysis when it attacks nerve centers (Plum 1975).

Most early childhood infections remain silent or mild, and result in lifelong immunity. A small percentage of infections can lead to inflammation of the membranes surrounding the spinal cord or brain (meningitis) with mild fever, headache, and general discomfort.

Sometimes the symptoms progress to severe muscle pain, plus stiff neck and back. Paralysis can follow within a few days when the infection attacks nerve cells in the spinal cord or brain that activate specific muscles. The location of nerve damage determines what part of the body becomes paralyzed. The legs incur damage more often than the arms, usually only on one side. Paralysis can be life-threatening when the muscles for breathing and swallowing weaken. Paralysis is actually an uncommon complication of poliomyelitis, occurring in less than 1 percent of infections (Benenson 1995).

Poliomyelitis has been just one of many silent natural gut infections in infants and young children (less than three years of age) in the Old World for centuries. It spread to the rest of the world through colonization and migration. The virus may have adapted to the human gut during the development of civilization when large urban populations facilitated circulation of the virus among the young.

Regardless of presence or absence of symptoms, individuals shed the virus in mouth secretions for about a week following infection. They then continue to shed the virus from the intestinal tract in feces for weeks. The virus can be transferred to others by mouth secretions or fecal contamination; infected babies and toddlers act as the best transmitters of the viruses.

As would be expected, evidence for paralytic poliomyelitis rarely occurs in ancient human remains, with only a few possible cases suggestive of the disease in the Old World from ancient Egypt (Aufderheide and Rodriguez-Martin 1998). In addition, the skeletal remains of a child eleven to twelve years of age from thirteenth-century Corinth, Greece, shows signs of paralysis most likely caused by poliomyelitis. The right leg appears abnormally thinner than the left leg, although both legs are the same length. The right hip joint had shrunk from disuse, and the thin bones of the right leg indicate that it had not been used for a long time. Bones shrink in size over time when not bearing weight regularly.

Symptoms of disease appear more frequently in older children and in adults acquiring the infection for the first time, and both have greater chances for developing serious complications, such as paralysis. The infection more likely will spread from the gut into the bloodstream and attack motor nerve cells in older individuals than in very young ones. The more mature immune system responds vigorously to the virus, and thus generates severe inflammation adding to the damage of nerve cells.

Epidemic poliomyelitis made its appearance when people tried to sanitize their environments to prevent other, more life-threatening infectious diseases. Improvements in public health and personal hygiene become a double-edged sword, reducing threats from invading pathogens while raising opportunities for indigenous microbes, such as the poliomyelitis viruses. Individuals protected from infection during infancy and early childhood become vulnerable to more serious infection in later years.

When the infection is introduced into a population where the majority have been sheltered from it since infancy, epidemics erupt with more cases of serious disease than when the infection occurs naturally during infancy among most individuals within a population. Studies of poliomyelitis infection in 1952 showed that young children in Cairo, Egypt, had been exposed to all three types of the virus by the age of two, while only a small percentage of those under two years of age in an American city of similar size and latitude had been exposed to the virus at all (Howe and Wilson 1959).

By the early twentieth century, epidemics of poliomyelitis made the rounds of vulnerable older children and young adults within modernizing regions of the world. The epidemics reached new highs during the late 1940s, when the disease struck U.S. troops sent to Southeast Asia and the eastern Mediterranean during World War II. Obviously, they had never before been exposed to the infection. Drastic measures were developed in the early 1950s to treat the surge of serious infections. Mechanical respirators, known as "iron lungs," kept victims with paralyzed respiratory muscles alive. Fortunately, up to 68 percent of iron lung patients were able to recover enough respiratory muscle power to breathe on their own and return to their lives (Howe and Wilson 1959).

The injectable Salk vaccine, introduced in 1955, contained all three types of killed poliomyelitis virus that stimulated immunoglobins in the bloodstream to provide protection against serious infection. However, the virus could continue to reside in the gut unharmed and hence continue to circulate in the population.

Another vaccine containing weakened live virus, the Sabin oral vaccine, gained popularity in 1962. It induces immunoglobin responses to kill the virus in the gut. This eliminates the virus from circulation within a population. The Sabin oral vaccine quickly replaced the Salk injectable vaccine to wipe out the virus from targeted populations (Cockburn 1963).

Over time, massive vaccination campaigns against poliomyelitis replaced any naturally acquired immunity in young children. Consequently, poliomyelitis epidemics in modernized nations faded into memory by the late twentieth century, with only occasional outbreaks of infection among unvaccinated children and adults. The World Health Organization began a global vaccination program in 1988 aimed at eliminating the virus from the world, hoping to reach that goal by 2010 (*International Herald Tribune*, 20 December 1999). While circulation of the wild virus has been reduced in many parts of the world, the virus continues to circulate throughout the Indian subcontinent and in parts of Africa (Benenson 1995).

Meningococcal Meningitis

Meningitis is a condition of inflammation of the membranes covering the brain and spinal cord. It can be caused by any infectious microbe that manages to reach them and cause harm. The most common microbe responsible for outbreaks of meningitis is the meningococcal bacterium *Neisseria meningitidis*, cousin to the bacterium responsible for gonorrhea (Benenson 1995; Moore and Broome 1994).

Like poliomyelitis, infection with *Neisseria meningitidis* commonly occurs in early childhood. While some variants of the bacteria possess the potential to cause blood-borne meningitis, most infections remain silent and localized in the mucosal lining of the nose and throat. The bacteria are shed in mucous secretions and are transmitted directly or through sneezed or coughed-up droplets (Baltimore 1998).

Infection brings immunity, but it applies only to the specific infectious serotype or strains children grow up with in the local environment. Such immunity does not provide protection from infection by other strains introduced from other areas. At least thirteen known major serotypes of this pathogen circulate throughout the world, and two or more often overlap in the same geographic area (Baltimore 1998).

Some strains can be dangerous when the infection does not stay confined to the mucosal lining of the nose and throat. Entry into the bloodstream causes systemic immune responses, and unless the invaders can be stopped immediately, the bacteria can wreak havoc on the circulatory system and attack the meningeal covering of the brain and spinal cord.

When the bacteria enter the bloodstream, fever and chills appear, along with rapid pulse and frequently some aching in the joints. Usually a red spotted rash also erupts on the skin and mucous membranes, lasting a few days before turning brown and fading. If the immune system cannot quickly halt the infection, intense headache, stiff neck, and sometimes vomiting signal the onset of meningitis. Delirium and coma can follow. Absence of early immune response can lead to overwhelming blood infection and collapse of the circulatory system with bleeding from the capillaries into the skin, septic shock, and rapid death (Schoenbach 1952). If left untreated, once the infection gains entry into the body, the fatality rate climbs higher than 50 percent (Benenson 1995).

The bacteria thrive in overcrowded, stressed groups of people with weakened immune systems. Outbreaks are not uncommon among crowded institutions and gatherings around the globe. Waves of epidemics have also raged for many years through poor crowded villages across sub-Saharan Africa and other poor regions of the world (Moore and Broome 1994). People with compromised immune systems from battling other diseases and malnutrition, as well as from the stress of social disruptions and living in overcrowded villages, appear to be the most vulnerable to meningitis.

Modernized countries not faced with the overcrowding and poverty that afflict underdeveloped parts of the world suffer only occasional isolated outbreaks of the disease. However, in the past, industrializing countries often did experience epidemics of this disease. Both Europe and North America reported epidemics matching this disease among the overcrowded urban poor during the nineteenth century. Four distinct epidemics occurred in North America between 1917 and 1945 among susceptible groups. Army recruits for World War I and World War II became targets for meningitis when they entered military training camps. The stress of preparing for war and the mixing of young men carrying different meningococcal strains from all over the country provided fertile ground for virulent strains to dominate and produce disease (Schoenbach 1952).

The great diversity within the meningococcal bacteria remained unknown until the 1950s, when four major serotypes came to be recognized. The dominant serotype circulating around the globe at that time and for more than a hundred years was identified as group A meningococci (Baltimore 1998).

Following World War II, epidemics throughout Europe and North America abated through restored social order and new public health measures. The drug sulfadiazine proved an effective treatment for meningococcal meningitis, and it was used to prevent the disease among army recruits and other susceptible groups of people (Baltimore 1998). Vaccines developed during the 1970s also helped prevent the disease (Moore and Broome 1994).

Similar preventive measures often were not used in underdeveloped parts of the world where the dominant group A meningococci continued to flourish among susceptible populations.

By the 1960s many strains of the bacteria gained drug resistance to sulfadiazine, forcing the use of large doses of other drugs to treat it. Eventually this enhanced bacterial resistance to these drugs also (Baltimore 1998).

While group A meningococci have dominated infections around the globe for the past century, other groups have been jockeying for dominance. Since 1990 group B and C infections have predominated among children and young adults in North America, while group B has generated epidemics in South America and Cuba (Benenson 1995). The vaccines developed in the 1970s only protect against strains in group A and C, and do not provide protection against group B strains (Baltimore 1998).

Perhaps the widespread use of vaccines and drugs has encouraged new strains to emerge. Generally, a single new strain arises followed by a chain of epidemics from one area to another. During the 1960s a new strain from Group A appeared in China, and then spread to Nepal, Tibet, northern India, and Pakistan by the 1980s. Muslim pilgrims carried it to Mecca in 1987 where it dispersed to sub-Saharan Africa (Moore and Broome 1994).

Alarmed at the rapid spread of the new strain from Mecca, millions of visiting pilgrims received vaccinations during the mid-1990s in an attempt to control the spread of the disease. This did not stop the appearance of a new variant of a vaccine-resistant strain known as W135 during the 2000 pilgrimage. This vaccine-resistant strain had been making occasional appearances around the world since 1970, but it reached an ideal breeding ground in the Muslim pilgrims at Mecca who in turn carried the bacteria with them to their home regions throughout the world (Mayer et al. 2002). The worldwide pattern of meningococcal infections is now changing, and we can only wait to see which variants gain dominance.

The Hepatitis World

Hepatitis literally means inflammation of the liver, and most inflammations result from viral infections. In the last twenty years medical research has shown that more than one type of virus can infect the liver, but they all produce similar symptoms of hepatitis, although most of the infections remain silent.

Hepatitis viruses acquired through the oral-fecal route generally produce short-term infection with full recovery and immunity. Viruses transmitted through blood or body fluids tend to produce chronic liver infections.

We know of only two types of hepatitis viruses transmitted by the oral-fecal route, RNA viruses type A and E. Hepatitis A has been the most commonly recognized liver infection for over a century in every part of the world, while hepatitis E has recently been identified as a separate type of infection. Like poliomyelitis, both virus types commonly produce silent infections among young children in underdeveloped parts of the world with poor sanitation.

Children growing up in modernized countries seldom become exposed to the viruses. If they contract one of the viruses for the first time as adults, they usually develop symptoms of disease. Outbreaks in modernized countries often can be traced to a common infectious source.

Discharged feces from infected individuals contain the viruses. Feces-contaminated drinking water, food handled by infected individuals with poor hygiene habits, and produce washed with contaminated water can transmit the viruses to others. Raw or undercooked mollusks harvested from contaminated waters can also transmit the viruses (Benenson 1995). The A type virus can survive in water and sediment for over three months, and it can survive on inert surfaces and in food for several days (Catton and Locarnini 1998).

Symptoms of hepatitis A and E usually appear abruptly three to four weeks after exposure, with fever, loss of appetite, a feeling of unwellness, and abdominal discomfort. Jaundice appears within a few days. The disease usually stays mild, lasting one to two weeks, with a prolonged convalescence that generally results in complete recovery with immunity. Occasionally there may be a relapse one to three months later before the virus clears from the host. Death occurs rarely, in less than 1 percent of infections (Benenson 1995; Sherlock 1998).

Chronic hepatitis differs from short-term hepatitis A and E in the causative agents and the route of infection. For years it has been known that hepatitis can be transmitted through blood transfusions. The major culprit for blood-borne transmission has been a DNA virus referred to as hepatitis B. The RNA virus hepatitis C often follows infection with type B (Sherlock 1998).

Modern medicine introduced blood transfusions, vaccinations, and injectable medications over a century ago. And unknowingly for more than a couple of generations, these procedures provided new and easy routes of transmission for blood-borne hepatitis viruses, spreading them throughout the world.

Recently a newly discovered blood-borne RNA virus, designated hepatitis G, has been identified. Modern medicine promoted this virus with organ transplant technology, since it commonly occurs with liver transplants (Karayiannis and Thomas 1998).

Blood transfusions; poorly sterilized needles and syringes used for injections and vaccinations; needles used for tattoos, body piercing, and acupuncture; and poorly sterilized dental and surgical tools have promoted transmission of the blood-borne viruses.

Modern countries began screening donor blood for hepatitis B virus during the second half of the twentieth century, along with improving the sterilizing techniques for surgical instruments. The introduction of disposable needles also helped reduce transmission of these viruses. However, many hospitals and clinics in underdeveloped countries continue to follow poor sterilization techniques, do inadequate testing of donor blood, and reuse contaminated needles.

Hepatitis B can also be transmitted through saliva, semen, and vaginal secretions with intimate contact from an actively infected individual. Shared objects contaminated with infected body fluids or blood, such as razors and toothbrushes, can also transmit infection. Similar transmission for hepatitis C has been suggested. Hepatitis B maintains endemic status in areas of Southeast and East Asia, where newborns of infected mothers commonly contract the virus around the time of birth (Benenson 1995).

Four major subtypes of hepatitis B with many variants circulate around the world. Fortunately, immunity gained from infection by one subtype protects against the others. Hepatitis B infection commonly occurs in infancy and early childhood throughout Africa as well as Asia, with most infections silent. Adults infected for the first time will be more likely than children to show symptoms and develop chronic disease. Beginning symptoms are similar to hepatitis A and E, but often with nausea and vomiting, and no fever. An attack of hepatitis B often appears more severe and lasts longer than an attack by hepatitis A or E. Host immune responses in a small percentage of infected individuals cannot stop the disease from progressing rapidly to fatal liver disease (Benenson 1995; Sherlock 1998).

Chronic infection occurs when the virus cannot be evicted from the liver cells. Most chronic infections remain low key, with few if any symptoms, while up to 25 percent of chronic infections by some variants of the virus can slowly progress to cirrhosis (Benenson 1995). Hepatitis B also serves as the major cause of liver cancer, which occurs in about 5 percent of those infected (Kann and Gerlich 1998).

Hepatitis C produces similar but less severe symptoms than hepatitis B, and only 25 percent of victims infected with hepatitis C develop jaundice. As with hepatitis B, the majority of infections are silent. Chronic infection without symptoms commonly occurs, with fluctuating or persistent high liver enzymes, often leading to cirrhosis or sometimes liver cancer (Benenson 1995; Sherlock 1998).

Sometimes a tiny RNA viral particle known as delta agent may be found with hepatitis B infection. This viral particle cannot replicate in liver cells unless the B virus is also present. As it completes its own replication cycle, B virus replication becomes temporarily suppressed (Benenson 1995). Combined infection with delta and B hepatitis can lead to more severe liver disease (Sherlock 1998).

New variants of the hepatitis B virus have been noted in recent years, particularly with the introduction and widespread use of a vaccine developed to prevent infection. This vaccine represents the first use of recombinant DNA technology for this purpose. About 3 percent of vaccinated infants born to infected mothers in Italy during the 1980s showed infection with a variant resistant to the vaccine. The variant had altered its antigens, allowing it to escape the effects of the vaccine, and so it was named a vaccine escape mutant (Lederberg et al. 1992). This raises the question of how routine vaccines may be affecting the evolution of infectious agents they were intended to control.

Obstreperous Strep and the Staph of Life

Staphylococcal and Streptococcal bacteria have interacted with human beings around the globe for millennia, mostly as harmless scavengers residing on skin or mucous membranes of the nose, mouth, and throat, living off sloughed dead skin and mucosal cells. Both bacteria consist of numerous diverse strains with several bags of tricks that help them survive changes in their microenvironment and changes in human behavior patterns. Some strains have managed to go beyond the status of harmless scavenger to become true pathogens, and some become pathogens by accident when introduced below the skin and mucous membrane barriers, or into the body interior (Burnet and White 1972). Both bacteria constantly upgrade and modify their defenses, and they can assimilate new information from other bacteria and viral bacteriophages.

Hospitals around the world often serve as unwitting swap meets and change agents for these bugs, and these bacteria have managed to adjust to the assaults of modern medicine, creating new disease patterns for modern times.

Staphylococcal Diseases

Staphylococci residing in the nose or on the skin can cause inflammatory responses from the immune system when they intrude below the skin surface. This can lead to pustules, boils, or highly contagious impetigo, a skin disease characterized by pustules that crust over, rupture, and spread. Insignificant scratches and nose picking can easily convey a staph skin infection. Untreated skin wounds can become contaminated with the bacteria. Some strains can produce a toxin (poison) that evokes a "scalded skin" reaction in susceptible persons.

Staphylococci can survive for a while on utensils, bedding, and other objects. The bacteria can also survive in food contaminated by infected food handlers, and with inadequate heating or refrigeration, the bacteria will multiply and produce toxins leading to food poisoning. Severe nausea, cramps, and vomiting, often with diarrhea, occur within a few hours after eating the contaminated food, lasting for one or two days (Benenson 1995).

Accidental introduction into the bloodstream can lead to bacteremia (blood poisoning). This allows pathological strains the opportunity to reach the lungs to cause pneumonia or lung abscess. They can also seed into bones to cause osteomyelitis (bone infection with pus formation), inflame joints, infect membranes surrounding the heart or brain, or lead to an abscess on the brain (Benenson 1995).

Hospitals have always provided a breeding ground for staphylococcal infections, particularly when sterile conditions have been marginal or nonexistent for surgeries (Krause 1991). Even today's modern hospitals, as well as poorly equipped hospitals in underdeveloped countries, still continue this tradition, and they have become centers for the spread of dangerous forms of staphylococcal infections. Furthermore, overuse of antibiotics has inspired new pathological strains more virulent than past strains, while lax sterile techniques and poor hand washing practices by staff have helped spread the antibiotic-resistant strains among patients, especially among vulnerable newborns and surgical patients (Ruben and Muder 1998).

Staphylococcal-induced toxic shock syndrome appeared suddenly in 1978 in North America, although the disorder had been alluded to back in the 1920s (Reingold 1998). Every system in the body reacts to a deadly toxin released by a virulent strain of *Staphylococcus aureus* that reaches the bloodstream. The bacteria usually do not invade the body, just the toxin. Symptoms include sudden high fever, vomiting, watery diarrhea, muscle aches, and low blood pressure, followed by a sunburn-like rash that later peels off (Benenson 1995; Schlievert et al. 1981). Severe reactions can cause fatal shock in 5–10 percent of cases (Garrett 1994).

Staphylococcal strains capable of producing the toxin appear to have increased during the 1970s, along with antibody resistance acquired from bacteriophages (viruses infecting bacteria). The newly modified strains often preside silently on the skin and mucous membranes of the nose, throat, and vagina without producing the toxins (Reingold 1998). Changes in their microenvironment or in host immunity apparently trigger the production of the damaging toxins.

Outbreaks of toxic shock syndrome appeared during the late 1970s and early 1980s, mostly among menstruating women in modernized countries around the world who used superabsorbent tampons just put on the market. Women carrying in their vaginas the staphylococcus capable of producing the deadly toxin placed themselves at risk by leaving the tampons in place for several hours. The superabsorbent tampon, left in place for long periods of time, alters the microenvironment of the vagina, triggering the staphylococcus to produce its deadly toxin. The toxin enters the bloodstream through abrasions caused by irritation of the vaginal wall from the tampons, and symptoms follow (Garrett 1994; Schlievert et al. 1981).

Following the removal from the marketplace of the superabsorbent tampons related to the incidence of toxic shock syndrome, the outbreaks stopped. Toxic shock rapidly retreated to sporadic incidents that include long-term use of some vaginal contraceptives and some invasive procedures in hospitals (Krause 1992).

Streptococcal Diseases

Streptococcus consists of a large group of diverse bacteria found throughout nature (Gray 1998; Swift 1952). Several strains reside on skin and mucous membranes of the mouth, nose, and throat of humans. Most of them do not cause harm, but they have the potential to cause disease if misplaced. And some have evolved into deadly strains capable of producing a wide variety of diseases (Burnet and White 1972). Descriptions of serious diseases associated with streptococcal infection have been known from the time of Hippocrates (Gray 1998; Low et al. 1998).

Three major groups of streptococci play significant roles in human disease: group A, group B, and the pneumoniae group. The resident oral streptococci, *S. mutans*, causes most of the dental caries in modernized nations. Group A streptococci are by far the most common bacteria known to cause infection in humans. Such infections vary from silent or temporary mild infections, to more severe disease that can threaten life, killing over 50 percent of victims (Medina et al. 2001; Stevens 2000a). Streptococcal infections can spread quickly in crowded, poor urban areas and within crowded institutions (Gray 1998).

Streptococci within group A exhibit genetic diversity, comprising over eighty different strains armed with various defensive weapons against the human immune system (Stevens 2000a). Most of the strains contain at least one bacteriophage that carries specific genes responsible for producing toxin (Cleary et al. 2000). Infection by one strain does not provide immune protection against another strain, so that repeated streptococcal infections often appear.

Activation of the microbe's defensive measures generally does not occur until changes in the microenvironment or host immune response trigger action. Getting past the skin or mucous membrane barriers into subsurface tissues, or into the bloodstream, and eventually arriving at different organs of the body constitutes a big microenvironmental change for the bacteria. Adaptive adjustments to the new microenvironments and to exposure to the host's internal immune system have to be made. Depending on the strain, the bacteria excrete various substances, including toxins, to ward off attack and help with adjustments to life inside the human body. The well-equipped invasive streptococci can change their arsenal as they move about within the body.

Group A streptococci living on the skin can cause skin diseases when allowed to enter skin tissue through abrasions, scratches, or wounds to the skin surface. Streptococcal impetigo, a pus-filled lesion that crusts over, similar to staphylococcal-caused impetigo, commonly affects young children during warm summers and in hot climates. Serious infection with potent strains entering the bloodstream can lead to inflammation of the kidneys (Benenson 1995).

One of the earliest known group A streptococcal infections, described by Hippocrates, was a skin disease known as erysipelas (Gray 1998). This same skin infection went by the name of "St. Anthony's fire" during the Middle Ages (Denny 2000). This form of streptococcal infection invades the tissue beneath the skin, creating a reddened, tender, swollen area that spreads outward from the site of entry. Infection usually appears on the face or legs, accompanied by fever, chills, nausea, and vomiting (Benenson 1995).

The most common group A streptococcal infection results in strep throat, a highly contagious disease that usually spreads by direct contact with secretions from the throat. Streptococci strains infecting the throat differ from those infecting the skin. The infection primarily attacks children, but adults can also be infected. Strep throat starts with fever and sore throat, and the throat becomes red and swollen, along with the tonsils. Lymph glands in the neck usually respond by swelling, and the tonsils may leak fluid filled with pus as the inflammatory process put into motion by the immune system tries to eliminate the culprit. Strep throat can range from mild to severe with complications, depending on host immune response and the streptococcal strain involved. Some strains infected with certain bacteriophages can produce toxins highly damaging to human tissues. Strains with the potential to be dangerous frequently infect individuals without signs of disease (Benenson 1995).

Recovery from strep throat does not always imply that the bacteria have been eliminated. The infection can reroute and persist in nearby tissues. Streptococci frequently journey up the short eustachian tube to the middle ear in children causing otitis media (middle ear infection). Infection in the middle ear can also move into the mastoid cells causing mastoiditis. Abscesses can form in the tissues around the tonsils, and in the past this was referred to as "quinsy" (Benenson 1995).

Some strains of group A streptococci that break through the mucosal barrier and into the bloodstream following strep throat or tonsillitis can seed out to connective tissues of joints, the heart, brain, or skin. Most of the victims are children. The microbes mimic antigenic components of cells within these tissues as they try to hide from the surveillance of the host immune system. When the host immune system fails to be fooled, it attacks not only the enemy but also its own cells that bear similar antigenic properties to the microbes (Ayoub et al. 2000; Cunningham 2000). The end result is rheumatic fever.

Following recovery from an attack of strep throat, usually ten to twenty days later (Markowitz and Kaplan 2000), symptoms of rheumatic fever appear: high fever, profuse sweating, rapid pulse, exhaustion, and painful, swollen joints appearing over a twenty-four-hour period. Joints on both sides of the body come under attack in sets, one set after another in rapid succession. Each time the bacteria assault a new set of joints, the fever spikes. Joint inflammation generally lasts four to six days, followed by complete recovery. Sometimes the cycle of attack on joints gets repeated, and this often indicates the heart will be a target. The heart valves can be permanently damaged when they become inflamed and scarred. The coronary arteries feeding blood to the heart tissue can also become inflamed and blocked by scar tissue (Swift 1951). Rheumatic fever remains one of the leading causes of heart disease in children worldwide (Cunningham 2000).

Sometimes rheumatic fever inflames blood vessels in the brain, leading to focal zones of encephalitis that can cause involuntary contraction or twitching of muscles of the trunk, arms, and legs, slurred speech, and faulty memory. This disorder goes by the rubric "Sydenham's chorea" (Swift 1951).

The skin can also show disturbances from rheumatic fever with various lesions, such as a red rash that tends to recur for weeks or months after the initial stages of the disease. Sometimes painful small red lumps appear on the legs, often in repeating crops, turning purple and greenish. Larger, painless swellings may form beneath skin along the spine and flat bony surfaces. These symptoms tend to disappear with recovery if the course of the disease does not become fatal (Swift 1951).

Rheumatic fever was well known throughout urban areas of the industrialized countries after World War II, becoming rare by the 1970s, until in the late 1980s isolated outbreaks began reappearing. The disease has always remained a threat in underdeveloped parts of the world (Denny 2000), and it occurs in high frequencies among Australian aborigines (Markowitz and Kaplan 2000).

Scarlet fever represents another group A streptococcal disease that also generally begins with the symptoms of strep throat. However, the strains causing this disease produce potent toxins that upon reaching the bloodstream trigger inflammatory reactions in the lining of blood vessels, often accompanied by nausea and vomiting. Inflamed blood vessels near the skin produce a swollen, bright red skin rash over the trunk, arms, and legs. Affected skin peels off when the rash disappears after the sixth to ninth day.

The disease can vary from mild symptoms, with a faint rash lasting only twenty-four hours, to severe life-threatening forms, with hemorrhagic skin rash, ending either in death within forty-eight hours or in prolonged infection that spreads through the bloodstream to other parts of the body. Scarlet fever affects mostly children over the age of three, and rarely appears in babies and adults (Keefer 1951).

Severe forms of scarlet fever disappeared from modernizing nations during the early twentieth century, long before antibiotics were introduced to fight the disease. Severe scarlet fever had haunted industrializing countries since the Middle Ages. The British physician Thomas Sydenham described the disease in 1675 and named it scarlet fever, and outbreaks continued for fifty years among urban populations in Britain before receding (Keefer 1951). Outbreaks of severe scarlet fever appeared often during the nineteenth century in urban populations of Europe and North America. Finally, milder forms of the disease began to take over after 1885 (Low et al. 1998).

Severe streptococcal infections nearly disappeared with the implementation of higher living standards and hygiene in modernizing countries following World War II. Penicillin treatment also helped prevent serious complications, such as rheumatic fever and scarlet fever.

Although streptococcal infections have dramatically declined in modern communities, many strains, like staphylococcal strains, continue to make rounds in hospital settings. Here they learn new tricks by exchanging information, and cause infections.

The best known group A streptococcal hospital-acquired infections date back to the nineteenth century when half of the women admitted to hospitals to bear their babies died from childbed fever due to streptococcal infection (Denny 2000). The lack of hand washing and poor hygiene inadvertently allowed attending physicians and their students to spread the infection among the new mothers (Gray 1998). The incidence of childbed fever dropped considerably once hospitals set standards for hygiene and hand washing. Soap and water can go a long way to prevent serious bacterial infections.

New strains of group B streptococci, including strains resistant to antibiotics, have been appearing in hospitals throughout North America and Europe to infect newborns. The bacteria can reside on the mucous membranes of a woman's vagina without causing harm. About 1 percent of newborns develop infection during birth from their infected mothers. The streptococci can spread through the infant's bloodstream causing pneumonia, shock, and meningitis, killing 10–50 percent of infected newborns. Sometimes the disease strikes after the time of birth with similar consequences but with better survival rates (Benenson 1995; Gray 1998; Nizet et al. 2000).

Streptococcal pneumoniae commonly reside harmlessly in the nose and throat of children throughout the world. Like group A streptococci, numerous strains exist with no cross-immunity. This allows a person to experience repeated disease-producing infections similar to those of group A, especially middle ear infections.

Most children in underdeveloped countries acquire pneumoniae before three years of age, while only about half of young children in modern countries are infected. Most infected young children become silent carriers and develop immunity to the infectious strain. However, pneumoniae-caused middle ear infections have become the most common infection occurring in children. *Streptococcal pneumoniae* have also become the leading cause of bacterial pneumonia in children and adults (Gray 1998), and form one of the leading causes of bacterial meningitis in young infants (Baltimore and Shapiro 1998), particularly in underdeveloped countries. Antimicrobial drug treatment has only offered temporary control of mucosal infections as the microbes have grown tolerant to the drugs, and symptoms return once treatment ceases (Syrjanen et al. 2001). Since the 1960s strains have emerged that resist penicillin, and in recent years strains have developed that are resistant to several other antibiotics (Hudspeth et al. 2001).

Strains of group A streptocococci, equipped with new capabilities for producing potent toxins once the bacteria invade the bloodstream, emerged during the 1980s. Some people are highly sensitive to their toxins, and their immune systems overreact with damaging inflammatory responses that lead to toxic shock with multi-system failure (Medina et al. 2001). One of the first victims of the deadly strains was Jim Henson, the puppeteer of television fame. He died in 1990 from a strep throat infection that quickly spread to his lungs and bloodstream, leading to irreversible toxic shock, despite antibiotic treatment (Krause 1992).

Another devastating disease caused by potent toxin-producing strains of group A streptococci attacks from the skin surface, penetrating through minor abrasions or wounds to tissues beneath the skin. The disease progresses rapidly with a destructive process of tissue known as necrotizing fasciitis, commonly known as "flesh eating bacteria" (Gray 1998). The affected area becomes swollen, red, and hot to the touch, and it spreads rapidly outward within twenty-four hours. The redness turns to dark purple, then to blue, and large blisters form containing yellow fluid by the fourth to fifth day, followed by tissue death and gangrene. From 20 percent to 50 percent of affected individuals die from the disease (Stevens 2000a).

The 1980s marked a turning point in streptococcal infections as newly formed strains with the capacity to produce harmful toxins spread around the world. Fortunately, only a small percentage of susceptible individuals have fallen victim to the new strains.

Similar toxin-producing streptococci that induce toxic shock and necrotizing fasciitis have existed in the past, with sporadic reports into the early twentieth century in Europe and China (Stevens 2000b). Descriptions of necrotizing fasciitis date back to Hippocrates in fifth-century B.C. Greece. This disease has been referred to as "phagedena," "malignant ulcer," "gangrenous ulcer," "putrid ulcer," and "hospital gangrene" (Low et al. 1998).

The remarkable capacity of streptococci to acquire toxin-provoking bacteriophages over the centuries has given them the power to produce devastating diseases. Hence, the recent surge in new strains containing powerful toxins represents nothing new, just a reminder from the past that scarlet fever and other toxic streptococcal infections can strike again.

Opportunistic Legionnaire's Disease

This disease received its name for a mysterious outbreak that occurred at an American Legion convention at a hotel in Philadelphia in 1976. Dozens of people became ill, with 221 hospitalized and 34 deaths. Researchers finally solved the mystery nearly a year later when they identified the cause—a bacterium commonly found in nature but never before associated with human disease. Soon, other outbreaks and sporadic cases of unknown cause that had occurred back to 1947 could be associated with *Legionella bacteria*.

Outbreaks of infection with this bacteria have been recorded in hospitals, office buildings, industrial plants, and hotels and resorts throughout the world (Butler and Breiman 1998). The last major outbreak of legionella infection in the twentieth century centered on a whirlpool spa exhibit at a flower show in the Netherlands in 1999. This outbreak involved 133 confirmed infections with 16 deaths (Boshuizen et al. 2001).

Legionella bacteria naturally thrive in pond and creek water. Lacking a cell wall but protected by a double membrane, they easily infect their natural prey, free-living one-celled amoebae. Human beings are rarely exposed to them in nature (Butler and Breiman 1998).

That situation changed with the introduction of evaporative coolers and air conditioners in closed modern buildings. This opened up a whole new environment and life style for these bacteria. Usually their numbers remain small in natural water settings, but when introduced into artificial water settings, free of natural enemies, they thrive and rapidly increase. Artificial water systems undergoing repeated use without cleaning can produce large numbers of bacteria that can ride water droplets through air ducts, coming into contact with human respiratory systems. The bacteria can also invade cold and hot water taps, and can travel in aerosol spray from showers and whirlpool spas. Improperly cleaned respiratory therapy equipment can also harbor the bacteria (Butler and Breiman 1998).

Bacteria breathed into the human respiratory system gravitate to macrophage-type cells that clean up debris and gobble up foreigners in air sacs deep inside the lungs. Most likely these cells resemble their natural prey, one-celled amoebae. The immune systems of most healthy individuals quickly respond to the foreign intruders within forty-eight hours before much damage can be done. The quick immune response triggers a transient, mild infection known as "Pontiac fever." The name originated from an outbreak in a building housing the Oakland County Health Department in Pontiac, Michigan, in 1968. Symptoms lasting less than a week begin with loss of appetite, fatigue, headache, and aching muscles, followed by a rapidly rising fever with chills. Some individuals also suffer a dry cough, abdominal pain, and diarrhea (Benenson 1995; Butler and Breiman 1998).

Delayed immune reactions unable to act quickly enough to prevent *Legionella bacteria* from invading and multiplying in macrophage cells lead to more serious disease. Crippling pneumonia, known as legionnaire disease, can develop within two to ten days, with up to 20 percent fatality rates. Smokers and older people with medical problems who usually have compromised immune responses, are most vulnerable to serious infection (Bulter and Breiman 1998).

Lyme Disease

In 1975 the town of Lyme, Connecticut, experienced a highly unusual outbreak of what appeared to be juvenile rheumatoid arthritis. The mystery was finally solved in 1982 when the spirochete *Borrelia burgdorferi*, transmitted by tick bites, proved to be the cause. The town of Lyme lies in a wooded area interrupted by grassland where the tick vector thrives on indigenous mammals, particularly the wild white-footed mouse. The area attracts all kinds of wildlife, particularly large numbers of deer, thus feeding and increasing the tick population. Residents of the town of Lyme gained constant exposure to the abundant tick population in the woods, parks, and even their own grassy yards (Daniels and Falco 1989; Kantor 1994).

The vector tick, *Ixodes scapularis*, undergoes a two-year life cycle beginning when the female drops from her animal host to lay eggs in the soil during the spring. Tiny, dot-size larvae emerge during the summer and attach to a passing small animal, such as the white-footed mouse, to feed on its blood. If the animal has been infected with the spirochete, the larvae become infected as they feed. The fed larvae drop back to the ground and molt into poppyseed-sized nymphs (Daniels and Falco 1989; Kantor 1974).

The nymphs wait until the next year's warm weather to search for another host to feed on before becoming adult ticks. They prefer the white-footed mouse, but will take any warm-blooded host that happens along. Infected nymphs can now infect new animal hosts. Humans often get caught in this part of the tick's life cycle with the hard- to-spot nymph using them for a blood feeding. The fed nymph falls back to earth to molt, emerging as an adult, less than sesame seed size, in early fall (Daniels and Falco 1989; Kantor 1974).

The adult has one more blood feeding before it mates by late spring, and infected nymphs carry the infection with them into adulthood. Adult ticks have a primary attraction to white-tailed deer for their final blood meal, but humans, dogs, cattle, horses, and other large animals can also serve at this stage. Male ticks die following mating, and females die after egg laying, completing the tick life cycle (Daniels and Falco 1989; Kantor 1994).

The bite of an infected nymph or adult tick can only transmit Lyme disease after it attaches to the host for thirty-six to forty-eight hours. Spirochetes waiting in the mid-gut of the tick only begin to multiply as the tick starts its blood meal. Then they migrate to the salivary glands where they are discharged into the host with the tick's saliva. It takes several hours before a large enough infectious dose of spirochetes can penetrate the new host. The blood meal usually lasts about a week before the blood-engorged tick drops off the host (Daniels and Falco 1989; Kantor 1994).

Symptoms that simulate juvenile rheumatoid arthritis do not represent the only symptoms of Lyme disease. Infection with the spirochete can cause a wide range of symptoms, ranging from mild to severe, and for some individuals the disease becomes chronic. The site of the tick bite often inflames within days to a month after the spirochetes enter the skin. The red area expands in a circular pattern up to several inches in diameter, clearing in the middle. It can fade within days or take several weeks to disappear. Flu-like symptoms develop when the spirochetes enter the bloodstream. Early symptoms include fatigue, fever and chills, headache, stiff neck, loss of appetite, and joint and muscle aches that can last for several weeks. If the immune response fails to stop them, they can disperse to any organ of the body, particularly the heart, nervous system, and joints (Benenson 1995; Kantor 1994).

The most common symptoms in the first weeks of the disease involve muscles and joints. Discomfort in one joint at a time is followed several months later with swelling and pain in some of the large joints, especially in one of the knees, that can develop into chronic arthritis. Unlike rheumatoid arthritis, Lyme arthritis does not affect sets of joints on both sides of the body (Benenson 1995). One knee often acts as the focal spot for Lyme arthritis, and its frequent appearance among people living near Montauk, New York, earned it the nickname "Montauk knee" (Kantor 1994).

The heart may suffer temporary disrupted rhythm, but this generally subsides within two weeks. Some individuals develop neurological symptoms within weeks or months after the tick bite. Affected cranial nerves can lead to paralysis of one or both sides of the face (Bell's palsy) lasting weeks or months. Meningitis, encephalitis, and involuntary muscle twitching can result. Tingling, pain, or numbness from nerve irritation, and defective muscle coordination from cerebellar involvement, can also occur. Symptoms can come and go, lasting months (Benenson 1995; Kantor 1994).

Lyme disease has not been confined to North America. The initial skin reaction of Lyme disease was first described in Sweden in 1909, followed by reports from France in 1922, and later from other European countries. The first recognized case of Lyme disease in North America occurred in 1969 in Wisconsin (Moore et al. 1998). Since worldwide recognition of the disease in 1985, reports of Lyme disease have surfaced from temperate regions around the world (Barbour 2000; Benenson 1995). Different geographic regions of the world house different variations of spirochetes, *Ixodes* ticks and animal hosts, giving rise to geographical variations of Lyme disease.

Infection has been found in migrating birds in Scandinavia, suggesting they help spread the disease. Deer flies, houseflies and mosquitoes can also carry the spirochetes, but their bites rarely produce infection in humans (Moore et al. 1998), though they do help spread the spirochetes in nature.

Since 1980 Lyme disease has become the most common insect-borne disease in North America, and it represents a growing problem in Europe, China, Japan, South Africa, and Australia. The increases in Lyme disease directly relate to changing land use patterns over the past two centuries (Lederberg et al. 1992).

Over two centuries ago many temperate forest lands throughout the world had been cleared, particularly those areas undergoing industrialization and massive reforms in agriculture. Increasing fuel demands for wood and charcoal by the new industries also depleted many forests. Deforestation disrupted the life cycle of the vector tick with the loss of animal host habitat, particularly deer, and Lyme disease became a rarity.

During the mid-nineteenth century in the eastern United States, farmers slowly but steadily abandoned farmland cleared from the eastern woodlands as Midwest farmland opened up. This paved the way for regeneration of the eastern woodlands, and by the mid-twentieth century dense regrowth forest offered shelter to a wide range of wildlife, including expanding populations of white-footed mice and white-tailed deer. Thus, the tick and spirochete population responsible for Lyme disease also increased and spread rapidly with their animal hosts.

The rejuvenated eastern woodlands attracted people for recreation and suburban development, bringing them directly into contact with large numbers of infected ticks. Similar situations exist in other reforested areas throughout the United States, and Lyme disease now has been identified in nearly every state. Europe is experiencing similar problems from Lyme disease through massive reforestation programs and increasing deer populations following World War II (Lederberg et al. 1992).

The dramatic increase in exposure to the spirochetes causing Lyme disease has also increased exposure to a protozoan parasite (Lederberg et al. 1992) infecting the same tick vector in North America, Mexico, and Europe. Deer play a major role in spreading the infected tick. *Babesia microti* is a blood-borne parasite that invades red blood cells to produce malaria-like disease lasting several days to a few months. Destruction of red blood cells by the invading parasite causes anemia, fever, chills, fatigue, jaundice, and muscle aches (Benenson 1995).

The Mystery of Chronic Diseases

While epidemic diseases have waned with modernization, chronic diseases have gained considerable prominence in modern countries. *Chronic disease* refers to a progressive disease of long duration. Chronic inflammatory reactions commonly accompany most chronic diseases. Inflammatory reactive processes normally set about to repair damaged tissues, but with chronic diseases, the damage appears to be an ongoing process. Chronic diseases can target specific organs or several different organs of the body. The cause may or may not be known. While some chronic diseases are related to some specific long-term infections, nutritional deficits, or genetic disturbances, too often the cause has remained a mystery to modern medicine.

Many chronic diseases have been defined as *syndromes*, groups of signs and symptoms that collectively characterize particular chronic disorders, such as chronic fatigue syndrome. Autoimmune disease represents another category of chronic disease. This type of disease results from apparent disorder in the body's immune response that causes it to attack the body's own tissues.

We know that certain infections can persist in various states within the human body, depending on host immune responses and internal environmental conditions. Some infections hide out and wait for a shift in the microenvironment, then reactivate under the right circumstances. Some immune responses cannot eliminate or control an infection, so it continues to smolder and activate immune inflammatory responses.

For too long, medical practitioners dismissed chronic peptic ulcer disease as related to type A personality and high stress, despite its recognized association to stomach infection as early as 1906. By 1984 Robin Warren of Perth, Australia, convinced medical science that bacteria caused the disease. *Helicobacter pylori* thrive on the mucosal lining of the stomach. Some variants can secrete an enzyme that damages the mucous membrane lining and provokes chronic inflammatory disease of the stomach (Smith and Parsonnet 1998).

Association of infection with many chronic diseases has often been dismissed for lack of evidence, but new research is beginning to uncover the truth behind chronic diseases and stealth infection (Lederberg et al. 1992; Mattman 1993). One major clue lies in the high levels of immunoglobins indicative of infection relative to various microbes frequently associated with autoimmune diseases (Isenberg and Morrow 1995).

Quite often the trail of a stealth infectious agent proves difficult to track as the agent changes form or shifts antigens to fool the immune system. The complex interaction between host immune responses, inflammatory reactions, and invading microbe can also obscure what is going on. Often drugs used to alleviate symptoms mask the culprit and exacerbate chronic disease (Isenberg and Morrow 1995). Perhaps long-term nutritional deficits and genetic predisposition contribute to weakened battle lines between stealth microbes and the immune system.

Two groups of bacteria, mycoplasma and chlamydia, can invade a wide variety of cells in stealth form, thus leading to "sleeper" infections that most often persist undetected. Both types of bacteria commonly occur throughout the world and infect a wide range of animals as well as human beings in either overt or covert disease form. Recent medical research has begun to expose the hidden nature of their involvement in chronic inflammatory diseases.

Mycoplasma are a divergent group of bacteria. They do not develop cell walls, a characteristic that enables them to easily act as stealth infections with or without symptoms of disease. They can be found throughout nature, some free living, others infecting plants as well as animals with a wide range of diseases. Humans frequently carry a harmless number of different types of mycoplasma within the normal flora living on the mucosal lining of the mouth, nose, and genital tract. Only one type, *Mycoplasma pneumoniae*, has proven links to human diseases involving the throat and bronchial tubes, frequently causing pneumonia (Couch 1975). Mounting evidence shows that mycoplasma may also be responsible for chronic inflammatory diseases of various bodily organs (Mattman 1993).

Chlamydia represents another diverse group of bacteria that cause a wide range of diseases in animals and humans. They can launch stealth attacks that may be responsible for a wide range of chronic diseases. The best known overt chlamydia infection is trachoma, the leading cause of blindness in underdeveloped parts of the world. Another type of chlamydia can cause pneumonia, while still another type forms one of the major causes of genital infections, and yet another causes Reiter's syndrome, a chronic form of arthritis (Dean 1997). Chlamydia has also recently been linked with chronic coronary heart disease (Lederberg et al. 1992; Mattman 1993; Mlot 1996).

Other bacteria in stealth forms, plus several viruses, appear to be involved in a wide array of chronic infections (Goedert 2000; Issenberg and Morrow 1995; Weetman 1996), such as multiple sclerosis, chronic fatigue syndrome, rheumatoid arthritis, insulin-dependent diabetes, fibromyalgia, Alzheimer's disease, Grave's disease, myasthenia gravis, pernicious anemia, sclerodoma, Behcet's syndrome, Crohn's disease, lupus erythematosus, Whipple's disease, and psoriasis, to name only a few.

Cancer Wars

In 1971 President Richard Nixon declared "war on cancer" in the United States. The war continues to this day, costing many millions of dollars each year in research and treatment, while overall cancer rates have not slowed in their continuous climb for the past hundred and fifty years. Actually, rates for some types of cancer have decreased in the last fifty years, but other types of cancer have increased greatly, pushing the overall cancer rate upward. Part of this growth correlates with increases in aging populations over the last fifty years, since the majority of cancers show up in older age (Tomatis 1990). However, the climbing rates, along with changing patterns of cancer, can also be attributed to changes within our environment and life styles that began with industrialization.

Lung cancer was rare before the introduction of habitual tobacco smoking in the twentieth century. Tobacco use in the form of snuff had already been associated with oral cancer in the eighteenth century, but cancer was not associated with tobacco smoking until the mid-twentieth century when the rate of lung cancer skyrocketed. Tobacco use is not the only cause of oral cancer. Habitual betel nut chewing in underdeveloped parts of Asia can also lead to oral cancer (Tomatis 1990). This shows that cultural habits do play a significant role in the development of various cancers.

Several chemical compounds introduced during the course of industrialization have also proved to be carcinogenic (cancer-promoting). Hints of repeated overexposure to chemical irritants leading to the development of cancers were noted early on. Continuous exposure to chimney soot was linked to scrotal cancer in chimney sweeps in the eighteenth century, and constant exposure to aromatic amines was linked to bladder cancer in perfume workers in the nineteenth century (Tomatis 1990).

Chemical production increased dramatically following World War II, with repeated overexposure to many different chemical irritants that have proven to be carcinogenic. Synthetic chemicals have seeped into water, air, and soil for a century, and now constitute a part of the global environment and our daily lives.

Manufactured chemicals are not the only carcinogenic agents. Radiation, natural toxins in foods, and microbes can also contribute to the development of cancer. Long-term absence of needed nutrients contributes to cellular and immune dysfunction that can predispose an individual to developing cancer. The development of cancer appears to be a complex process or series of events, with more than one factor involved, including the underlying genetic basis that determines susceptibility of damaged cells to transform into cancer cells and how the immune system will react to malignant cells (Tomatis 1990).

Cancers have been around as long as humankind, and cancers can be found in all animal species. Cancerous tumors have been discovered in extinct animal remains, and they have also been recorded in ancient human bones throughout time and around the world (Strouhal 1993). Cancer frequencies are much higher today than in the past. This shift correlates with the population explosion, huge increases in older populations, changing life styles, and industrialization.

Cancer is a catchall term that covers a wide range of abnormal new growths, called *malignant neoplasms*, that tend to seed out to new sites in the body. The site of origin can be anywhere, in any tissue. Cancer has been referred to as a disease of DNA, since the cell's DNA becomes altered to create an abnormal cell reproducing clones capable of infinite new growth.

The role that microbes play, especially viruses, in the development of many cancers is far more important than was realized in the past. Most likely, infection constitutes the major external factor leading to the development of cancer. Exposure to other carcinogenic substances with long-term irritation of certain body tissues may provide the right opportunity for a virus or other microbe to invade a damaged, genetically susceptible cell and transform its DNA. Links between chronic diseases and cancer have been noted (Issenberg and Morrow 1995), with chronic disease setting up the opportunity for cancer to develop.

As noted above, the bacteria *Helicobacter pylori* causes chronic peptic ulcers and stomach infections, but infection can also progress to stomach cancer in genetically susceptible individuals. Stomach cancer remains common in modern Japan, while decreasing in modern Europe and North America, suggesting the involvement of carcinogenic factors within the environment, or pertaining to life style or food choices (Smith and Parsonnet 1998).

Herpes viruses can remain inactive in the body for years before some stimulus that weakens immune responses stimulates viral activity. Most people around the world naturally acquire the Epstein-Barr virus in early childhood, but if the infection occurs during adolescence, the usually asymptomatic infection from early childhood triggers immune responses that produce mononucleosis. Early childhood infection happens much less frequently in modern countries, while mononucleosis occurs much more often than in underdeveloped countries (Seemayer et al. 2000). The virus invades the epithelial layer covering the nose and throat, and immune responses generally stop the infection here. Otherwise it can go on to infect nearby B lymphocytes, spawning a wide variety of chronic diseases that in turn can lead to B lymphocyte cancers, such as Hodgkin's disease, polyclonal B-cell lymphocytosis, Burkitt's lymphoma, and nasopharyngeal carcinoma (Jenkins and Hoffman 2000).

Burkitt's lymphoma is primarily endemic among young children living in equatorial Africa and Papua New Guinea who have a high susceptibility to Epstein-Barr virus activity. Since chronic malaria infection also frequents these regions, malaria infection may allow the virus to transform the DNA of infected B cells (de The 2000). Nasopharyngeal carcinoma rates appear highest in south China, suggesting a particularly virulent form of Epstein-Barr virus, or some environmental or genetic factor, that favors cancer development. The cancer evolves in the large number of B lymphocytes present in the depression leading to the opening of the eustachian tubes within the passageway from nose to throat (Roab-Traub 2000).

Chronic infection with sexually transmitted *Herpes simplex* type 2 virus, and the papilloma virus, causes cervical cancer. Chronic infection with schistosomiasis can lead to bladder cancer (Tomatis 1990). Retrovirus infection can transform helper T lymphocytes into cancer cells to produce adult T-cell leukemia, lymphotrophic virus type 1 (HTLV-1). This type of leukemia is endemic in southwest Japan, areas in the Caribbean, central Africa, parts of Melanesia, Papua New Guinea, Solomon Islands and among Australian aborigines (Matsuoka 2000). Chronic infection of the gallbladder with *Salmonella typhi* has been linked to a rare form of cancer of the gallbladder (Goedert 2000).

Liver cancer (hepatocellular carcinoma) represents one of the most common cancers worldwide, with the highest rates in Southeast Asia and sub-Saharan Africa. Chronic infection of the liver with certain variants of hepatitis B or C is the major precursor to developing liver cancer (Kao and Chen 2000).

The evidence for infectious causes of various cancers may be just the tip of the iceberg. The link between chronic infection and cancer, interwoven with changes that human beings have forced upon the world, along with changing lifestyles, most likely gives the clue to eventual victory in the cancer wars.

CONCLUDING COMMENTS

Rapid modernization during the twentieth century severely affected populations and environments around the globe. During this process, disease patterns underwent a dramatic shift. Progressive changes in all aspects of human life have affected human interaction with both the environment and the microbial world. At the same time, the global population has exploded, reaching 6 billion by the end of the twentieth century, despite huge losses of human lives from wars, famines, diseases, and other human-engineered catastrophes.

Modernization developed unevenly throughout the twentieth century, leaving many areas lagging behind and creating a checkerboard pattern of progress. This uneven development contributed to the shift in patterns of disease as old diseases continued to fester in some parts of the world while modern medicine and public health measures put controls on infectious diseases in other regions. Modern medicine's successes have often been counterbalanced by the inadvertent promotion of rapid evolution among infectious microbes and the opening up of new opportunities for other potentially dangerous pathogens.

Selected populations have received protection from many infectious diseases through vaccination, antibiotics, and chemical control of disease vectors. But several microbes have learned new tricks to get around these defenses, while becoming more deadly in the process. We have also learned that many infectious microbes can transform themselves into stealth infections, either from necessity when attacked or as part of their natural life cycle, leading to the development of chronic diseases and cancer. Ironically, as epidemic diseases have waned in modernized countries, chronic diseases and cancer rates have increased in these countries.

Manipulation of our environments and burgeoning human populations encroaching into wilderness areas have brought human beings into close contact with wild infections that rarely afflicted humans in the past. One of the greatest threats to people throughout the world today comes from exposure to dangerous pathogens, either as new variants of old infections or new infections never encountered before (Mitchison 1993). This threat has been magnified by rapid global travel and commerce that can quickly move diseases around the world.

Toward the end of the twentieth century, global illness and death rates from infectious diseases began to climb to new levels, and they continue to rise (Koenig 1996) with the waning of antibiotic effectiveness, disrupted vaccination programs, vectors resistant to insecticides, and the emergence of new patterns of disease. Many old diseases, such as tuberculosis and malaria, have developed drug resistance and have returned with a vengeance wherever public health measures and hygiene have fallen into disorder. Social upheavals, population dislocations, wars, economic collapses, political mismanagement, and natural disasters have all contributed to the latest increases in infectious diseases.

Infectious disease is now recognized as the leading cause of death worldwide (Conner et al. 1997).

The New Viral Wars and Sleeping Dragons

CHAPTER 22

THE NEW VIRAL WARS AND
SLEEPING DRAGONS

The rapidly growing populations of today's world face many challenging environmental, economic, and geopolitical problems. There are simply too many people pressing for finite land and water resources for survival and economic gain. Human populations are spilling over and settling into one-time wilderness areas. Major rain forests are being destroyed. Giant dams are being built to control water sources, thereby upsetting local ecological zones. Huge numbers of refugees fleeing famine and social, economic, and political turmoil find themselves displaced and barely surviving in a marginal existence, often living in makeshift camps or megacity slums.

Turmoil around the globe has presented us with new challenges from the microbe world. We keep stirring the pot, mixing germs from all over the planet as we break down geographic barriers that once kept them localized and separated. The constant global movements of people and commerce have been acting as conduits for infectious microbes to travel from one place to another.

Today, maverick viruses pose a new threat to human populations. They can arise basically in one of three ways: evolutionary production of a new variant of a recognized virus; a virus jumping from an animal species to human beings; or relatively unknown viruses existing in small isolated populations entering larger populations with first-time recognition. Maverick viruses usually emerge with environmental disturbances or changes in human behavior patterns (Morse 1993). Current environmental and social upsets around the world have provoked the appearance of many such viruses.

The HIV/AIDS Pandemic

The human immunodeficiency virus (HIV) infecting humans originated as a natural infection of chimpanzees. The virus evolved into a silent infection causing no harm within its natural host. Chimpanzees that were hunted and slaughtered for food by rural peoples gave the virus the opportunity to jump species and infect humans during the butchering process. It would only take a skin scratch or nick in contact with infected blood or other body fluids of the animal to permit infection. Most likely the virus sporadically infected rural people in isolated areas of the Congo with deadly results for many years before its escape from rural central Africa during the latter half of the twentieth century (Kanki and Essex 2000). The virus quickly adapted to human beings to become a human disease transmitted through blood and sexual contact.

Many Africans' lives were disrupted as colonial Africa began to nationalize during the second half of the twentieth century. A chain of destabilizing events took place across the continent, facilitating the spread of both old and new infectious diseases, including HIV. Between 1970 and 1975 sub-Saharan Africa saw itself torn apart by ruthless rulers, civil wars, and tribal conflicts augmented by severe drought and famine. Hardest hit was the Congo area of central Africa, especially Uganda under Idi Amin's rule. By the end of the 1970s, HIV and the disease it caused, acquired immune deficiency syndrome (AIDS), had radiated outward from the eastern shores of Lake Victoria to become endemic throughout the region (Garrett 1994). The virus, once confined to isolated rural villages, escaped into the general population of the region as rural people were driven from their homes to more populated areas. Military troops moving through the area also picked up the virus and carried it back to their home regions. Regional truck drivers and prostitutes further contributed to the spread of the virus into urban areas.

Spread of the virus was facilitated by the constant reuse of contaminated needles both within medical facilities and on the street. Routine vaccinations for many children, and the uncontrolled use of injectable medications adapted by street entrepreneurs, turned deadly when contaminated needles were reused. Children and adults treated for malaria with contaminated blood transfusions in clinical facilities also became easy prey for the virus (Garrett 1994). The virus probably would not have been able to spread so quickly throughout Africa if needle use and blood transfusions had taken place under stringent controls.

The world did not know what was happening in central Africa. People outside Africa mostly ignored reports of the mysterious "slim" disease and the surge of rare cancers and diseases related to AIDS killing tens of thousands of people in this part of the world. Many Africans blamed witchcraft for the carnage, and African governments denied the seriousness of the epidemic (Garrett 1994). While the continent of Africa endured the rage of this unknown virus, it managed to leave its homeland and spread around the world. The global blood market and illicit heroin traffic greatly facilitated movement of the virus to different parts of the globe.

The recognition of AIDS in 1981 finally put the world on notice of the impending HIV pandemic. The syndrome was first described in an unusual cluster of rare diseases among young homosexual men in the United States. Soon it became apparent that this syndrome resulted from destruction of the immune system by an unknown virus. Medical researchers quickly set to work to learn about this new virus and how to combat it. New drugs were soon developed in an attempt to control the progression of the disease, and attempts to find drug cures and a preventive vaccine continue to this day. The virus has proven to be an elusive target, capable of rapid evolution, allowing it to maneuver around the arsenal of drugs used to fight it.

Human Immunodeficiency Virus (HIV)

Human immunodeficiency virus (HIV) comprises a complex of related RNA lentiviruses within the retrovirus family that can rapidly evolve into many variants within the individual host. Retrovirus genomes contain two copies of RNA. When HIV gains entry into the cytoplasm of the target cell, it forms two copies of double-stranded DNA that become integrated into the host cell chromosome DNA. The integrated viral DNA, known as a provirus, directs replication of the virus within the host cell. New viruses, known as *virions*, form near the plasma membrane where they bud out of the host cell. Conversion of the two strands of viral RNA to provirus DNA to produce new viral RNA allows the virus to mix and match its genetic code and produce a wide range of variants (Guatelli et al. 2002).

The original virus complex, known as simian immunodeficiency virus (SIV), naturally infects chimpanzees in central Africa. Similar SIVs exist as natural infections among several different kinds of monkeys in west Africa. These viruses are unique to African primates, and do not cause them any harm, but when introduced to non-African primates, they produce deadly disease similar to HIV infection in humans (Kanki and Essex 2000). Obviously, SIVs have existed in their natural hosts for millennia.

HIV coming from central Africa has been labeled HIV-1 to distinguish it from another HIV type from west Africa, HIV-2, first identified in 1985 (Marlink 2001). The virus from west Africa bears a close relationship to SIVs in mangabey monkeys, macaques, green monkeys, and mandrills (Strauss and Strauss 2002). This indicates that humans picked up HIV-2 from monkeys in west Africa separately from transmission of HIV-1 in central Africa from chimpanzees to humans. Like HIV-1 viruses, HIV-2 viruses probably jumped species from monkeys to humans in isolated rural areas more than once over many years.

HIV-2 mostly remains confined to west Africa, and it follows a far less virulent path in humans than HIV-1. Human-to-human transmission is significantly lower, disease progresses at a much slower pace, and only a small number of infected individuals develop AIDS after several years. HIV-1 and HIV-2 usually do not overlap, but when they do, lab studies suggest that HIV-2 may act as a deterrent to HIV-1 (Kanki and Essex 2000).

The human immunodeficiency viruses responsible for the pandemic belong to the HIV-1 complex. Different subtypes have developed as HIV-1 has spread around the world. Subtype B emerged in North America and Western Europe in the early 1980s, while subtype E appeared in Southeast Asia about ten years later. Two other major subtypes, A and D, emerged in east and central Africa during the early 1980s. Currently, another subtype known as subtype C is raging across southern Africa, causing the largest epidemic of HIV/AIDS to date. This HIV-1 type appears to be far more virulent than other types and more easily transmitted heterosexually than the others. The virus has spread so rapidly that in some areas over half of the young adult population have been infected (Essex 1999).

HIV-1 Infection

HIV-1 infection presents a work in progress since the virus continuously changes as the infection develops. Like all other infectious agents, HIV-1 represents a mixed population of variants jockeying for dominance. Generally, a variant known as R5 serves as the initial infecting virus invading the human host. This form of the virus targets specific sentry cells of the immune system in order to infiltrate the body of the host. Usually, various macrophage-type cells guarding portals of entry into blood and tissues serve as the major attraction to R5 variants. The virus takes these cells hostage by locking in on specific receptors on their surface. The CD4 receptor allows the virus to grab the targeted cell, but entry via fusion with the hostage cell can only take place when the R5 virus simultaneously locks into an adjacent receptor or coreceptor known as the chemokine CCR5 receptor (Rizzardi and Pantaleo 2002). Chemokine receptors on the host cell function to bind specific proteins involved in signaling various immune and inflammatory responses (Michael 2002).

The invasion triggers the hostage macrophage-type cells to migrate to the nearest lymph node site to alert other immune cells to act. The lymph node then becomes the primary site of infection, where the virus finds a rich source of young new host cells more to its liking, the helper T cells that also have CD4 receptors and CCR5 coreceptors. Helper CD4 T cells rush to the infected cells to pick up identifying antigens of the virus in order to relay antigen code signals to B cells and killer CD8 T cells so they can identify and kill the virus and infected cells. In the process the CD4 T cells get infected by the virus and become the primary focus for HIV infection (Abbas et al. 1997).

The virus frequently changes antigens to thwart attacks by killer T cells and B cells throughout the course of infection. The defending immune cells fail to recognize mutated viral antigenic forms without the proper identification signals from CD4 T cells. As the destruction of infected CD4 T cells increases, mutant viruses continue to escape defenders of the immune system (Rizzardi and Pantaleo 2002).

When the immune response first goes on alert, it attempts to contain and destroy the identified virus and infected cells within the lymphoid tissue before the virus mutates and escapes. The virus replicates very quickly within vulnerable CD4 T cells, and if the immune response cannot act just as quickly to destroy it within the lymph nodes, the virus mutates and disperses throughout the body. Within forty-eight hours after exposure the virus can spread throughout the lymphoid system and enter the bloodstream and other body fluids (Rizzardi and Pantaleo 2002).

HIV infection commonly is transmitted by sexual contact as the virus moves into vaginal secretions and semen. Any damage to the mucosal linings of the genitalia from other infections or irritations greatly facilitates the movement of HIV through the mucosal barrier. The virus goes for macrophage-type cells, known as dendritic or Langerhans's cells, found just below mucosal surfaces of the genitalia. The dendritic cells normally capture microbe invaders, sound the alarm to T cells, and carry the invaders to the nearest lymph node site. These cells have CD4 receptors and CCR5 coreceptors that the R5 virus favors for hostage taking. The virus can also be transmitted via oral sex, as vulnerable dendritic cells lie beneath the mucosal surface of the tonsils (Rizzardi and Pantaleo 2002).

Blood-borne transmission primarily happens through sharing of contaminated needles as well as through contaminated blood products. The R5 virus in blood searches out vulnerable immune cells with the right receptors in blood and lymph tissues (Rizzardi and Pantaleo 2002). The virus can also pass through amniotic fluid and breast milk from infected mothers to their newborns (Guatelli et al. 2002).

The immune system declares allout war to eradicate the terrorist attack. Alerted B cells and other phagocytic cells gobble up any free virions, while killer CD8 T cells destroy recognizable infected CD4 T cells and macrophage-type cells. The allout immune response can appear to win the war when the virus disappears from detection by activated immune cells. However, the virus just retreats into the genome of resting CD4 T cells. These cells contain the memory of the virus, but in their resting state do not activate against it. Here the virus waits as a nonreplicating provirus in the chromosome of the cell for the right opportunity to reactivate and begin a new round of replication and dispersal.

The provirus can hide in the nucleus of resting host cells and regenerate along with them, and it can wait years before reactivating. The key trigger for reactivation of the virus comes with activation of the immune response to another infective agent. This causes the resting CD4 T cells containing the provirus to go into action, and in the process the provirus also activates and begins another cycle of HIV replication. Also, virions held prisoner within the follicular dendritic cell network inside lymph nodes, designed to capture pathogens, manage to infect newly activated CD4 T cells and impair lymph node functions (Rizzardi and Pantaleo 2002). Consequently, the immune system becomes its own worst enemy.

Reactivated late-stage HIV infection in some individuals may be dominated by another variant of the virus, known as X4. This form of the virus prefers to use the chemokine coreceptor CXCR4, most often found on CD4 T cell lines produced to combat the R5 variant. The X4 form of the virus cannot target macrophage-type cells, and relies strictly on the CD4 T cell–adapted line of cells for invasion and replication. R5 virus variants continue to be produced to use CCR5 coreceptors, but they cannot use the CXCR4 coreceptor. While the X4 virus dominates during the later stages of infection for some individuals, the majority of reactivated HIV infections generally continue to allow the R5 virus to dominate throughout the course of the infection (Michael 2002).

We are still learning about the virus and how it interacts with the immune system. Underlying genetic factors influence the immune responses to HIV infection, as does virulence of the virus type, and the general state of health of the individual, including existence of other infections and nutritional status. Damage to the immune system occurs more quickly when poor health compromises immune responses, or when other infections, such as malaria, are present, provoking the virus to remain active and continue to mutate.

Immediate or quick immune responses to the invading virus can determine the course of the infection. A small percentage of HIV-1–infected individuals manage to fend off infection and never develop AIDS. Studies of prostitutes in Nairobi show that regardless of repeated exposure to HIV-1, some of the women failed to develop HIV-1 infection. Most of these women were related, suggesting shared genetic factors that work to prevent infection by invoking a quick immune response to the virus. Their immune systems must be attacking the infected dendritic cells underlying the vaginal mucous layer before they become stimulated to migrate to the lymph nodes (Martin and Carrington 2002).

Another form of resistance has been found in individuals born without the gene that creates the CCR5 cytokine coreceptor on vulnerable cells. They show resistance to HIV-1 infection if they receive the defective gene from both parents. The R5 invading virus cannot invade targeted immune cells if the CCR5 coreceptor is missing. Individuals receiving the gene from only one parent can still be infected but with slower than usual progression to AIDS (Martin and Carrington 2002).

The defective gene for CCR5 occurs only in Indo-European populations. Some have suggested that the defective gene arose long ago in response to another viral infection using the same CCR5 receptor. The defective gene may have been selected to resist the smallpox virus that uses CCR5 receptors on targeted cells when smallpox epidemics ravaged populations of Indo-European descent from Western Asia to northern Europe for centuries. The frequency of the defective gene has reached 15 percent of the population of northwestern Europe, where epidemics raged intensely throughout the Middle Ages (Martin and Carrington 2002).

AIDS

Acquired immune deficiency syndrome (AIDS) marks the final outcome of HIV infection through destruction of the immune system. The harmful effects of other microbes can no longer be contained. The battle ceases when the immune system becomes disarmed, allowing enemy microbes freedom to invade and conquer all parts of the body. Infections normally contained and rendered harmless by an effective immune system can no longer be restrained from causing harm. Opportunistic microbes suddenly find easy pickings with a nonresistant host. Diseases considered rare because of effective immune responses find a safe haven in the host who has AIDS. Infections run rampant with the lack of adequate host immune responses, inevitably ending in the death of the host within a few years (Strauss and Strauss 2002).

Most adults show few symptoms of disease when they first acquire HIV-1. Mild flu-like symptoms can appear from two to six weeks following exposure, and can last up to four weeks as the immune system carries out large-scale attacks on the virus. Early symptoms that endure longer indicate unusually rapid progression of the infection. Common early symptoms can include fever, sore throat, headache or stiff neck, nausea, diarrhea, rash, general aches, and fatigue (Guatelli et al. 2002; Martin and Carrington 2002; Strauss and Strauss 2002).

Once the virus disappears from the radar of the immune sensors, the infection goes stealth in provirus form for a long period of time without showing any symptoms of disease. The infection will remain quiet for eight to ten years in most individuals. Less than 5 percent of those infected will remain free of symptoms for several more years. Unfortunately, some individuals have less than two or three years of respite. How long the latency period lasts depends on the various factors mentioned earlier (Guatelli et al. 2002; Martin and Carrington 2002; Strauss and Strauss 2002).

AIDS appears following the latency period when opportunistic infections take over as CD4 T cells become too few and far between to initiate adequate immune responses, and many of the lymphoid cells have been destroyed. Symptoms of disease appear as other infections move in. In some highly susceptible individuals, HIV-1 takes this opportunity to invade macrophages and microglia cells in the brain to produce mental deterioration known as AIDS-related dementia (Guatelli et al. 2002).

Chronic fatigue, night sweats, chronic diarrhea, loss of appetite, malabsorption of nutrients from the gut, and rapid weight loss leading to wasting syndrome (known as "slim" disease in Africa) appear as the immune system deteriorates. These symptoms relate to activation of other resident stealth microbes moving freely about in the host in addition to the ravages of HIV-1. Old infections, such as tuberculosis, once sealed off from harm, break loose and wreak havoc on vulnerable tissues. Skin disorders usually develop as the immune system shuts down. The affected host now becomes extremely vulnerable to unusual opportunistic infections plus the development of rare cancers caused by viruses in any system within the body (Guatelli et al. 2002).

Non-Hodgkin's lymphoma and Kaposi's sarcoma are the most frequently occurring virus-caused cancers associated with severe AIDS. The B cell cancer called non-Hodgkin's lymphoma relates to the unregulated replication of Epstein-Barr virus, which usually remains quiescent in healthy individuals. Kaposi's sarcoma, a rare skin cancer, has links to the unbridled replication of herpesvirus-8, which normally causes no harm in healthy individuals. Ano-genital cancer, caused by human papilloma virus, can also appear (Guatelli et al. 2002; Strauss and Strauss 2002).

Opportunistic infections can come from a wide variety of microbes, including pneumonia-causing *Pneumocystitis carnii*, a rarely seen bacteria, and fungus infections that take advantage of weakened immunity (Guatelli et al. 2002). Different populations around the world vary in exposure to a wide array of microbes capable of infecting humans. These differences determine the pattern of AIDS opportunistic infections that will appear within each population. *Pneumocystitis carnii* infection appears often in North American and European AIDS victims but only rarely in African AIDS victims. African AIDS victims will far more likely succumb to reactivated tuberculosis than will North American and European AIDS victims (Farmer et al. 2000).

The course of HIV infection in infants and children proceeds at an accelerated pace. Less than half of infants born to HIV-1–infected mothers acquire the infection, and about 20 percent develop AIDS in their first year. Breast-fed infants also become vulnerable to infection leading to AIDS. The most obvious sign of AIDS in babies shows up as failure to thrive. They readily develop serious illness from common childhood infections, and become vulnerable to opportunistic infections, particularly those causing pneumonia (Guatelli et al. 2002).

The Spread of HIV-1

HIV-1 made its way outside Africa sometime between the 1950s and 1970s before it was recognized. By the early 1980s it had reached North America by way of Haiti and entered Europe from Africa through contaminated needles tied to illegal drug use, the homosexual trade, and contaminated blood supplies. By the mid-1980s it reached Thailand by similar routes, and then India via illegal drug users, where it quickly spread by way of the sex trade, and on to Burma, Vietnam, Laos, Cambodia, China, and the Philippines (Essex 2000; Farmer et al. 2000).

The virus continues to race around the world, often introduced to a new area through illegal injectable drug use and the medical use of untested blood and blood products. Following blood-borne introductions, the virus often moves through the general population by sexual transmission. Human sexual behavior patterns and socioeconomic conditions often influence the rate of HIV-1 infection within a population.

The estimated number of people infected with HIV-1 around the world by the end of 2001 ranged from around 34 million to 43 million with at least 15 million to 20 million AIDS deaths. The majority of HIV infections occur in sub-Saharan Africa, followed by much lower but rising rates in Southeast Asia and India (Michael 2002; Strauss and Strauss 2002). By the end of the twentieth century over 70 percent of HIV infections in the world occurred in young adults in sub-Saharan Africa as truck drivers, migrant workers, soldiers, and prostitutes spread the infection along with contaminated blood and needle use (Farmer et al. 2000). The number of infected adults in some large African cities was estimated in 2001 to be between 20 percent and 40 percent (Strauss and Strauss 2002). By comparison, less than 1 percent of the adult populations of Europe and North America had been infected with HIV-1 at that time (Guatelli et al. 2002).

The current HIV-1 outbreaks, coupled with famine, malaria, and tuberculosis in southern Africa, have had a devastating effect on the populations in this part of the world. Life expectancy has dropped as more and more young adults die from AIDS-related disorders (Michael 2002).

High infection rates can be attributed to traditional sexual practices, encouraging men to have many sex partners, along with traditional migration patterns of young men searching for wage work. Women have become easy prey for the virus passed to them from their male sex partners. Large numbers of young women, farmers, laborers, teachers, businessmen, and government employees infected with HIV-1 continue to die, leaving large gaps in the social and economic fabric of their countries. Corrupt governments and wars continue to facilitate the spread of HIV-1 as they tear apart the daily lives of millions of people throughout Africa.

China now faces serious HIV-1 outbreaks compounded by uncontrolled blood-collecting methods used to harvest plasma, the liquid part of blood, for manufacturing blood-derived medical products during the early 1990s. Officials solicited rural villagers for their blood with the promise of cash and the return of their blood following extraction of the plasma. They pooled the drawn blood for easier plasma extraction. Once the plasma had been removed, they divided up the remaining blood and returned it the donors. In this process, HIV from a single donor infected all of the other donors. HIV-1 has reached infection rates as high as 80 percent in some rural villages in China's Hunan province (Rosenthal 2001).

The mix of drugs developed to combat HIV-1 infection has become very expensive, and they have to be adjusted to meet differing individual responses to control the course of the infection. Such a medical regime requires the intake of several pills each day with constant monitoring by physicians for side effects for the lifetime of the patient, or for as long as the individual can tolerate them. When the right mix can be tolerated by an individual with HIV-1, the latency period dramatically lengthens. However, the right mix of drugs can only control the virus, not eradicate it. Furthermore, we cannot overlook the ever present danger that the virus will mutate to avoid the action of the drugs. And if drug treatment is interrupted, the virus resumes its activities (Rizzardi and Pantaleo 2002; Strauss and Strauss 2002). No magic bullet exists to end the infection at this time, and no vaccine has been developed to prevent it.

The best way to control HIV infection comes through education to help people overcome their own cultural bias and understand how they themselves can prevent the infection and keep it from spreading. The infection thrives on ignorance, superstitions, and human behavior. Campaigns to teach people about HIV and how to prevent infection have proven successful in slowing the spread of the disease in Uganda (Strauss and Strauss 2002) where HIV-1 once ran rampant and killed tens of thousands.

HIV Postscript

Chronic infection with other viruses, such as Epstein-Barr, cytomegavirus, and *Herpes simplex*, can remain quiet for life without showing any symptoms. They have reached a state of fluctuating equilibrium within the human population. This means that the infecting virus never gets completely eradicated but is held in check by a healthy immune system (Walker

2001). The infecting virus can get out of control whenever the equilibrium established between individual host immunity and the virus gets upset by factors that weaken the immune system, such as another infection, poor nutrition, or other stresses. Perhaps in time, as HIV settles into the global population, it will come to behave in a similar compromise within the human population, held in check. This would render it a harmless infection for most people, becoming active only when the established balance breaks down.

Hemorrhagic Fevers

Some local viruses linked to specific natural hosts and confined to certain geographic regions can produce deadly hemorrhagic fevers in humans. They can be found in every part of the world, and most of them thrive among wild rodents. Some use ticks or mosquitoes for transmission and some have a natural host that is yet unknown. Human beings become accidental hosts whenever they intrude into the natural cycle between the virus and its natural host (Johnson 2002).

The dramatic population explosion of the latter half of the twentieth century placed heavy demands on local environments. Increasing human disturbance of delicate ecological balances has exposed more and more people to deadly viruses. The viruses have always been there, with occasional attacks on humans who get in their way, while remaining relatively unknown to the rest of the world. Our awareness of these viruses grows as more and more people fall victim to them. We often refer to these newly recognized diseases caused by rogue viruses as "emerging diseases."

All hemorrhagic viruses consist of RNA viruses, but they do not all belong to the same family of viruses. They can be *Arenaviruses, Bunyaviruses, Filoviruses,* or *Flaviviruses.* Most hemorrhagic fevers do not produce obvious bleeding but instead cause capillary leaks with the liquid part of the blood, plasma, seeping out of the blood vessels into adjacent tissue spaces. This causes severe pain and can rapidly lead to shock from sudden collapse of blood volume, and death (Johnson 2002). Some viruses focus primarily on the kidneys, liver, or lungs; some cause nerve damage; others target all organs. The viruses can quickly replicate and move throughout the body in a hit-and-run mode before sufficient immune reactions have a chance to respond. Quick and efficient immune responses can limit viral damage.

Insect-borne Infections

Ticks can carry a few *Flaviviruses* causing hemorrhagic fevers in remote areas of Western Asia and Siberia. In the 1940s a tick flavivirus producing Omsk hemorrhagic fever gained identity in western Siberia. Most often found among muskrat hunters, the infection can lead to hearing loss. The death rate from the Omsk virus is between 0.5 and 3 percent. Another tick virus, Kyasanur Forest disease, became recognized in Karnataka state in western India in 1957, with fatality rates between 3 percent and 5 percent. A related tick virus has recently been discovered in Saudi Arabia (Monath and Tsai 2002).

The phlebovirus causing Crimean-Congo hemorrhagic fever, carried by ticks, operates widely throughout rural areas of Africa, Eastern Europe, and Asia, but this virus rarely causes human disease. When it does infect people, up to 50 percent of victims die from it (Mertz 2002). Several cases with thirty-four reported deaths have been reported in recent years among Afghan refugees along the Afghanistan-Pakistan border (Frantz 2001).

Aedes mosquitoes transmit Rift Valley fever, caused by another phlebovirus, throughout Africa, and it has recently spread to the Arabian Peninsula. The disease first came to notice in domestic sheep and cattle introduced from Europe. Human infections remained sporadic until 1977 when the disease struck Egypt in the area near the Aswan Dam for the first time. The newly constructed dam provided a haven for breeding mosquitoes carrying the virus. Over 200,000 people contracted the infection with 598 deaths (0.3 percent) from hemorrhagic fever and liver damage. Similar outbreaks have been reported around other newly constructed dams in Africa (Garrett 1994; Lederberg et al. 1992).

Ebola Virus

Ebola constitutes one of the most frightening hemorrhagic diseases to emerge on the world scene. Fortunately, the virus remains isolated in mostly rural parts of central Africa, and only a few thousand individuals have been infected by it. Most likely, the virus has been around for quite some time with isolated infections going unnoticed throughout rural central Africa. The virus is transmitted through direct contact with infected blood and body fluids, such as urine, vomitus, watery feces, and probably sweat introduced through a cut, scratch, abrasion, or injection (Bray 2002). Sexual transmission and infection from mother to the unborn infant can also occur (Lederberg et al. 1992).

The virus gained its name from the Ebola River in Zaire (now the Democratic Republic of Congo) where it first became recognized in 1976. The missionary hospital at Yambuku near the river suffered a severe outbreak of hemorrhagic disease following the admission of an individual who had the infection. Reuse of needles and syringes and poor nursing care allowed the virus to spread quickly among patients, staff, and their families. Eighty-eight percent of the 318 infected victims died from the disease before the outbreak ended when the hospital was abandoned. The virus would probably not have been noticed by the world community if traditional African quarantine practices had been observed, isolating the sick from their home villages. Instead, the villagers brought their sick to the mission hospital where it would take only one infected individual to transmit the disease to many others (Bray 2002).

A similar outbreak of ebola occurred that same year 500 miles away in the regional hospital at Maridi in Sudan. Again, poor nursing care and reuse of needles spread the disease throughout the hospital, resulting in 284 infections with 53 percent dying from the disease. The infection arose from another variant of the virus brought to the hospital from a cotton factory in Nzara, where some of the workers had become so ill that they had to be taken to the hospital for medical care. Another outbreak in 1979 followed with thirty-four people infected, twenty-two of whom died. In Gabon between 1994 and 1996, three small outbreaks of ebola appeared among hunters and workers in logging camps. Ebola also struck the Kikwit hospital in Zaire in 1995, infecting 315 people and killing 244 (77 percent), including eighty medical staff workers, and family members caring for dying loved ones and preparing them for burial. In 2000 an outbreak of ebola in the hospital at Gulu in Uganda infected 425 individuals, causing 224 deaths (53 percent) (Bray 2002). Sporadic outbreaks continue to be reported in the Congo region, including cases in northern Gabon.

Another variant of ebola, capable of infecting humans, and closely related to the other African variants in Sudan and Zaire, killed a number of chimpanzees in Ivory Coast in 1994. Again, the source of the infecting virus remains unknown (Bray 2002).

Outbreaks of yet another variant of ebola that does not affect humans has been identified in groups of monkeys, the cyno molgus macaques from the Philippines, placed in primate facilities in the United States. Infected monkeys die from the disease, while their human handlers resist the infection. The variant received its name, "Reston ebola," from the first recognized outbreak, which occurred at the Reston primate facility in Virginia in 1989. Similar outbreaks occurred in primate facilities in Pennsylvania in 1990, and Texas in 1992, and at a primate facility in Italy in 1996. All of the infected monkeys received by these facilities came from the same supplier in the Philippines, yet the source of the virus remains unknown (Bray 2002).

Ebola is an RNA filovirus that comes out of the Congo area of Africa from an unknown source. The virus initially targets macrophage-type cells throughout the body and in the blood and lymph systems, damaging lymph nodes and creating chaos in the blood. Survivors of ebola infection possess immune systems able to activate a strong immune response that initially slows down viral replication until specific immune responses can attack and contain the virus. Otherwise the infected individual is doomed (Bray 2002).

Ebola appears to block the initial immune response in susceptible individuals so that the virus can replicate quickly and overwhelm the immune system. Newly released virions attack a broad range of cells throughout the body, including endothelial cells lining blood vessels. In addition, infected macrophage cells release large quantities of cytokines and chemokines and other mediating factors that contribute to tissue damage and that may increase the permeability of infected blood vessels, causing them to leak fluid. The immune system responses fall into turmoil as tissue damage increases with internal hemorrhaging. Tissues die from lack of oxygen, as capillaries collapse and become blocked by masses of virions. Severe pain with bleeding into the skin, mucous membranes, gastrointestinal tract, liver, and spleen follows, usually culminating in death (Bray 2002).

Symptoms of ebola can show up between four days and three weeks, but usually around six days, after infection. Abrupt fever, headache, weakness, abdominal pain, muscle pains, diarrhea, nausea, and vomiting appear. About half of infected individuals will also exhibit bloodshot eyes and sore throat. A rash appears within a week, beginning on the flanks, and spreading all over the body except the face. Internal hemorrhage may not always be evident. Tiny pinpoint bruises, as well as large bruised areas, reflect hemorrhaging beneath the skin, along with bleeding from the eyes and from needle punctures. Death from shock and dysfunction of multiple organs usually occurs within six to nine days following the onset of symptoms in severely ill individuals. Those who survive take weeks to recover; the recovery period is marked by weakness, weight loss, joint aches, hair loss, and skin sloughing. They can retain the virus in some parts of the body for two to three months (Bray 2002).

Marburg Virus

Marburg represents another filovirus closely related to Ebola virus, attacking the body in a similar manner and with similar symptoms. Marburg virus received its name from the city of Marburg, Germany, where it was first identified in 1967. The virus had been shipped to a vaccine facility in Marburg from Uganda among a batch of green monkeys. Laboratories in Frankfort and Belgrade also received infected green monkeys from the same supplier. Thirty-one people working with the monkeys became ill, and seven died from the disease (Bray 2002).

The virus did not appear again until 1975 in a hitchhiker from Zimbabwe, followed by a few other human infections in west Kenya in 1980, 1982, and 1987. The first major outbreak among humans occurred in 1998 among gold miners at Durba in the Democratic Republic of Congo, following four smaller outbreaks in the same area since 1983. The last outbreak infected 141 individuals and killed 82 percent of them (Bray 2002).

Hemorrhagic Fever with Renal Syndrome

Several localized hantaviruses within the *Bunyaviridae* family, which extend across a wide temporal forest belt from northeastern China, Korea, Siberia, and Central Asia into Scandinavia, and down into the Balkans, can produce hemorrhagic fevers that cause kidney damage. Each localized virus has a specific rodent for its natural host, and humans become infected by breathing in the virus that rides dust particles contaminated by infected rodent feces and urine. Most of these viruses and their rodent hosts reside in rural areas. When human beings, particularly agricultural and forest workers, and even soldiers on bivouac, intrude into these creatures' territory, they run the risk of exposure to the viruses. Rodents attracted to grain storage areas also expose rural farmers to infection.

The disease was first recognized in 1912 in Vladivostok, Siberia. Physicians in the Soviet Union and Japan identified several cases during the 1930s along the Amur River in Manchuria. The disease came to world attention in the early 1950s during the Korean War. Several thousand United Nations soldiers suffered from a viral hemorrhagic disease affecting the kidneys, with 15 percent of them dying from the viral infection, which was referred to as Hantaan virus (Benenson 1995; Johnson 2002; Mertz 2002).

Early symptoms include fever, headache, muscle pains, bloodshot eyes, pinpoint hemorrhages under the skin, red rash affecting the face and upper trunk, abdominal or lower back pain, and often nausea and vomiting. This lasts for three to seven days, followed by low blood pressure for several hours to three days that can progress to shock accompanied by more symptoms of capillary leaking. Blood pressure returns to normal following this phase of the disease, but nausea and vomiting may persist. Severe infections induce kidney damage with hemorrhaging and a severe drop in urinary output. Those who recover from the illness take weeks to months to recover (Benenson 1995; Johnson 2002).

Field mice carry hantaan virus throughout Korea, northeastern China, eastern Russia, and the Balkans. The virus poses a major health threat in rural northeastern China, where thousands of cases are reported each year. A similar virus known as Puumala virus, associated with bank voles, occurs west of the Ural Mountains and into Scandinavia. Puumala virus usually causes milder forms of the disease known as "nephhropathia epidemica," with less than 1 percent dying from it (Benenson 1995; Lederberg 1992). Puumala virus has also been identified in the common house mouse in Belgrade, Serbia (Grady 1993).

Another variant of the virus, known as Seoul virus, also produces mild symptoms with less than a 1 percent death rate. This virus is associated with rats. It probably originated in field rats around Seoul and was later transferred to city brown rats, the same rats that have traveled by ship all over the world. The virus has shown up in major seaport cities around the globe, and it has even been found in laboratory rats (Benenson 1995; Mertz 2002).

Studies of rats and people in poor areas of central Baltimore, Maryland, have revealed that infection with Seoul virus is not unusual and that people infected with the virus do not show any of the typical symptoms of the infection. The study does raise the question of whether or not human infection by the virus leads to high blood pressure and kidney failure since a number of individuals with natural antibodies to the virus suffer from these conditions (Strauss and Strauss 2002).

Hantavirus Cardiopulmonary Syndrome

While hantaviruses in the Old World focus on the kidneys, hantaviruses found in the New World focus on the lungs and heart. Various types of rodents throughout the Americas carry hantaviruses. The first hantavirus to be identified, "Sin Nombre" virus, is associated with deer mice in North America, and it can cause human infections, especially in the West. Another variant, known as "Black Creek Canal" virus, associated with the cotton rat, thrives in Florida. The white-footed mouse carries the virus in New York and Rhode Island. Rice rats in Louisiana carry a variant known as "Bayou" virus. Pack rats, chipmunks, and other rodents can also carry the virus throughout North America. Humans get exposed to the virus when rodents move in with them and into their outbuildings. Cleaning areas where the mice have left droppings or urine can stir up contaminated dust particles carrying the virus (Mertz 2002).

Other variants have been found throughout South America, associated with a wide range of different rodents and named for the regions they inhabit. Strong evidence suggests that a variant found along the southern Andes can be transmitted from person to person (Mertz 2002).

The medical community first recognized the disease in 1993 during an outbreak among young adults from the Navajo Nation in the Four Corners region of northeastern Arizona and northwestern New Mexico. Since then, sporadic cases have been reported throughout North America (Benenson 1995; Mertz 2002).

Symptoms begin to develop approximately two weeks following exposure with fever, muscle pains, and gastrointestinal upsets. Abrupt onset of severe respiratory failure follows, as the lungs fill up with plasma from massive capillary leakage, blocking oxygen uptake and sending the heart into shock. Death results in approximately 50 percent of infected individuals. Those who survive recover rapidly with no long-lasting effects (Benenson 1995).

The disease caused by "Sin Nombre" virus has been known to the Navajo and other Native Americans from the Southwest for some time. Navajo traditions dictate avoidance of mice and burning items soiled by them, with the knowledge that they carry sickness that can spread through the air (Grady 1993).

Lassa and Other Related Arenaviruses

Lassa virus first came to the world's attention in 1969 with an outbreak at a mission hospital in Nigeria near its border with Cameroon. After one American nurse died, a second American nurse became ill and eventually had to be airlifted to a New York hospital for treatment in isolation. She recovered, but the virus infected a physician researching her disease. He survived after he received serum filled with immunoglobins against the virus from the recovered nurse. Then, one of the lab technicians also became infected, but the technician died before antiserum could be administered (Garrett 1994).

Lassa virus is carried by wild rodents throughout west Africa's savannas and wherever forests have been cleared for farming. Rural villages are generally surrounded by agricultural fields, and the houses attract infected rodents. Lassa virus has been infecting rural people in west Africa for a long time, and it has been estimated that the infection strikes tens of thousands each year with hundreds or thousands of deaths. Infection rates go up when social unrest accompanies political turmoil (Peters 2002).

Not only can this virus be carried on dust particles contaminated with rodent droppings and urine, it can also travel by aerosol particles exhaled by individuals suffering from the disease. Infected blood and body fluids also contain the virus. Hospitals in west Africa can quickly become foci of the disease with death rates from 15 percent to 60 percent (Mertz 2002; Peters 2002).

This hemorrhagic virus focuses on the throat and upper respiratory system, but it can also damage lymph nodes and organs throughout the body. Symptoms develop gradually five to sixteen days following exposure to the virus. Fever, headache, muscle pains, fatigue, chest pain, and sore throat signal the beginning of the disease, sometimes accompanied by abdominal pain, diarrhea, nausea, and vomiting. The eyes redden and the throat becomes swollen and congested with mucous, making it difficult to swallow. Severe infection leads to low blood pressure, capillary leakage into the lungs, hemorrhaging into tissues, facial and neck swelling, and seizures prior to death. Most infections in pregnant women bring about fetal death, especially during the last three months of pregnancy. Victims carry the virus for several weeks following infection. Recovery from the disease can take one to three months, with hair loss and disturbed muscle coordination. Survivors commonly suffer permanent hearing loss due to damage of the eighth cranial nerve (Benenson 1995; Peters 2002).

Several arenaviruses harbored among wild rodents and producing hemorrhagic fevers similar to Lassa virus have been identified in South America. Scattered outbreaks in rural areas have been noticed since the 1950s, as more people have moved into wilderness areas to clear land for agriculture and settlements. Settlers moving into territory occupied by wild Calomys mice disturb their habitat and bring themselves into contact with the virus carried by the mice.

Between 1959 and 1962 scattered reports of *el typho negro* (black typhus) with symptoms of hemorrhagic fever began coming from eastern rural areas of Bolivia. The small frontier town of San Joaquin, with 3,000 people, had

637 infections within two years, and 113 people (18 percent) died from the disease. The virus came to be called "Machupo" virus after the river near the town that flowed into the Amazon Basin (Peters 2002).

Other arenaviruses identified in South America, and named for localities where they were first identified, include "Junin" virus found in rural areas of the pampas of Argentina, which has a 25 percent fatality rate. Hemorrhagic fever caused by "Junin" virus first received notice among corn harvesters in 1955. In 1989 outbreaks of another hemorrhagic disease caused by "Guanarito" virus centered on a small town in Venezuela, killing just over 25 percent of those infected. Another virus named "Sabin" has been identified in a few individuals near São Paulo in Brazil (Benenson 1995; Lederberg 1992; Peters 2002).

Arenaviruses that can give rise to hemorrhagic fevers have been identified in wild rodents in western North America since 1995. "Whitewater Arroyo" virus carried by wood rats claimed the lives of three people in California between 1999 and 2000 (Mertz 2002; Peters 2002).

Viral Encephalitis

Three groups of hit-and-run viruses can attack the brain and spinal cord if they are not stopped as soon as they enter the host. Fortunately, most people possess sufficient and immediate immune responses to the viruses, and symptoms of disease never develop. Some individuals may develop mild symptoms of fever and headache for a few days. In some people signs of meningitis will develop. A small percentage of susceptible individuals develop severe infections leading to encephalitis that can bring about death (Benenson 1995).

Mosquitoes, primarily Culex but also some Aedes mosquitoes, function as the major vector carriers of the viruses causing encephalitis. Wild birds act as natural hosts for many of these viruses, and every part of the world contains some kind of virus capable of producing the disease.

People become infected when they intervene between the natural host and the mosquito cycle. Horses have a high susceptibility to many of the viruses, and some other animals, such as pigs, rodents, and bats, also get infected. Birds not accustomed to some of the viruses succumb to disease brought on by infection.

Sporadic infections and occasional small outbreaks of viral encephalitis have been associated with mosquito-carried bunyaviruses in North America,

China, and Russia. Some tick-carried flaviviruses in Central Asia and parts of Europe also can produce encephalitis, but most of these viruses are confined to rural areas with only occasional encounters with humans (Benenson 1995).

Generally outbreaks of mosquito-borne viral infections will strike horses, pigs, or susceptible bird populations before they strike people in the same area. Only a small proportion, often less than 1 percent, of mosquitoes carry the viruses during their natural cycle with wild birds (Strauss and Strauss 2002). Horses and pigs can amplify the number of infected mosquitoes since they attract large numbers of the insects to feed on them, which then pick up the viruses. This amplification of the viruses increases the chances for human infections in the same area.

Outbreaks of viral encephalitis have slowly increased over the past century as urban sprawl, horse farms, and large pig farms intrude into mosquito territories. Some of these viruses have been able to spread outside their geographic boundaries by way of rapid travel and global transport (Marra 2000).

Western and Eastern Equine Encephalitis

Urban growth in North America throughout the twentieth century sparked outbreaks of viral encephalitis caused by alphaviruses known as western (WEE) and eastern (EEE) equine encephalitis viruses attacking both humans and horses. The eastern virus circulates in eastern and north-central portions of North America with scattered cases exported to the Caribbean islands, Central America, and South America. The western virus operates throughout the western and central portions of North America and portions of South America (Benenson 1995).

Symptoms of western equine encephalitis appear within two to four days after a mosquito bite, producing fever, severe headache, and muscle aches. Stiff neck indicates progression to encephalitis. Drowsiness and disorientation follow, leading to coma. Children often have convulsions and symptoms of paralysis. Around 10 percent of individuals developing western equine encephalitis die from the disease, and children recovering from encephalitis may suffer permanent neurological damage (Johnson 1975c).

Eastern equine encephalitis can be more severe than its western cousin, particularly among horses. Over half of infections in horses develop into symptomatic disease, and deaths among horses showing symptoms can reach as high as 90 percent. Up to 50 percent of humans developing encephalitis die from the EEE disease. The incubation period for eastern equine encephalitis lasts a little longer than the western virus, around seven to ten days before symptoms develop. Nausea and vomiting accompany the headache, fever, and muscle aches. Progress to encephalitis moves rapidly with drowsiness, irritability, muscle spasms, sometimes inability to speak or swallow, delirium, and coma. Recovery takes a long time, and there may be permanent neurological damage (Johnson 1975c).

St. Louis Encephalitis

Another type of viral encephalitis is caused by a flavivirus known as St. Louis encephalitis (SLE) virus because it was first recognized in the suburbs of St. Louis, Missouri, in 1933. No more than 1–2 percent of infections produce symptoms of encephalitis, and then it usually hits older adults with fatality rates from 10 percent to 25 percent. Tremors of the hands and face, and light sensitivity accompany stiff neck, fever, severe headache, and muscle ache symptoms (Johnson 1975c). The virus has also been found in other parts of North America, parts of the Caribbean region, and South America (Benenson 1995).

Japanese Encephalitis

St. Louis encephalitis virus belongs to a large complex of flaviviruses known as Japanese encephalitis (JE) virus complex circulating throughout Asia and the Pacific region. Outbreaks of Japanese encephalitis have been recognized since 1871 in Japan, and annual outbreaks of JE have appeared throughout East Asia since the 1920s, with most infections inconsequential (Olitsky and Clarke 1959). Pigs, herons, and egrets serve as intermediate hosts for these viruses. Symptoms of JE resemble those of St. Louis encephalitis, but neurological damage can be more severe in 45–70 percent of survivors. Death rates are as high as 40 percent of individuals suffering encephalitis (Johnson 1975c; Strauss and Strauss 2002).

Murray Valley Encephalitis

Australia and New Guinea have experienced sporadic outbreaks of encephalitis caused by a JE complex variant known as Murray Valley encephalitis (MVE). The disease first gained recognition in 1917–18, with 134 cases of encephalitis and 70 percent fatality in the Murray and Darling River Valleys of Victoria and New South Wales, Australia. Over half the victims had not reached five years of age. The disease reappeared in 1922, 1925, and 1926. The cause of this unknown disease puzzled physicians who referred to it as the "X disease" until the virus was isolated during another outbreak in 1951. The virus naturally cycles among wild birds of northern Australia and New Guinea, occasionally getting carried to the south of Australia by migratory waterfowl (Johnson 1975c; Olitsky and Clarke 1959).

West Nile Virus

Another flavivirus belonging to the JE complex circulates among wild birds throughout Africa, southern Europe, the Middle East, and West Asia. It was first isolated in Uganda in 1937. Domestic stock, especially horses, appears to draw infected mosquitoes. The virus has been labeled West Nile virus since it represents a common infection among children in the Nile River delta of Egypt. Most infections remain silent without consequence among children. Older adults appear to be the most susceptible to the virus (Johnson 1975c; Monath and Tsai 2002).

Symptoms of disease follow three to six days of incubation with fever, headache, back and muscle aches, and light sensitivity. Symptoms usually disappear rapidly in about a week. Some individuals also develop a pink rash, sore throat, nausea, vomiting, and abdominal pain. A small proportion of symptomatic infections progress to encephalitis with tremors, altered consciousness, and paralysis, with fatality rates around 33 percent (Johnson 1975; Monath and Tsai 2002).

Various strains of West Nile virus have managed to spread throughout Europe, Russia, Indonesia, and Australia over the nineteenth and twentieth centuries. The virus reached North America by the end of the twentieth century. Horses have become the main victims, followed by humans. Susceptible bird species, such as crows and jays, have proven to be highly susceptible to the virus. Dogs and cats can also be infected and can suffer from this viral disease (Monath and Tsai 2002).

The first outbreak of West Nile virus in North America appeared in New York City in 1999. Thousands of crows died, and sixty-two people developed encephalitis with seven deaths (11 percent). Within a year the virus had spread all along the eastern Atlantic coast (Strauss and Strauss 2002). Firmly entrenched in the wild bird and mosquito populations of eastern North America, the virus quickly spread westward throughout most of the United States by 2002. Between 1999 and 2002 there were nearly 3,000 human infections resulting in 146 deaths (5 percent), and at least 40 percent of infected horses died from the disease (McConnaughey 2002).

Despite the media-driven scare of West Nile virus in the United States, the human fatality rate for this imported virus falls far below the fatality rates for encephalitis-causing viruses indigenous to North America.

Nipah Virus

Encephalitis caused by this virus was first detected in the village of Nipah, Malaysia, in 1997 (Uppal 2000), followed by three separate outbreaks in other areas between September 1998 and April 1999 (CDC bulletin MMWR 4-9-1999/48[13]:265–69). Symptoms suggested that the mosquito-borne Japanese encephalitis virus (JE) caused the disease. Human infections primarily occurred among workers on pig farms. This suggested amplication of the suspected JE virus by infected pigs, a process that often occurs prior to outbreaks of human infections.

In these cases, the infected pigs suffered severely with rapid breathing and explosive coughing as well as neurological symptoms that often caused death. Infected humans displayed three to fourteen days of fever and severe headache followed by drowsiness, disorientation, and coma within twenty-four to forty-eight hours. A few individuals also developed respiratory symptoms. All together, 229 cases of encephalitis developed with 111 (48 percent) deaths. Eleven abattoir workers having contact with infected pigs imported from Malaysia into Singapore in March 1999 came down with similar symptoms and one died. The governments of both countries and the surrounding areas quickly quarantined all pigs and banned movement of the animals. Over 1 million pigs had to be destroyed to end the outbreaks (MMWR 4-9-1999/48[13]: 265–69).

The virus turned out not to be part of the JE complex. Previously unknown, this virus belongs to the paramyxovirdae family of viruses, and it is closely related to another virus causing similar symptoms in horses and their human handlers in Australia. The disease first captured attention there in 1994 at Hendra in Queensland. Thirteen of twenty horses suffered from an outbreak of the disease, and one of the two human handlers infected with the Hendra virus died from it (MMWR 4-9-999/48[13]: 265–69).

The Hendra and Nipah viruses naturally infect fruit bats or flying foxes (Pteropid bats) found from Australia to India. Ecological upsets associated with farming and animal husbandry have brought the bats increasingly into contact with domestic animals (Field et al. 2001). Bat droppings and urine transmit the viruses, contaminating areas used by pigs and horses. Infected animals most likely transmit the virus to humans in close contact with them through the respiratory route, since the virus has been isolated in the respiratory tract of infected animals (Hooper et al. 2001).

Concluding Comments

The world has become a very crowded place just in the last half-century. Increasing populations around the world are pressuring global environments with increasing demands for more space and resources. Add rapid global transit and sociopolitical turmoil, and the microbe pot is stirred faster and faster. Global warming with changes in weather patterns allows tropical and subtropical insect vectors of disease to establish colonies beyond their geographic limits.

Sleeping dragons in secluded rural areas have been awakened to find new opportunities to attack human beings and animals outside their niches. HIV/AIDS leads the way among these emerging maverick viruses, showing us just how quickly a dangerous virus can rouse out of its containment and rapidly spread throughout the world, especially with the help of human behavior.

CHAPTER 23

BACK TO THE FUTURE

Human beings have come a long way over the last ten thousand years, moving from hunting and foraging to modern high-tech living. Rapid changes spawned by industrialization and globalization throughout the last century have accelerated exponentially by the twenty-first century. These changes have affected the entire global community regardless of regional developmental status.

Rural populations have outnumbered urban populations for centuries, but by the close of the twentieth century more people resided in cities and towns than in rural areas. Travel at the beginning of the twentieth century relied on horse power, steamship, and train. The automobile soon took over from the horse, and later jet air travel became king of both domestic and international travel.

The modern life style has introduced humanity to a fast-paced way of life as people hurry to reach daily commitments, gobble highly processed foods, breathe polluted air, and get little exercise. Social skills are diminishing from hours spent watching television, playing computer games, or surfing the Internet. Modern life insulates people from nature with only occasional holiday ventures out into the natural world. Nature has become secondary to the demands of high-tech living.

Regardless of the many evolutionary cultural changes humanity has passed through, the human body and its elaborate immune system remain essentially unchanged from those of our earliest ancestors. And we still inhabit a microbial soup despite our efforts to sterilize our modern world.

As human beings have rapidly evolved from nomadic hunters and for-agers, through early agriculturalists and early civilizations, to industrialization and modernization, we have made changes in our relationships with the environment, and the microbial world has adjusted to our every change. Regardless of our efforts to insulate ourselves from nature, we still belong to the natural order of life, and the rules of nature still apply to us.

Whenever we alter the natural landscape to suit our desires, we alter our interaction with the microbial world. Clearing of rain forests, dam building, strip mining, plantation agriculture, industry, chemical and garbage dumping, fossil fuel use, modern transport systems, large-scale immigration, war destruction, and urban sprawl have created tremendous upheavals in global environments. In the process we have unwittingly teased out hidden microbes and allowed once isolated microbes to meet and exchange survival information among them.

The uneven pace of modern development has left major areas of the globe in limbo or turning backward in the struggle against dangerous microbes. Public health safety nets for fighting off many infectious diseases have been lost or were never fully attained in many underdeveloped countries. Sociopolitical turmoil, poverty, and famine, with or without natural disasters, set the stage for outbreaks of infectious diseases that can now spread far more quickly around the world than ever before.

Welcome to the latest paradigm shift in the relationship between humans and the microbial world as we begin the twenty-first century.

SARS: The Warning Shot Heard around the World

We continue to face dangers from a variety of pathogens lurking in the animal kingdom that until recently had little chance of becoming human diseases. The ever growing numbers of people crowding together in areas where wild and domesticated animals are concentrated offer increasing opportunities for animal pathogens to jump the species barrier into human populations. Constant human and animal interaction under crowded circumstances can foster emergence of a mutant strain of a pathogen capable of producing zoonotic infection in humans to convert to a human-transmitted disease.

Severe acute respiratory syndrome (SARS), first recognized in Vietnam in February 2003, represents an example of this threat. This disease is caused by a unique coronavirus with similar RNA viruses circulating among wild animals in southeastern China. The outbreak among humans began in Guangdong province and spread to Hong Kong, Beijing, Vietnam, Taiwan, and other areas of China and Asia primarily via infected airline travelers. It even spread to Toronto, Canada. Hospital workers and family members in close contact with the victims proved to be the most vulnerable to infection since the virus is carried in droplets coughed up by the victims. Death rates from severe pneumonia can be as high as 50 percent among the most vulnerable individuals, older people and the immune-compromised, while children are less severely affected (Whitby and Whitby 2003).

As the SARS outbreak receded in July 2003 (Liu 2003), researchers sought the source of the infection. Studies of wild animal markets in Guangdong province suggest that the virus has been infecting human handlers of wild animals as a mild zoonotic infection for some time (Pearson 2004). Researchers found that the DNA sequence of SARS virus matches the coronavirus DNA infecting wild palm civets commercially raised and sold in live animal food markets in southeastern China (Nomile 2004). The custom of keeping these animals alive in crowded markets and restaurants until diners select them for their dinner presented opportunity for a mutant strain to jump the species barrier and spread among humans.

Pollution's Progress

As modern human populations have reshaped much of the global environment over the past hundred years, thousands of manufactured chemical substances have been added to the global environment. Pollution is everywhere, both in modern and underdeveloped countries. No nation is spared. No ocean is spared. Every major city around the world suffers from pollution, particularly in the air. Smoke from massive burnings of tropical forests in Indonesia, combined with urban pollution, have blanketed Southeast Asia in recent years. Dust storms laden with industrial pollution and smoke have left Inner Mongolia to cross over Bejing, the Korean Peninsula and even the Pacific Ocean to western North America. Wind currents know no national boundaries. Pollutants dumped into rivers and oceans do not stop at national borders. The Chernobyl nuclear plant melt-down left its mark across Europe. Like it or not, we all inhabit this planet together, and we all pay the price one way or another for reckless behavior.

The most pressing need for burgeoning human populations, particularly in poor countries around the world, is for safe drinking water. There is just not enough to go around. Underground water tables are falling to precipitous levels. Most rivers around the world are polluted, and many of them are being diverted or are drying up. Runoff from agricultural fields and animal feed lots add pollutants to reservoirs built to hold drinking water. Rainfall patterns are shifting while enormous amounts of water are being wasted or contaminated. Loss of water also causes loss in food supplies with less water for crops and livestock.

Not all underground water can be assumed to be safe. Villagers lacking access to clean drinking water in rural parts of West Bengal, India, and neighboring Bangladesh were encouraged to sink pipes into underground aquifers starting in the 1960s. Unfortunately, the underground water naturally contains high levels of arsenic that slowly poisoned over 1 million villagers through time. Similar water problems exist elsewhere around the world. The northern coast of Chile, parts of Taiwan, and Mongolia have a similar problem with underground water containing high levels of arsenic (Bagla and Kaiser 1996; Bearak 1998).

Many chemical pollutants that enter land and water ultimately pass up the food chain through plants and animals to humans. Insecticides used to protect grain crops fed to cattle come to us in meat products. Mercury filters up to us through fish. Many of the fruits, vegetables, and grains we eat directly contain chemical residues. We not only live in a microbial soup, we have added thousands of chemicals to that soup. What is amazing is how much chemical assault the human body can take without showing serious effects. However, long-term exposure to a variety of chemical pollutants in food, drinking water, or air not only can directly damage our health, but also can encourage infectious agents to move in or allow cancers to develop.

Air pollution poses the most urgent pollutant problem around the globe. Many people develop chronic nasal congestion and cough from constant exposure to irritants in the air. Habitual cigarette smoking only intensifies the amount of pollution entering the respiratory system. Repeated chemical irritation of the bronchial tubes causes increased mucous production as the body's defense mechanism tries to dissolve, dilute, and remove the irritants that in turn trigger coughing to rid them from the respiratory system.

Excessive mucous production and irritation to the bronchial tubes offers an invitation to infectious microbes and recurring respiratory infections. Chronic bronchitis results. Continued assault on the bronchial tubes can lead to permanent damage of the air passageways, particularly to the tiny air sacs where oxygen enters the body and carbon dioxide leaves the body. Continuous increased pressure inside these air sacs from chronic obstruction of the bronchial tubes often leads to emphysema. This build-up of pressure comes from repetitive excessive mucous build-up plugging the bronchial tubes, along with repeated contraction of bronchial muscles trying to expel the mucous plugs. The tiny air sacs balloon and lose their elasticity or break, unable to expel carbon dioxide. They can take air in but cannot expel it. This also places stress on the heart.

When nitrogen oxides and hydrocarbons produced by automobile exhaust, particularly diesel fuel, and industrial emissions react chemically in sunlight, they produce ground-level ozone (Regush 1992). As ozone levels rise dramatically in major cities around the world, the incidence of breathing disorders among susceptible individuals, particularly young children, also begin to rise. We are all affected by high ozone levels, but some people are hurt more than others. The most vulnerable individuals already suffer chronic obstructive lung disorders, such as emphysema, bronchitis, and asthma.

Asthma has become the fastest growing health problem in major cities and urban areas throughout the modern world. Once considered a disorder among children, initial onset of the disease now appears in adults of all ages as well. Within a ten-year period from 1979 to 1989, severe asthma attacks requiring hospitalization increased 43 percent in the United States. From 1982 to 1992 deaths from asthma increased 50 percent in North America, Great Britain, Sweden, and New Zealand. Ozone by itself does not present the major problem, but it acts as a catalyst for reactions to allergens that trigger an asthma attack. It takes only small amounts of allergens to trigger a wave of asthma attacks when ozone levels rise (Regush 1992).

Individuals with air passageways overly sensitive to specific particles in the air can develop asthma. Allergens can range from cat dander, dust mites, cockroach excrement, pollen, and molds to a variety of chemicals released by hundreds of materials used in the home, schools, offices, and industry. More than sixty thousand new chemicals have been introduced into the commercial market over the last fifty years. Chemical fumes released by artificial carpet fibers, paints, glues, and household cleaners represent just a few examples of the new chemical air pollutants.

The dramatic increase in asthma cases and other lung disorders followed the introduction of closed indoor environments to save energy costs during the 1970s. Builders of homes, schools, and office buildings moved to total enclosure, recycling indoor air that greatly increases indoor pollution. At the same time, people began spending most of their time indoors, gaining greater exposure to indoor pollutants. The combination of indoor and outdoor pollution can be overwhelming to asthma sufferers. They become so overcome by air pollutants that even the stress of exposure to cold air or exercise can trigger an attack. Even the medications used by asthmatics can have an adverse affect with overuse (Regush 1992).

Asthma follows previous exposure to the offending allergen. The immune system develops an acute sensitivity to the allergen by preparing itself for future contacts with the mobilization of specialized immunoglobins known as IgE. For some unknown reason, the sensitized immune system considers the offending allergen extremely dangerous, and allout war preparations develop for any future encounters. Circulating IgE molecules attach to mast cells in the connective tissues of the body and basophils (specialized white blood cells) circulating in the bloodstream, waiting for the next encounter.

The next exposure to the allergen meets a rapid response from the sensitized immune system as the IgE molecules act quickly to bind with the offender. This triggers the allergic sequence, releasing histamine, cytokines, and other agents to force the allergen away and protect irritated tissues. Sneezing, congested runny nose, wheezing, and shortness of breath herald the immune reaction. The immediate release of histamine stimulates the production of mucous, followed by constriction of bronchial muscles and leakage of fluid in small blood vessels causing tissue swelling. Symptoms disappear within an hour only to return a few hours later with an influx of inflammatory cells rushing in to clean up the damage (Lichenstein 1993). Symptoms of asthma can vary from mild to severe, depending on individual responses and length of exposure to allergens. Severe attacks can be deadly as the victim literally suffocates.

A Word about Fungus

Today's changing patterns of disease include changes in the way fungal infections operate. Fungi take advantage of immune-compromised individuals, such as people suffering from AIDS and other debilitating diseases. Fungal infections have been increasing along with modern medical interventions (Richardson and Warnick 1997), and increasing numbers of people moving into new areas and disturbing the land where fungi abound in nature.

Only a few fungi have adapted to living harmlessly on human skin and mucosal surfaces, such as athlete's foot, ringworm fungus, and fungal infection of the nails. The fungus *Candida albicans* has achieved status as a commensal within the human digestive tract, capable of surviving on mucous membranes from the mouth to the anus (Richardson and Warnick 1997). It can turn into a nasty infection, commonly known as thrush, with overuse of antibiotics or other medications, or illnesses that compromise natural immunity (Benenson 1995).

Most fungi exist in nature, not dependent on any kind of host for survival, absorbing nutrients from living or dead organic matter. They can appear in vegetative states known as molds, as reproductive spores, and as budding yeasts. Most prefer moist soil containing decaying organic material.

The vast majority of fungal infections acquired by humans arise from human disturbance of the environment. Fungal infections acquired from the environment have mostly been sporadic throughout human history around the globe. Environmental infections can be contracted by traumatic implantation through a contaminated wound in the skin. Most environmental infections derive from breathing in fungal spores arising from disturbed land areas (Richardson and Warnick 1997). Some fungi contaminate grain crops and peanuts under moist field conditions to produce a toxin that can lead to toxic reactions when ingested by people (Aufderheide and Rodriguez-Martin 1998).

As more people crowd into areas and disturb the land where environmental fungal spores have reached endemic levels, increasing numbers of people become exposed to the spores. While the majority of infections remain silent or mild, some susceptible individuals respond with significant lung disease, such as coccidioidomycosis (valley fever), found throughout arid and semiarid areas of the Western Hemisphere, and histoplasmosis, found throughout the Americas, East Asia, Africa, and Australia. Histoplasmosis can become a chronic lung disease similar to tuberculosis. Sometimes a fungal infection proves fatal when it manages to spread throughout the body of a susceptible host (Benenson 1995).

Germs and Chemicals Designed for War

The terrorist attacks of September 11, 2001, put the world on notice of the dangerous threat of bioterrorism. Anthrax-laden letters mailed to U.S. congressional leaders in Washington, D.C., and news media outlets in Florida and New York killed five people and sickened twenty-three others. Was the intent to kill many more, shut down the government, and spread panic? The anthrax spores used in the bio-letter bombs had been cultured, refined, and mixed with an additive in a laboratory to make them stay airborne for longer periods of time. What if the refined anthrax spores had been delivered by crop dusters? If weather conditions cooperated, chances are that hundreds of thousands of people would have inhaled the spores and most of them would have died.

The use of toxic mustard and chlorine gas as subtle agents for warfare during World War I set in motion ideas for chemical and biological weaponry for the future. The Japanese conducted a secret research program for use of anthrax, as well as smallpox, other germs, and toxins, as weapons during the late 1930s in Harbin, the capital city of old Manchuria, using Chinese prisoners as guinea pigs. The Japanese initiated biological warfare in China at the battle for Chekiang in 1942, by contaminating waterways and wells with various microbes and dropping porcelain bombs filled with anthrax spores over the area. The loss of Chinese lives was never calculated, but an estimated ten thousand Japanese soldiers in the battle zone died from the biological attack (Brookesmith 1997). Biological warfare can be a two-way street with exposure to both sides.

Britain, the United States, and the former Soviet Union carried out their own biological and chemical weapons programs following World War II (Brookesmith 1997). Anthrax served as one of the favored germs studied for use as a biological weapon. How many other countries carried out their own secretive research programs remains unknown.

The Biological Weapons Convention of 1972, signed by Britain, the United States, the Soviet Union, and over a hundred other nations, was supposed to have put an end to research and development of biological and toxic weapons. However, the Soviet Union ignored the accord, and Russian scientists continued their research programs and stockpiling of dangerous microbes and toxins until the collapse of communist control in 1991. The Soviets developed and refined methods and equipment for fermentation, production, and weaponizing of biological and toxic weapons. They researched at least seventy different types of microbes for use as biological weapons. They focused on those that have no cure or preventive vaccine, and when the programs stopped they were busy modifying and splicing microbes to create more deadly artificial mutants (Alibek 1999).

Anthrax has proved to be one of the top deadly contenders for use as a biological weapon, capable of killing up to 90 percent of attacked individuals within days. Smallpox gained attention for use as a biological weapon when the World Health Organization declared its eradication in 1980. Only two laboratories, one in the Soviet Union and one in the United States, had permission to hold samples of the virus for future research. Vaccination for smallpox ceased, and the potential for its use as a biological weapon was soon realized by the Soviet Union and other nations operating secretive research programs. The Soviet scientists managed to increase the virulence of smallpox viruses grown in their laboratories in order to cut short the incubation period and raise death rates above the known 30–50 percent fatality range (Alibek 1999).

Anthrax and smallpox form the major biological weapons threat in the world today. Both can be transmitted through the air. Anthrax spores have proven to be more deadly than the smallpox virus, and they can contaminate an attack area for years. Although less deadly than inhaled anthrax, the smallpox virus can be transmitted by sick individuals, while anthrax cannot be transmitted from person to person. Thus, smallpox can spread through the infected population by human-to-human contact, while inhalation anthrax relies on wind currents to carry its spores to new victims in contaminated areas.

Unfortunately, international commercial enterprise has allowed a number of biological and chemical agents, along with laboratory equipment for modifying them into weapons, to be sold on the international market. Iraq managed to buy highly lethal strains of anthrax by mail order from the United States. We now know that over seventeen nations around the world possess biological and toxic weapons. This includes North and South Korea, China, Taiwan, Vietnam, Laos, India, South Africa, Libya, Iraq, Syria, Iran, Israel, Bulgaria, Cuba, and Russia (Alibek 1999). Research programs in themselves present a constant danger of possible accidents releasing dangerous microbes into the environment.

The multinational military effort Operation Desert Storm, waged against Saddam Hussein in 1991, left thousands of military personnel suffering from a variety of unexplained illnesses. Questions have been raised about whether or not they encountered contamination by biological and/or chemical agents stored in Iraq (Brookesmith 1997).

Chemical and toxin weapons also pose a threat to the world community. Botulinum, a neurotoxin produced by the bacteria *Clostridium botulinum*, and ricin, a toxic protein derived from castor beans, have been refined for use as toxin weapons. Saddam Hussein revived chemical warfare when he used poisonous gases during his war with Iran and against the rebellious Kurds in northern Iraq between 1983 and 1988. Serin, a deadly nerve gas released by terrorists on a crowded subway train in Tokyo in 1995, sickened over five thousand people and killed twelve (Brookesmith 1997). Recent counterattack using the gas Fentanyl, a common anesthetic, against terrorists holding hundreds of people hostage in a Moscow theater, killed not only the terrorists but also 117 of the hostages (Glasser 2002). Obviously. uncontrolled dosages of this gas can be deadly.

Subtle attacks employing biological or chemical agents can be carried out by terrorists anywhere in the world at any time, and by the time an attack is recognized, it could be too late. The terrorists aim to cause panic, and sociopolitical and economic disruption rather than allout war. They have no regard for whether or not the weapons they employ affect them, and they either don't know or don't care how these weapons contaminate the world we all share. Other weapons, such as "dirty bombs," nuclear devices, and biological and chemical weapons aimed at agriculture, food, and water supplies, also threaten human lives in the twenty-first century.

Recent laboratory synthesis of the polio virus from basic chemicals provokes alarm. The synthetic polio virus proved capable of inducing infection. This raises questions of how this new knowledge can be used to create more lethal weapons for bioterrorism. We human beings appear to be our own worst enemies.

Mad Cows, Designer Pigs, and Fancy Plants

Whenever human beings tinker with nature, we inadvertently rearrange the order of certain biological interactions. Feeding animal byproducts to herbivores is certainly not what nature had intended. The idea of making money from rendered animal carcasses by grinding them up for use as "protein" supplements to add to feed for other animals became popular during the 1970s.

This moneymaking venture caused British cattle that were fed animal protein supplements to be exposed to a little known disease, transmissible spongiform encephalopathy, often referred to as "mad cow disease." The scientific name reflects the damage to the brain, which takes on the appearance of a sponge as it becomes riddled with holes. More than 170,000 cattle in Britain came down with the disease. Over 3 million cattle had to be destroyed by the 1990s when the British discovered that the disease had spilled over into the human population.

Sheep carcasses proved to be the original culprit in the spread of this unusual disease. Some breeds of sheep—not all breeds—and goats can contract a disease known as scrapie, a form of spongiform encephalopathy. Sheep infections have been recognized in the British Isles and throughout Europe since the eighteenth century. Infected animals develop chronic neurological symptoms with restlessness, apprehension, tremors, unsteady gait, skin irritations called "scrapie," stupor, and eventual death several months after onset of symptoms (Craighead 2000).

Cows fed protein supplements developed from rendered infected sheep carcasses develop a disease similar to scrapie, transmissible bovine spongiform encephalopathy (mad cow disease). People who eat meat products, especially brain and other neurological tissue, from infected cows also develop a similar spongiform encephalopathy known as Creutzfeldt-Jakob disease (Chesebro and Caughey 2002).

Creutzfeldt-Jakob disease was rarely reported among human beings until the recent outbreak in Britain. The disease first gained recognition during the 1920s. Another form of the human disease became known in 1936 as Gerstmann-Strausstler-Scheinker syndrome (Craighead 2000), and heredity appears to play a role in most of those cases. Otherwise the cause of many of the early cases remains unknown.

In 1957 Gajdusek (1979) discovered another form of this disease, which he named kuru, among the Fore, an indigenous group of people in the highlands of New Guinea. Gajdusek suspected ritual cannibalism as the cause, but the disease may well have been acquired from handling infected brain tissue of deceased relatives during macabre mortuary practices. Once the government stopped traditional mortuary practices, the disease disappeared. The origin of this transmissible form of the disease has never been identified.

The disease has also been found in zoo animals and farm-raised mink that have been fed protein supplements from infected animals. Animals in the wild can also be affected by the disease. For the past twenty-five years mule deer and elk in the western Rocky Mountains of the United States have been known to develop a chronic wasting disease similar to scrapie. The source of the disease remains unknown (Cheseboro and Caughey 2002).

Whatever the cause, all forms of spongiform encephalopathy have similar pathogenesis and symptoms caused by damage to certain membrane proteins known as prions. Prions exist primarily in the brain. They also appear in the heart, lungs, and activated lymphocytes. Their normal function remains unknown. The true nature of the infective agent remains elusive. Some researchers suggest that an unknown virus or viral particle alters the form of normal prions in brain tissue (Chesebro and Caughey 2002), while others believe that transmissible defective prions damage normal prions (Prusiner 1995).

Defective prions take on a different configuration from normal prions. Unlike normal prions sensitive to digestive juices, defective prions can resist the digestive enzymes in the gut. They also resist breakdown by irradiation, heat, and harsh chemicals (Craighead 2000).

Modern medicine has inadvertently introduced the disease to some patients. Pituitary glands harvested during autopsies and refined for medical use to treat pituitary dwarfism in children generated over a hundred cases of Creutzfeldt-Jakob disease. Over eighty cases of the disease have appeared following neurosurgery and corneal transplants (Craighead 2000), bringing into question just how widespread the disease may be. Some forms of progressive dementia and shaking in the elderly often get dismissed as part of aging. Dementia, along with loss of coordination, is a sign of spongiform encephalopathy.

The disease appears slowly. Symptoms generally take from two to ten years to develop as the defective prions spread and damage the brain. The incidence of British mad cow disease peaked in cattle during the early 1990s after large numbers of cattle had been exposed to the disease in previous years. The outbreak of the human Creutzfeldt-Jakob disease followed the cattle outbreak in Britain with over 113 reported cases by 2001. The disease has also been reported in other parts of Europe (Cheseboro and Caughey 2002).

Most of the victims of this outbreak have been young adults. Older people were the usual victims of Creutzfeldt-Jakob disease in earlier times and also in cases reported elsewhere in the world. Symptoms of transmissible spongiform encephalopathy related to mad cow disease include behavioral changes, followed several weeks or months later by muscle spasms, lack of coordination, memory disturbances, and mental impairment (dementia). Death follows within one to twelve months (Cheseboro and Caughey 2002).

The mystery of the spongiform encephalopathies has not been resolved. Cause and effects remain a riddle for scientists to ponder. This disease provides just a reminder of how little we do know about the invisible world around us. The danger of unknowingly transmitting or amplifying an infectious agent continues whenever we experiment with novel ways of medical intervention and genetic manipulation of plants, animals, and insects. We may unknowingly be opening a "Pandora's box."

The biotechnology industry has introduced several biogenetic manipulations affecting our food supplies. Genetically modified plants and animals, along with cloning, have raised concerns about how nature will react to these artificial manipulations.

Infectious agents can sneak through screening tests if not targeted by the testing apparatus. We have seen this happen with HIV and the hepatitis viruses in donated blood used for transfusions and blood products. Organ transplant recipients risk acquiring a hidden infection. The agent behind transmissible spongiform encephalopathy proved to be capable of surviving modern sterilization of surgical equipment to cause infection (Craighead 2000).

The increasing need for transplant organs has spawned a new industry known as xenotransplants. Pig organs are strikingly similar to human organs, suggesting that they may be ideal for transfer to humans in need of replacing malfunctioning organs. Commercially designed pigs have been cloned to produce organs suitable for human transplants. The pigs have been genetically altered so that their organs will not be rejected by the human immune system. Concern has been expressed that the pigs may be carrying silent retroviruses native to pigs that could be detrimental to humans once introduced directly into the human body (Goedert 2000).

The Greatest Danger: A Crowded World

Today, severe overpopulation poses the greatest threat to global human health. There are just too many people pressing on finite resources of food and water. The global population topped 6 billion at the turn of the twenty-first century, having dramatically climbed from a global population of 1.6 billion at the turn of the twentieth century, despite millions of deaths from wars, purges, massacres, attempted genocides, famine, and disease. Continued population growth at its present rate will lead to a global increase of at least another 3 billion by 2050 (Small 2002).

We have already passed the global carrying capacity for sustainable human populations. This was reached in the mid-twentieth century at 2.5 billion. Since then we have been pushing the limits of global resources with staggering human population growth around the world (Small 2002). The current pace of global population growth cannot be sustained (Coale 1975).

For most of human existence, the estimated global population remained below 10 million. Population increases remained at a minimum until the rise of civilization. After that, gradual increases raised global population to around 300 million by the first century A.D.. From that time on, an exponential human population growth rate allowed global numbers to double about every five hundred years, to reach 1 billion for the first time by 1800 (Coale 1975). This phenomenal growth stems from progressive improvements in survival rates of infants and breeding-age females along with increasingly longer lifespans.

Population growth in many poor areas of the world hovered around zero until the eighteenth century when the introduction of new food staples, such as the potato, maize, and the sweet potato, stabilized diets. Coale (1975) claims that the new foods promoted gradual population increases into the twentieth century. Throughout the last century, introduced modern medical practices and some public health measures also helped increase survival and longevity rates of both infants and adults, promoting increased population growth in poor countries.

In 1974 the United Nations foresaw that most of the global population growth by 2000 would be in underdeveloped countries (Coale 1975). Spiraling population growth pressing dwindling local resources in these countries, coupled with sociopolitical unrest, has led to millions of migrants pouring into other, more affluent parts of the world. Most of them wind up in cities already stretched to provide for the growing numbers of inhabitants.

Out of Order

Nature has rules for keeping order and balance among all living things. Whenever the balance is upset, the laws of nature see to it that the balance gets restored to equitable levels. We humans have broken the rules. The human population is horribly out of balance with nature. We will either run out of water and food to sustain our large numbers or we will try to kill each other off. The most likely scenario will be that our natural predators in the microbe world will quickly restore human populations to more sustainable levels. That means reducing the global population by more than half its present size of over 6 billion, to less than 3 billion.

One of nature's rules provides that no microbic predator will completely annihilate its prey. There must always be at least a few resistant survivors to re-create the delicate balance between them. In some instances, survivors may move away from an area under siege, leaving the false impression that a population has been wiped out.

The best example of breaking the balance with nature comes from what happened to the rabbit population in Australia. Rabbits were introduced into Australia from Europe in 1859. Lacking significant natural predators, they quickly adapted to their new environment and rapidly reproduced until the country was overwhelmed with rabbits. The rabbit population reached an estimated 600 million by the 1940s. They eventually would have eaten themselves and all other plant-eating animals out of sustainable food supplies if not stopped by some predator. One had to be imported.

The myxoma virus, native to rabbits in Brazil and causing them little harm, proved to be lethal to European rabbits. The Australians introduced the virus to rabbits in the Murray Valley of southeastern Australia in 1950, in the hopes that it would eradicate, or at least drastically reduce, their numbers. Mosquitoes feeding on infected rabbits picked up the virus and transmitted it to other rabbits without becoming infected with it themselves. Within three months, the virus killed over 95 percent of the rabbits, thus nearly wiping out the rabbit population of Australia.

However, the small number of survivors of this viral onslaught possessed inherent resistance to the virus. Year by year the virus and its new host population jockeyed back and forth in the dance of survival. Virulent forms of the virus remained lethal to some genetically weak and sick rabbits, while less virulent forms allowed their victims to survive infection, and inherited resistance in some rabbits kept the virus from taking over completely. Eventually a balance was struck between prey and predator populations, and deaths from the viral infection declined to 20–30 percent of the rabbit population following the initial drastic reduction of their numbers with introduction of the virus (Andrewes 1967; Ryan 1997; Strauss and Strauss 2002).

Human history is riddled with accounts of epidemics wreaking similar havoc among human populations around the world, though not as severe as the rabbit myxomatosis introduced to Australia. Even the great influenza pandemic in the early twentieth century did not come close to killing off a significant portion of the global population. However, a more deadly influenza pandemic is all too likely.

Influenza virus exemplifies the ideal predator for reducing human populations. It is airborne and travels the globe easily and quickly, capable of infecting all age groups in repeated waves within a short time span.

Influenza type A viruses are unstable and continuously evolving. Global movements of people and viruses at a rapid pace make gene swapping possible among previously isolated strains. Hybrid virus produced by such gene swapping could result in a deadly strain that targets the lower branches of the bronchial tubes and the lungs. Severe viral pneumonia and death within twenty-four hours would follow. The new influenza virus could easily move around the globe within days and kill over half the human population (Ryan 1997). Crowded cities, especially megacities, could suffer up to 90 percent fatalities within days or weeks.

CONCLUDING COMMENTS: IGNORANCE IS NOT BLISS

The evolution of diseases among human beings has always depended on human cultural evolution. Changes in human behavior patterns over the centuries have actually promoted changes in human disease patterns. Instead of conquering infectious diseases in the modern world, we have only altered the pattern of infectious diseases around the globe, and we now face greater interaction with more microbes than ever before (Lederberg et al. 1992).

Complacency regarding the dangers we face appears to be common throughout the world. We do not want to face the fact that we have too many people, and we tend to ignore threats we cannot visualize from the microbial world. Faith that medical intervention will save us makes many of us feel invulnerable to infectious diseases.

We have passed through the ages of ignorance and the arrogance of the twentieth century regarding our knowledge of the microbial world around us (Gillett 1971). We have defied our place in the natural world and we are quickly using up the vital natural resources needed to sustain current population growth.

Humankind can no longer afford to ignore the facts of life on this planet. Population growth has to be controlled. We need to take better care of our environment and protect our natural resources. We need to stop stirring the microbial soup.

By design, accident, or natural intent, the next pandemic will most likely be the deadliest one in human history. It is not a question of if, but when.

WORKS CITED

Abbas, Abul K., Andrew H. Lichtman, and Jordan S. Pober
  1997 *Cellular and Molecular Immunology*. Philadelphia: W. B. Saunders.
Adams, Junius G. III
  1986 The Genetics of Human Hemoglobin. In: *Hemoglobin Variants in
        Human Populations*, Volume 1, edited by William Winter. Boca
        Raton, Fla.: CRC Press, pp. 3–15.
Adams, Robert M.
  1979 The Origin of Cities. In: *Readings from Scientific American*.
        San Francisco: W. H. Freeman, pp. 11–18.
Adler, Jack J., and David N. Rose
  1996 Transmission and Pathogenesis of Tuberculosis. In: *Tuberculosis*,
        edited by William N. Rom and Stuart M. Garay. Boston:
        Little, Brown, pp. 129–40.
Ahuja, M. L.
  1958 Rabies in India. *Journal of Tropical Medicine and Hygiene*
        61: 95–99.
Alibek, Ken
  1999 *Biohazard*. New York: Random House.
Allison, Marvin J, and Enrique Gerszten
  1982 *Paleopathology in South American Mummies*. Richmond:
        Medical College of Virginia.
Allison, Marvin J., Enrique Gerszten, Juan Munizaga, Calogero Santoro,
    and Daniel Mendoza
  1981 Tuberculosis in Pre-Columbian Andean Populations. In: *Prehistoric
        Tuberculosis in the Americas*, edited by Jane E. Buikstra. Evanston, Ill.:
        Northwestern University Archeological Program, pp. 49–61.
Anderson. John Y.
  1995 Paleopathology in Oceana: Evidence for Pre-Contact Treponematosis
        from Navatu, Fiji. In: *Papers of the 22nd Paleopathology Association
        Meeting* (Oakland, Calif.), p.18. Published by the Paleopathology
        Association.
Andrewes, Christopher H.
  1967 *The Natural History of Viruses*. New York: W. W. Norton.

Angel, J. Lawrence
    1966 Porotic Hyperostosis, Anemias, Malarias and Marshes in the
          Prehistoric Eastern Mediterranean. *Science* 153: 760–63.
Antonarakis, Stylianos E., Haig H. Kazazian, and Stuart H. Orkin
    1986   DNA Polymorphism in the A- and B-globin Gene Clusters and
          Molecular Etiology of the Thalassemia Syndromes in Man. In:
          Hemoglobin Variants in Human Populations, Volume 1, edited
          by William P. Winter. Boca Raton, Fla.: CRC Press, pp. 29–45.
Arriaza, Bernardo T.
    1995 *Beyond Death*. Washington, D.C.: Smithsonian Institution Press.
Arriaza, Bernardo T., Wilmar Salo, Arthur C. Aufderheide, and Todd A. Holcomb
    1995 Pre-Columbian Tuberculosis in Northern Chile: Molecular
          and Skeletal Evidence. *American Journal of Physical
          Anthropology* 98: 37–45.
Ashmead, Albert S.
    1901 Testimony of the Bones from the Madeleines of the Middle Ages
          on Confusion of Leprosy with Syphilis in Precolumbian Europe.
          St. Louis Medical and Surgical Journal 80 (2): 65–80.
Associated Press
    2001 Migrating Birds Spreading Nile Virus. *Arizona Daily Star*,
          11 September.
Aufderheide, Arthur C., and Conrado Rodriguez-Martin
    1998 *The Cambridge Encyclopedia of Human Paleopathology*. Cambridge:
          Cambridge University Press.
Ayoub, Elia M., Malak Kotb, and Madeleine W. Cunningham
    2000 Rheumatic Fever Pathogenesis. In: *Streptococcal Infections*,
          edited by Dennis L. Stevens and Edward L. Kaplan. New York: Oxford
          University Press, pp.102–32.
Azad, Abdul Farhang
    1988 Relationship of Vector Biology and Epidemiology of Louse-
          and Flea-borne Rickettsioses. In: *Biology of Rickettsial Diseases*,
          Volume 1, edited by David H. Walker. Boca Raton, Fla.:
          CRC Press, pp. 51–61.
Bagla, Pallava, and Jocelyn Kaiser
    1996 India's Spreading Health Crisis Draws Global Arsenic
          Experts. *Science* 274: 174–75.
Baker, Brenda J., and George J. Armelagos
    1988 The Origin and Antiquity of Syphilis. *Current Anthropology*
          29 (5): 703–37.
Baker, J. R.
    1974 Epidemiology of African Sleeping Sickness. In: *Trypanosomiasis and
          Leishmaniasis*. Ciba Foundation Symposium 20 (New Series).
          Amsterdam: Associated Scientific Publishers, pp. 9–43.
Baker, Steven K., and Jeffrey Gassroth
    1996 Miliary Tuberculosis. In: *Tuberculosis*, edited by William N.
          Rom and Stuart M. Garay. Boston: Little, Brown, pp. 493–511.

Baltimore, Robert S.
    1998 Meningococcal Infections. In: *Bacterial Infections of Humans*, edited
        by Alfred S. Evans and Philip S. Brachman. New York: Plenum
        Medical Book Co., pp. 459–79.

Baltimore, Robert S., and Eugene D. Shapiro
    1998 Pneumococcal Infections. In: *Bacterial Infections of Humans*, edited
        by Alfred S. Evans and Philip S. Brachman. New York: Plenum
        Medical Books, pp. 559–82.

Barbour, Alan G.
    2000 Borrelia Infections: Relapsing Fever and Lyme Disease. In: *Effects
        of Microbes on the Immune System*, edited by Madeleine W.
        Cunningham and Robert S. Fujinam. Philadelphia: Lippincott
        Williams & Wilkins, pp. 57–70.

Barinaga, Marcia
    1996 A Shared Strategy for Virulence. *Science* 272: 1261–63.

Barnes, Gina L.
    1993 *China, Korea, and Japan: The Rise of Civilization in East Asia.*
        London: Thames & Hudson.

Barr, David P.
    1951 Simple Goiter. In: *Textbook of Medicine*, edited by Russell L. Cecil
        and Robert F. Loeb. Philadelphia: W. B. Saunders, pp. 1218–19.

Barriga, Omar O.
    1981 *The Immunology of Parasitic Infections.* Baltimore: University
        Park Press.

Barrow, P. A.
    1986 Physiological Characteristics of the Mycobacterium TB-M, Bovis
        Group of Organisms with Particular Reference to Heterogeneity
        within M. Bovis. *Journal of General Microbiology* 132: 427–30.

Barua, Dhiman
    1992 History of Cholera. In: *Cholera*, edited by Dhiman Baruga and
        William B. Greenough III. New York: Plenum Medical Books,
        pp. 1–36.

Basch, Paul F.
    1991 Schistosomes: *Development, Reproduction, and Host Relations.*
        Oxford: Oxford University Press.

Bates, Marston
    1949 *The Natural History of Mosquitoes.* New York: Macmillan.

Beadle, Muriel
    1977 *The Cat: History, Biology, and Behavior.* New York: Simon & Schuster.

Bearak, Barry
    1998 A Safe-Water Plan Poisonous in Bangladesh. *International Herald
        Tribune*, 11 November, pp. 1, 5.

Beaver, Chester Paul, and Rodney Clifton Jung
    1985 *Animal Agents and Vectors of Human Disease.* 5th ed. Philadelphia:
        Lea & Febiger.

Beck, J. Walter, and John E. Davies
    1981 *Medical Parasitology.* 3rd ed. St. Louis: C. V. Mosby.

Benenson, Abram S.
    1970 *Control of Communicable Diseases in Man.* 11th ed.
        Washington, D.C.: American Public Health Association.

Benenson, Abram S.
    1981a Plague. In: *Communicable and Infectious Diseases*, edited by Paul F.
        Wehrle and Franklin H. Top. St. Louis: C. V. Mosby, pp. 473–78.

Benenson, Abram S.
    1981b Smallpox. In: *Communicable and Infectious Diseases*, edited
        by Paul F. Wehrle and Franklin H. Top. St. Louis: C. V. Mosby,
        pp. 577–88.

Benenson, Abram S.
    1995 Control of Commincable Diseases Manual. 16th ed. Washington D.C.:
        American Public Health Association.

Bisseru, B.
    1967 *Diseases of Man Acquired from His Pets.* Philadelphia: J. B. Lippincott.

Bitton, Gabriel, James E. Maruniak, and William F. Zettler
    1987 Virus Survival in Natural Ecosystems. In: *Survival and Dormancy
        of Microorganisms*, edited by Yigel Henis. New York: John Wiley &
        Sons, pp. 301–32.

Black, Francis L.
    1975 Infectious Diseases in Primitive Societies. *Science* 187: 515–18.

Black, Francis L.
    1980 Modern Isolated Pre-agricultural Populations as a Source of
        Information on Prehistoric Epidemic Patterns. In: *Changing Disease
        Patterns and Human Behavior*, edited by N. F. Stanley and R. A. Joske.
        New York: Academic Press, pp. 37–54.

Blake, Leslie A., Burton C. West, Cynthia H. Lary, and John R. Todd
    1987 Environmental Nonhuman Sources of Leprosy. *Reviews of
        Infectious Diseases* 9 (3): 562–77.

Blank, Harvey, and Geoffrey Rake
    1955 *Viral and Rickettsial Diseases of the Skin, Eye, and Mucous
        Membranes of Man.* Boston: Little, Brown.

Blerkom, Linda M.
    1991 Zoonoses and the Origins of Old and New World Viral Diseases.
        In: *The Anthropology of Medicine: From Culture to Method*, edited by
        Lola Romanucci-Ross, Daniel E. Moerman, and Laurence R. Tancred.
        2nd ed. New York: Bergin & Garvey, pp. 196–218.

Blount, Joseph H., and King K. Holmes
    1976 Epidemiology of Syphilis and the Non-Venereal Treponematoses. In:
        The Biology of Parasitic Spirochetes, edited by Russell C. Johnson.
        New York: Academic Press, pp. 157–61.

Bollet, Alfred J.
    1987 *Plagues and Poxes: The Rise and Fall of Epidemic Disease.*
        New York: Demos.

Boshuizen, Hendriek C., Sabine E. Neppelenbroek, Hans van Vliet,
    Joop F. P. Schellekens, Jeroen W. den Boer, Marcel F. Peeters, and
    Marina A. E. Conyn-van Spaendonck
    2001 Subclinical Legionella Infection in Workers near the Source
        of a Large Outbreak of Legionnaires Disease. *Journal of Infectious
        Diseases* 184: 515–18.

Bradbury, Phyllis C.
    1987 Protozoan Adaptations for Survival. In: *Survival and Dormancy
        of Microorganisms*, edited by Yigel Henis. New York: John
        Wiley & Sons, pp. 267–300.

Bray, Mike
    2002 Filovividae. In: *Clinical Virology*, edited by Douglas D. Richman,
        Richard J. Whitely, and Frederick G. Hayden. Washington, D.C.:
        ASM Press, pp. 875–90.

Brookesmith, Peter
    1997 *Biohazard: The Hot Zone and Beyond*. New York: Barnes &
        Noble Books.

Brothwell, Don R.
    1991 On Zoonoses and Their Relevance to Paleopathology. In: *Human
        Paleopathology: Current Syntheses and Future Options*, edited
        by Donald J. Ortner and Arthur C. Aufderheide. Washington, D.C.:
        Smithsonian Institution Press, pp. 18–22.

Brothwell, Don, and Richard Spearman
    1963 The Hair of Early Peoples. In: *Science in Archaeology*, edited
        by Don Brothwell and Eric Higgs. London: Thames & Hudson,
        pp. 427–36.

Bryceson, Anthony D. M.
    1975 Leishmaniasis. In: *Textbook of Medicine*, edited by Paul B.
        Beeson and Walsh McErmott. 14th ed. Philadelphia: W. B.
        Saunders, pp. 490–95.

Buckley, H.
    1998 Subadult Skeletal Pathology at a Prehistoric Site on Taumako
        Island, Solomon Islands, Melanesia. *American Journal of Physical
        Anthropology* Supplement 26: 115.

Buikstra, Jane E., and Sloan Williams
    1991 Tuberculosis in the Americas: Current Perspectives. In: *Human
        Paleopathology: Current Syntheses and Future Options*, edited by
        Donald J. Ortner and Arthur C. Aufderheide. Washington, D.C.:
        Smithsonian Institution Press, pp. 161–72.

Burgos, J. D., G. Correal-Urrego, and C. Arregoces
    1994 Treponematosis en Restos Oseos Pre Ceramicos de Colombia.
        Revista Academie Colombia Ciencias 19 (73): 237–41.

Burnet, Sir MacFarlane, and David White
    1972 *Natural History of Infectious Disease*. Cambridge: Cambridge
        University Press.

Bussell, Robert H., and David T. Karzon
    1966 Measles-Canine Distemper-Rinderpest Group. In: *Basic Medical Virology*,
        edited by James E. Prier. Baltimore: Williams & Wilkins, pp. 313–36.

Busvine, James R.
    1980 The Evolution and Mutual Adaptation of Insects, Microorganisms
    and Man. In: *Changing Disease Patterns and Human Behavior*, edited
    by N. F. Stanley and R. A. Joske. New York: Academic Press, pp. 55–68.

Butler, Jay C., and Robert F. Breiman
    1998 Legionellosis. In: *Bacterial Infections of Humans*, edited by
    Alfred S. Evans and Philip S. Brachman. New York: Plenum
    Medical Books, pp. 355–75.

Butzer, Karl W.
    1964 *Environment and Archeology*. Chicago: Aldine Press.

Caffey, John
    1957 Cooley's Anemia: A Review of the Roentgenographic Findings in
    the Skeleton. *American Journal of Roentgenology* 78 (3): 381–91.

Campitelli, Laura, Concetta Fabiani, Simona Puzelli, Alessandro Fioretti, Emanuela
    Foni, Alessandro DeMarco, Scott Krauss, Robert G. Webster, and Isabella
    Donatelli
    2002 H3N2 Influenza Viruses from Domestic Chickens in Italy:
    An Increasing Role for Chickens in the Ecology of Influenza?
    Journal of General Virology 83: 413–20.

Canci, Alessandro, Simona Minozzi, and Silvana M. Borgognini
    1996 New Evidence of Tuberculosis Spondylitis from Neolithic Liguria
    (Italy). *International Journal of Osteoarchaeology* 6: 497–501.

Carpenter, Kenneth J.
    1986 *The History of Scurvy and Vitamin C*. Cambridge: Cambridge
    University Press.

Carter, Richard, and Kamini N. Mendis
    2002 Evolutionary and Historical Aspects of the Burden of Malaria.
    Clinical Microbiology Reviews 15 (4): 564–94.

Cartwright, Frederick F., and Michael Biddiss
    2000 *Disease and History*. London: Sutton Publishing.

Catton, M. G., and S. A. Locarnini
    1998 Epidemiology: Hepatitis A (HAV). In: *Viral Hepatitis*, edited
    by Arie J. Zuckerman and Howard C. Thomas. London:
    Churchill Livingstone, pp. 29–41.

Chandler, Asa C.
    1945 *Introduction to Parasitology*. 7th ed. New York: John
    Wiley & Sons.

Chang, Kwang-Chih
    1986 *The Archaeology of Ancient China*. 4th ed. New Haven:
    Yale University Press.

Chesebro, Bruce, and Byron Caughey
    2002 Transmissible Spongiform Encephalopathies (Prion Protein
    Diseases). In: *Clinical Virology*, edited by Douglas D. Richman,
    Richard J. Whitely, and Frederick G. Hayden. Washington,
    D.C.: ASM Press, pp. 1241–62.

Chopra, Deepak
    1994 *Alternative Medicine: The Definitive Guide*. Fife: Future Medicine
    Publishing.

Cipolla, Carlo M.
1978 *The Economic History of World Population.* Sussex: Harvester Press.

Claas, Eric C. J., Albert D. M. E. Osterhaus, Ruud van Beek, Jan C. DeVong, Gus F. Rimmelzwaan, Dennis A. Senne, Scott Krauss, and Kennedy F. Shortage
1998 Human Influenza A H5N1 Virus Related to Highly Pathogenic Avian Influenza Virus. *Lancet* 351: 472–77.

Clark, G. A., M. A. Kelley, J. M. Grange, and C. Hill
1987 Evolution of Mycobacterial Disease in Human Populations: A Reevaluation. *Current Anthropology* 28: 45–62.

Cleary, P. Patrick, Kristen H. Pritchard, W. Michael McShan, and Joseph K. Ferretti
2000 Group A Streptococcal Genetics and Virulence. In: *Streptococcal Infections*, edited by Dennis L. Stevens and Edward L. Kaplan. New York: Oxford University Press, pp. 37–56.

Clemments, A. N.
1992 *The Biology of Mosquitoes*, Volume 1: *Development, Nutrition, and Reproduction.* London: Chapman & Hall.

Cloudsley-Thompson, J. L.
1976 *Insects and History.* New York: St. Martin's Press.

Clutton-Brock, Juliet
1981 *Domesticated Animals from Early Times.* Austin: University of Texas Press.

Coale, Ansley J.
1974 The History of the Human Population. In: *Biological Anthropology: Readings from Scientific American.* San Francisco: W. H. Freeman, pp. 459–70.

Cockburn, Aidan
1963 *The Evolution and Eradication of Infectious Diseases.* Baltimore: Johns Hopkins University Press.

Cockburn, Aidan
1980 The Marquise of Tai. In: *Mummies, Disease and Ancient Cultures*, edited by Aidan Cockburn and Eve Cockburn. Cambridge: Cambridge University Press, pp. 233–34.

Cockerell, Clay J.
1997 Poxvirus Infections. In: *Pathology of Infectious Diseases*, Volume 1, edited by Daniel H. Conner, Francis W. Chandler, David A. Schwartz, Herbert J. Manz, and Ernest E. Lack. Stamford, Conn.: Appleton & Lange, pp. 273–79.

Cohen, Mark Nathan, and George J. Armelagos
1984 *Paleopathology at the Origins of Agriculture.* Orlando, Fla.: Academic Press.

Collins, Frank M.
1996 Pathogenicity of M. Tuberculosis in Experimental Animals. In: *Tuberculosis*, edited by William N. Rom and Stuart M. Garay. Boston: Little, Brown, pp. 259–68.

Colwell, Rita R., and William M. Spira
  1992 The Ecology of Vibrio Cholerae. In: *Cholera,* edited by Dhiram Baura
        and William B. Greenough III. New York: Plenum Medical Books, pp.
        107–27.

Congressional Subcommittee on Oversight, Permanent Select Committee of
        Intelligence, U.S. House of Representatives
  1980 *Soviet Biological Warfare Activities.* Washington, D.C.: U.S.
        Government Printing Office. Report 64-540-0.

Conner, Daniel H., Francis W. Chandler, David A. Schwartz, Herbert J.
        Manz, and Ernest E. Lack
  1997 *Pathology of Infectious Diseases,* Volume 1. Stamford, Conn.:
        Appleton & Lange.

Cooper, J. I., and F. O. MacCallum
  1984 *Viruses and the Environment.* London: Chapman & Hall.

Couch, Robert B.
  1975 Mycoplasmal Diseases. In: *Textbook of Medicine,* edited by
        Paul B. Beeson and Walsh McDermott. 14th ed. Philadelphia:
        W. B. Saunders, pp. 270–74.

Councilman, Morgan
  1970 The Ultrastructure of the Host Cell in Viral Infection. In:
        Infectious Agents and Host Reactions, edited by Stuart Mudd.
        Philadelphia: W. B. Saunders, pp. 440–65.

Coura, J. R., A. C. Junqueira, C. M. Giordano, and R. K. Funatsu
  1994 Chagas' Disease in the Brazilian Amazon. *Review of the
        Institute of Medicine of the Tropics, São Paulo* 36 (4): 363–68.

Cox, N. J., and K. Subbarao
  2000 Global Epidemiology of Influenza: Past and Present.
        Annual Review of Medicine 51: 407–21.

Craighead, John E.
  2000 *Pathology and Pathogenesis of Human Viral Disease.* San Diego:
        Academic Press.

Crawford, Gary W.
  1992 Prehistoric Plant Domestication in East Asia. In: *The Origins of
        Agriculture,* edited by C. Wesley Cowan and Patty Jo Watson.
        Washington, D.C.: Smithsonian Institution Press, pp. 7–38.

Crosby, Alfred W.
  1969 The Early History of Syphilis: A Reappraisal. *American
        Anthropologist* 71: 218–27.

Crosby, Alfred W.
  1976 *Epidemic and Peace, 1918.* Westport, Conn.: Greenwood Press.

Cuff, Leighton E.
  1975 Shigellosis. In: *Textbook of Medicine,* edited by Paul B. Beesen and
        Walsh McDermott. 14th ed. Philadelphia: W. B. Saunders, pp. 371–73.

Cunningham, Madeleine W.
  2000 Streptococcal Sequelae and Molecular Mimicry. In: *Effects of
        Microbes on the Immune System,* edited by Madeleine W. Cunningham
        and Roberts S. Fujinami. Philadelphia: Lippincott Williams & Wilkins,
        pp. 123–49.

Daniels, Thomas J., and Richard C. Falco
    1989 The Lyme Disease Invasion. *Natural History* 7 (89): 4–10.

Davis, Kingsley
    1972 The Urbanization of the Human Population. In: *Biology and Culture in Modern Perspective: Readings from Scientific American.* San Francisco: W. H. Freeman.

Dean, Deborah
    1997 Chlamydial Infections: Chlamydia Trachomatis. In: *Pathology of Infectious Diseases,* Volume 1, edited by Daniel H. Conner, Francis W. Chandler, David A. Schwartz, Herbert J. Manz, and Ernest E. Lack. Stamford, Conn.: Appleton & Lange, pp. 473–90.

Deane, Phyllis
    1996 The British Industrial Revolution. In: *The Industrial Revolution in National Context,* edited by Mikulas Teich and Roy Porter. Cambridge: Cambridge University Press, pp. 13–35.

DeGroot, Leslie J.
    1975 Endemic Goiter. In: *Textbook of Medicine,* edited by Paul B. Beeson and Walsh McDermott. 14th ed. Philadelphia: W. B. Saunders, pp. 1727–28.

Delamater, E. D., Haanes, M., Wiggal, R. H., and D. M. Pillsbury
    1951 Studies of the Life Cycle of Spirochetes. VIII. Summary and Comparison of Observations on Various Organisms. *Journal of Investigative Dermatology* 16: 231–56.

De Lumley, Henry
    1972 A Paleolithic Camp at Nice. In: *Old World Archaeology: Foundations of Civilization: Readings from Scientific American.* San Francisco: W. H. Freeman, pp. 33–48.

Dennel, Robin W.
    1992 The Origins of Crop Agriculture in Europe. In: *The Origins of Agriculture,* edited by C Wesley Cowan and Patty Jo Watson. Washington, D.C.: Smithsonian Institution Press, pp. 71–100.

Denny, Floyd W.
    2000 History of Hemolytic Streptococci and Associated Diseases. In: *Streptococcal Infections,* edited by Dennis L. Stevens and Edward L. Kaplan. New York: Oxford University Press, pp. 1–18.

Desowitz, Robert S.
    1981 *New Guinea Tapeworms and Jewish Grandmothers.* New York: W.W. Norton.

De The, Guy
    2000 Epstein-Barr Virus and Burkitt's Sarcoma. In: *Infectious Causes of Cancer,* edited by James J. Goedert. Totowa, N.J.: Humana Press, pp. 77–92.

De Zuleta, Julian
    1973 Malaria and Mediterranean History. *Parasitologia* 15: 1–15.

De Zuleta, Julian
    1980 Man and Malaria. In: *Changing Disease Patterns and Human Behavior,* edited by N. F. Stanley and R. A. Joske. New York: Academic Press, pp. 176–86.

Dixon, Bernard
   1978 *Beyond the Magic Bullet*. New York: Harper & Row.
Dixon, C. W.
   1962 *Smallpox*. London: J. & A. Churchill.
Downies, Allen W.
   1959 Smallpox, Cowpox, and Vaccinia. In: *Viral and Rickettsial Infections
         of Man*, edited by Thomas M. Rivers and Frank L. Horsfall, Jr. 3rd ed.
         Philadelphia: J. B. Lippincott, pp. 673–700.
Downs, Wilbur G.
   1975   Yellow Fever. In: *Textbook of Medicine*, edited by Paul Beeson
         and Walsh McDermott. 14th ed. Philadelphia: W. B. Saunders,
         pp. 238–40.
Dubos, René
   1980 *Man Adapting*. New Haven, Conn.: Yale University Press.
Dubos, René, and Jean Dubos
   1952 *The White Plague: Tuberculosis, Man and Society*. Boston:
         Little, Brown.
Duvette, Jean-François, and Loel Blondiaux
   1993 Two Early Cases of Leprosy from Northern and Southern France.
         In: *Papers on Paleopathology, 20th Annual Meeting of the
         Paleopathology Association* (Toronto), p. 20. Published by the
         Paleopathology Association.
Eagle, Harry
   1952 The Spirochetes. In: *Bacterial and Mycotic Infections of Man*,
         edited by René J. Dubos. 2nd ed. Philadelphia: J. B. Lippincott,
         pp. 572–607.
Eaton, John W.
   1994 Malaria and the Selection of the Sickle Gene. In: *Sickle Cell
         Disease: Basic Principles and Clinical Practice*, edited by
         Stephen Embury, Robert P. Hebbel, Narla Mohandas, and
         Martin H. Steinberg. New York: Raven Press, pp. 13–18.
Edman, John D.
   1991 Biting the Hand That Feeds You. *Natural History* 7: 8–9.
Eisenberg, Henry, Frederick Plotke, and Amelia H. Baker
   1949 Asexual Syphilis in Children. *Journal of Venereal Disease
         Information* 30: 7–11.
El-Najjar, Mahmoud Y.
   1979 Human Treponematosis and Tuberculosis: Evidence from the New
         World. *American Journal of Physical Anthropology* 51: 599–618.
Embury, Stephen H., and Martin H. Steinberg
   1994 Genetic Modulators of Disease. In: *Sickle Cell Disease: Basic
         Principles and Clinical Practice*, edited by Stephen Embury,
         Robert P. Hebbel, Narla Mohandas, and Martin Steinberg.
         New York: Raven Press, pp. 279–98.

Erasmus, David A.
    1987 The Adult Schistosome: Structure and Reproductive Biology.
        In: *The Biology of Schistosomes: From Genes to Latrines*,
        edited by David Rollinson and Andrew J. G. Simpson. London:
        Academic Press, pp. 51–82.

Erlich, Henry L.
    1985 The Position of Bacteria and Their Products in Food Webs.
        In: *Bacteria in Nature*, Volume 1: *Bacterial Activities in Perspective*,
        edited by Edward R. Leadbetter and Jeanne S. Poindexter. New York:
        Plenum Press, pp. 199–219.

Esch, Gerald W., and Jacqueline C. Fernandez
    1993 *A Functional Biology of Parasitism*. London: Chapman & Hall.

Essex, Myron
    1999 The New AIDS Epidemic. *Harvard Magazine*, September–
        October, pp. 35–39.

Esslinger, J. H.
    1985 Insects. In: *Animal Agents and Vectors of Human Disease*,
        edited by Paul C. Beaver and Rodney C. Jung. Philadelphia:
        Lea & Febiger, pp. 206–27.

Fagan, Brian M.
    1996 *World Prehistory: A Brief Introduction*. 3rd ed. New York:
        Harper Collins College.

Farmer, Paul E., David A. Walton, and Jennifer J. Furin
    2000 The Changing Face of AIDS: Implications for Policy and
        Practice. In: *The Emergence of AIDS*, edited by Kenneth H.
        Mayer and H. F. Pizer. Washington, D.C.: American Public
        Health Association, pp. 139–61.

Faust, Ernest Carroll
    1951 Toxoplasmosis. In: *Textbook of Medicine*, edited by Russell L.
        Cecil and Robert F. Loeb. Philadelphia: W. B. Saunders, pp. 402–3.

Fenner, Frank
    1980 Smallpox and Its Eradication. In: *Changing Disease Patterns and
        Human Behavior*, edited by N. F. Stanley and R. A. Joske. London:
        Academic Press, pp. 215–29.

Field, H., P. Young, J. M. Yob, L. Hall, and J. MacKenzie
    2001 The Natural History of Hendra and Nipah Viruses. *Microbes and
        Infection* 3 (4): 307–14.

Fine, Paul E. M.
    1982 Leprosy: The Epidemiology of a Slow Bacterium. *Epidemiologic
        Reviews* 4: 161–88.

Finnegan, John
    1993 *The Facts about Fats*. Berkeley, Calif.: Celestial Arts.

Forbes, Charles D., and William F. Jackson
    1993 *Color Atlas and Text of Clinical Medicine*. St. Louis: C. V. Mosby.

Ford, John
    1971 *The Role of the Trepanomiases in African Ecology*. Oxford:
        Clarendon Press.

Formicola, Vincenzo, Quinzio Milanesi, and Caterina Scarsini
    1987 Evidence of Spinal Tuberculosis at the Beginning of the Fourth
        Millennium B.C. from Arene Candide Cave (Liguria, Italy).
        American Journal of Physical Anthropology 72: 1–6.
Francis, John
    1958 *Tuberculosis in Animals and Man.* London: Cassell.
Frantz, Douglas
    2001 Deadly Virus Strikes Refugees in Pakistan. *International Herald
        Tribune,* 5 October, p. 3.
Fribourg-Blanc, A.
    1972 Treponema. In: *Pathology of Simian Primates, Part II,* edited
        by R. N. T. Fiennes. Basel: Karger, pp. 255–62.
Fried, Michael, and Patrick E. Duffy
    1996 Adherence of Plasmodium Falciparum to Chondroitin Sulfate A
        in the Human Placenta. *Science* 272: 1502–4.
Gajdusek, D. Carlton
    1979 Observations on the Early History of Kuru Investigation. In: *Slow
        Transmissible Diseases of the Nervous System,* Volume 1, edited by S.
        Prusiner and W. Hadlow. New York: Academic Press, pp. 7–35.
Garay, Stuart M.
    1996 Pulmonary Tuberculosis. In: *Tuberculosis,* edited by William N.
        Rom and Stuart M. Garay. Boston: Little, Brown, pp. 373–412.
Garrett, Laurie
    1994 *The Coming Plague.* New York: Farrar, Straus & Giroux.
Gatner, E. M. S., E. Glatthaar, F. M. J. Himkamp, and S. H. Kok
    1980 Association of Tuberculosis and Leprosy in South Africa.
        Leprosy Review 51: 5–10.
Gerras, Charles
    1977 *The Complete Book of Vitamins.* Emmaus, Pa.: Rodale Press.
Gibbs, Mark J., John S. Armstrong, and Adrian J. Gibbs
    2001 Recombination in the Hemagglutinin Gene of the 1918
        "Spanish Flu." *Science* 293: 1842–45.
Gillett, J. D.
    1971 *Mosquitos.* London: Weidenfeld & Nicolson.
Glader, Bertil E.
    1994 Anemia. In: *Sickle Cell Disease: Basic Principles and Clinical
        Practice,* edited by Stephen H. Embury, Robert P. Hebbel,
        Narla Mohandas, and Martin H. Steinberg. New York:
        Raven Press, pp. 545–53.
Glass, Roger I., and Robert E. Black
    1992 The Epidemiology of Cholera. In: *Cholera,* edited by Dhiram
        Barua and William B. Greenough III. New York: Plenum
        Medical Books, pp. 129–54.
Glasser, Susan B.
    2002 Moscow Names Gas Used in Theater Siege. *International
        Herald Tribune,* 31 October, p. 3.

Goedert, James T.
    2000 Preface. In: *Infectious Causes of Cancer*, edited by James T. Goedert.
          Totowa, N.J.: Humana Press, pp. v–ix.
Goodwin, C. S.
    1984 *Microbes and Infections of the Gut*. Melbourne: Blackwell Scientific
          Publications.
Gottfried, Robert S.
    1983 *The Black Death*. New York: Free Press.
Gowlett, John A. J.
    1992 Tools—The Paleolithic Record. In: *The Cambridge
          Encyclopedia of Human Evolution*, edited by Steve Jones, Robert
          Martin, and David Pilbeam. Cambridge: Cambridge University Press,
          pp. 350–60.
Grady, Denise
    1993 Death at the Corners. *Discover* 14 (12): 84–91.
Graham, S. V., and J. D. Barry
    1995 Transcriptional Regulation of Metacyclic Variant Surface Glycoprotein
          Gene Expression during the Life Cycle of Trypanosma Brucei.
          Molecular Cell Biology 15 (11): 5945–56.
Grange, John M.
    1980 *Mycobacterial Diseases*. New York: Elsevier/North-Holland.
Graves, William
    1990 *National Geographic Atlas of the World*. 6th ed. Washington,
          D.C.: National Geographic Society.
Gray, Barry M.
    1998 Streptococcal Infections. In: *Bacterial Infections in Humans*,
          edited by Alfred S. Evans and Philip S. Brahman. New York: Plenum
          Medical Books, pp. 673–711.
Greene, Lawrence S.
    1993 G6PD Deficiency as Protection against Falciparum Malaria:
          An Epidemiologic Critique of Population and Experimental
          Studies. *Yearbook of Physical Anthropology* 36: 153–78.
Grin, E. I.
    1956 Endemic Syphilis and Yaws. *W.H.O. Bulletin* 15: 959–73.
Grmek, Mirko D.
    1989 *Diseases in the Ancient Greek World*. Baltimore: Johns Hopkins
          University Press.
Grove, David I.
    1980 Schistosomes, Snails and Man. In: *Changing Disease Patterns
          and Human Behavior*, edited by N. F. Stanley and R. A. Joske.
          New York: Academic Press, pp. 187–204.
Guan, Y., K. F. Shortridge, S. Krauss, and R. G. Webster
    1999 Molecular Characterization of H9N2 Influenza Viruses: Were
          They the Donors of the "Internal" Genes of H5N1 Viruses
          in Hong Kong? *Proceedings of the National Academy of Sciences
          of the United States of America* 96 (16): 9363–67.

Guatelli, John C., Robert F. Silicano, Daniel R. Kuritzes, and
    Douglas D. Richman
    2002 Human Immunodeficiency Virus. In: *Clinical Virology*,
        edited by Douglas D. Richman, Richard J. Whitley, and
        Frederick G. Hayden. Washington, D.C.: ASM Press, pp. 685–729.

Guggenheim, Karl Y.
    1981 *Nutrition and Nutritional Diseases*. Lexington, Mass.: Collamore
        Press, D. C. Heath.

Guhl, Felipe, Carlos Jaramillo, Roxan Yockteng, Gutavo Adolfo Vallejo,
    Felipe Cardenas-Arroyo
    1997 Trypanosoma Cruzi DNA in Human Mummies. *Lancet* 349: 1370.

Gust, Ian
    1980 Acute Viral Hepatitis. In: *Changing Disease Patterns and Human
        Behavior*, edited by N. F. Stanley and R. A. Joske. New York:
        Academic Press, pp. 85–113.

Guthe, Thorstein
    1975 Treponemal Diseases. In: *Textbook of Medicine*, edited by Paul B.
        Beeson and Walsh McDermott. 14th ed. Philadelphia: W. B. Saunders,
        pp. 416–34.

Guthe, Thorstein, and A. Luger
    1957 Epidemiological Aspects of Non-Venereal "Endemic" Syphilis.
        Dermatologica 115: 248–72.

Guthe, Thorstein, and R. R. Wilcox
    1954 Treponematosis: A World Problem. *W.H.O Chronicle* 8 (2–3): 7–113.

Gutteridge, W. E., and G. H. Combs
    1977 *Biochemistry of Parasitic Protozoa*. Baltimore: University
        Park Press.

Haas, François, and Sheila Sperber Haas
    1996 The Origins of Mycobacterium Tuberculosis and the Notion of Its
        Contagiousness. In: *Tuberculosis*, edited by William N. Rom and
        Stuart M. Garay. Boston: Little, Brown, pp. 3–20.

Hackett, C. J.
    1963 On the Origin of the Human Treponematoses. *W.H.O. Bulletin* 29: 7–41.

Hackett, C. J.
    1976 *Diagnostic Criteria of Syphilis, Yaws, and Trepinarid (Treponematoses)
        and of Some Other Diseases in Dry Bones*. Berlin: Springer Verlag.

Hagen, Paul
    1987 The Human Immune Response to Schistosome Infection. In:
        The Biology of Schistosomes: From Genes to Latrines, edited by
        David Rollinson and Andrew J. G. Simpson. London: Academic Press,
        pp. 295–320.

Hale, T. L., and D. F. Keren
    1992 Pathogenesis and Immunology in Shigellosis: Application for
        Vaccine Development. In: *Pathogenesis of Shigellosis*, edited
        by P. J. Sansonetti. Berlin: Springer Verlag, pp. 117–37.

Hanney, Peter W.
    1975 *Rodents: Their Lives and Habits*. New York: Taplinger.

Hardy, Paul H.
1976 Pathogenic Treponemes. In: *The Biology of Parasitic Spirochetes*, edited by Russell C. Johnson. New York: Academic Press, pp. 107–19.

Hare, Ronald
1967 The Antiquity of Diseases Caused by Bacteria and Viruses, a Review of the Problem from a Bacteriologist's Point of View. In: *Diseases in Antiquity*, edited by Don Brothwell and A. T. Sandison. Springfield, Ill.: Charles C. Thomas, pp. 115–31.

Harlan, Jack A.
1967 A Wild Wheat Harvest in Turkey. *Archaeology* 20: 197–201.

Harlan, Jack A.
1992 Indigenous African Agriculture. In: *The Origins of Agriculture*, edited by C. Wesley Cowan and Patty Jo Watson. Washington, D.C.: Smithsonian Institution Press, pp. 59–70.

Harrison, L. W.
1959 The Origin of Syphilis. *British Journal of Venereal Diseases* 35: 1–7.

Hawley, William A.
1991 Adaptable Immigrant. *Natural History*, July, pp. 55–59.

Hay, Alan J.
1998 The Virus Genome and Its Replication. In: *Textbook of Influenza*, edited by K. G. Nicholson, R. G. Webster, and A. J. Hay. Oxford: Blackwell Science, pp. 43–53.

Heilbroner, Robert L.
1975 *The Making of Economic Society*. Englewood Cliffs, N.J.: Prentice Hall.

Hemmer, Helmut
1990 *Domestication*. Cambridge: Cambridge University Press.

Hendrickson, Robert
1983 *More Cunning Than Man*. New York: Kensington.

Henig, Robin Marantz
1993 *A Dancing Matrix*. New York: Vintage Books.

Henis, Yigel
1987 Survival and Dormancy of Bacteria. In: *Survival and Dormancy of Microorganisms*, edited by Yigel Henis. New York: John Wiley & Sons, pp. 1–108.

Henneberg, Renata J., and Macicej Henneberg
1993 Possible Occurrence of Treponematosis in the Ancient Greek Colony of Metaponto. *American Journal of Physical Anthropology* Supplement 16: 107–8.

Henneberg, Macicej, Renata J. Henneberg, and Joseph Coleman Carter
1992 Health in Colonial Metaponto. *National Geographic Research and Exploration* 8 (4): 446–59.

Henry, Donald O.
1989 *From Foraging to Agriculture: The Levant at the End of the Ice Age*. Philadelphia: University of Pennsylvania Press.

Hepstein, H.
1971 *The Origin of the Domestic Animals of Africa*, Volume 1. New York: Africa Publishing.

Herlihy, David
    1997 *The Black Death and the Transformation of the West.*
          Cambridge, Mass.: Harvard University Press.

Herre, Wolf
    1969 The Science and History of Domestic Animals. In: *Science
          in Archaeology: A Survey of Progress and Research*, edited
          by Don Brothwell and Eric Higgs. 2nd ed. London: Thames &
          Hudson, pp. 257–72.

Hershkovitz, I., and G. Edelson
    1991 The First Identified Case of Thalassemia? *Human Evolution*
          6 (1): 49–54.

Higginson, John
    1980 Cancer and the Environment. In: *Changing Disease Patterns and
          Human Behavior*, edited by N. F. Stanley and R. A. Joske. London:
          Academic Press, pp. 447–66.

Holcomb, R. C.
    1941 The Antiquity of Congenital Syphilis. *Bulletin of the History of
          Medicine* 10: 148–77.

Holmgren, Jan
    1992 Pathogenesis. In: *Cholera*, edited by Dhiram Barua and William B.
          Greenough III. New York: Plenum Medical Books, pp. 199–208.

Holzman, Robert S.
    1997 Infection by M. Avium-Intracellulare Complex in the Acquired
          Immunodeficiency Syndrome. In: *Pathology of Infectious Disease*,
          Volume 1, edited by Daniel H. Conner, Francis W. Chandler,
          David A. Schwartz, Herbert J. Manz, and Ernest E. Lack. Stamford,
          Conn.: Appleton & Lange, pp. 711–20.

Honess, R. W., and D. H. Watson
    1977 Unity and Diversity in the Herpes Viruses. *Journal of General
          Virology* 37: 15–37.

Hooper, P., S. Zaki, P. Daniels, and D. Middleton
    2001 Comparative Pathology of the Diseases Caused by Hendra and
          Nipah Viruses. *Microbes and Infection* 3 (4): 315–22.

Hope-Simpson, R. Edgar
    1992 *The Transmission of Epidemic Influenza.* New York: Plenum Press.

Hopkins, Donald R.
    1983 *Princes and Peasants: Smallpox in History.* Chicago: University
          of Chicago Press.

Horsfall, William R.
    1962 *Medical Entomology: Arthropods and Human Disease.* New York:
          Ronald Press.

Horsfall, William R.
    1972 *Mosquitoes: Their Bionomics and Relation to Disease.* New York:
          Hafner.

Howe, Howard, and James L. Wilson
    1959 Poliomyelitis. In: *Viral and Rickettsial Infections of Man*, edited
          by Thomas M. Rivers and Frank L. Horsefall. Philadelphia:
          J. B. Lippincott, pp. 432–78.

Hudson, Ellis Herndon
   1958 *Non-Venereal Syphilis.* Edinburgh: E. & S. Livingstone.
Hudson, Ellis Herndon
   1965 Treponematosis in Perspective. *W.H.O. Bulletin* 32: 738–48.
Hudson, Ellis Herndon
   1968 Christopher Columbus and the History of Syphilis. *Acta Tropica* 25:
        1–16.
Hudspeth, Marie K., Tyler C. Smith, Christopher P. Barrozo. Anthony W.
   Hawksworth, Margaret A. K. Ryan, and Gregory C. Gray
   2001 National Department of Defense Surveillance for Invasive Streptococcal
        Pneumoniae: Antibiotic Resistance, Serotype Distribution, and
        Arbitrarily Primed Polymerase Chain Reaction Analysis. *Journal of
        Infectious Diseases* 184: 591–96.
Hughes, Jonathan
   1970 *Industrialization and Economic History: Theses and Conjectures.*
        New York: McGraw-Hill.
Hull, Thomas G.
   1941 *Diseases Transmitted from Animals to Man.* Springfield, Ill.:
        Charles C. Thomas.
Hyams, Edward
   1972 *Animals in the Service of Man.* Philadelphia: J. B. Lippincott.
Isenberg, David, and John Morrow
   1995 *Friendly Fire: Explaining Autoimmune Disease.* Oxford: Oxford
        University Press.
Ito, Toshihiro
   2000 Interspecies Transmission and Receptor Recognition of Influenza
        Viruses. *Microbiology and Immunology* 44 (6): 423–30.
Ito, Toshihiro, and Yoshihiro Kawaoka
   1998 Avian Influenza. In: *Textbook of Influenza,* edited by K. G. Nicholson,
        R. G. Webster, and A. J. Hay. Oxford: Blackwell Science, pp. 126–36.
Jaax, Nancy K., and David L. Fritz
   1997 Anthrax. In: *Pathology of Infectious Diseases,* Volume 1, edited by
        Daniel H. Conner, Francis W. Chandler, David A. Schwartz, Herbert J.
        Manz, and Ernest E. Lack. Stamford, Conn.: Appleton & Lange,
        pp. 397–415.
Jackson, George Gee
   1975 The Common Cold. In: *Textbook of Medicine,* edited by Paul B.
        Beeson and Walsh McDermott. 14th ed. Philadelphia: W. B. Saunders,
        pp. 184–86.
Jaffe, Henry L.
   1972 *Metabolic, Degenerative, and Inflammatory Diseases of Bones and
        Joints.* Philadelphia: Lea & Febiger.
James, Maurice T., and Robert F. Harwood
   1969 *Herm's Medical Entomology.* London: Macmillan.
Janeway, Charles A., Jr.
   1993 How the Immune System Recognizes Invaders. *Scientific American*
        269 (3): 73–79.

Janssens, Paul A., Antonia Marcsik, Christel de Meyere, and Guy de Roy
    1993 Qualitative and Quantitative Aspects of Scurvy in Ancient Bones.
        Journal of Paleopathology 5 (1): 25–36.
Jenkins, Frank J., and Linda J. Hoffman
    2000 Overview of Herpes Viruses. In: *Infectious Causes of Cancer*, edited
        by James J. Goedert. Totowa, N.J.: Humana Press, pp. 33–49.
Johnson, Karl M.
    1975a Dengue. In: *Textbook of Medicine*, edited by Paul B. Beeson
        and Walsh McDermott. 14th ed. Philadelphia: W. B. Saunders,
        pp. 224–25.
Johnson, Karl M.
    1975b Hemorrhagic Fever Caused by Dengue Viruses. In: *Textbook of
        Medicine*, edited by Paul B. Beeson and Walsh McDermott.
        14th ed. Philadelphia: W. B. Saunders, pp. 241–43.
Johnson, Karl M.
    1975c Arthropod-Borne Viral Fevers, Viral Encephalitides, and Viral
        Hemorrhagic Fevers. In: *Textbook of Medicine*, edited by Paul B.
        Beeson and Walsh McDermott. 14th ed. Philadelphia: W. B. Saunders,
        pp. 223–36.
Johnson, Karl M.
    2002 Viral Hemorrhagic Fevers: A Comparative Appraisal. In: *Clinical
        Virology*, edited by Douglas D. Richman, Richard J. Whitely, and
        Frederick G. Hayden. Washington, D.C.: ASM Press, pp. 135–44.
Jones, Thomas C.
    1975a Malaria. In: *Textbook of Medicine*, edited by Paul B. Beeson
        and Walsh McDermott. 14th ed. Philadelphia: W. B. Saunders,
        pp. 472–80.
Jones, Thomas C.
    1975b Toxoplasmosis. In: *Textbook of Medicine*, edited by Paul B. Beeson and
        Walsh McDermott. 14th ed. Philadelphia: W. B. Saunders, pp. 502–6.
Jones, W. H. S.
    1909 *Malaria and Greek History*. New York: Ames Press.
Jourdane, Joseph, and Andre Theron
    1987 Larval Development: Eggs to Cercariae. In: *The Biology of Schistosomes:
        From Genes to Latrines*, edited by David Rollinson and Andrew J. G.
        Simpson. London: Academic Press, pp. 83–113.
Kanki, Phyllis J., and Myron E. Essex
    2000 The Past and Future of HIV. In: *The Emergence of AIDS*, edited by
        Kenneth H. Mayer and H. F. Pizer. Washington, D.C.: American Public
        Health Association, pp. 2–22.
Kann, M., and W. Gerlich
    1998 Structure and Molecular Virology: Hepatitis B (HBV). In: *Viral Hepatitis*,
        edited by Arie J. Zuckerman and Howard C. Thomas. London: Churchill
        Livingstone, pp. 77–105.
Kantor, Fred S.
    1994 Disarming Lyme Disease. *Scientific American* 271 (3): 34–39.

Kao, Jia-Horng, and Ding-Shinn Chen
    2000 Overview of Hepatitis B and C Viruses. In: *Infectious Causes of Cancer*, edited by James J. Goedert. Totowa, N.J.: Humana Press, pp. 313–30.

Kaplan, Martin M., and Hilary Koprowski
    1980 Rabies. *Scientific American* 242 (1): 121–31.

Karayiannis, P., and H. C. Thomas
    1998 Disease Association and Treatment of HGV (GBV-C). In: *Viral Hepatitis*, edited by Arie J. Zuckerman and Howard C. Thomas. London: Churchill Livingstone, pp. 437–41.

Kawaoka, Yoshihiro, and Robert G. Webster
    1988 Molecular Mechanism of Acquisition of Virulence in Influenza Virus in Nature. *Microbial Pathogenesis* 5: 311–18.

Kazazian, Haig H., Carol E. Dowling, Corinne D. Boehm, Tina C. Warren, Effrossini P. Economou, Joel Katz, and Stylianos E. Antonarakias
    1990 Gene Defects in B-Thalassemias and Their Prenatal Diagnosis. In: *6th Cooley's Anemia Symposium*, edited by Arthur Bank. Annals of the New York Academy of Sciences, Volume 612. New York: New York Academy of Sciences, pp. 1–14.

Keefer, Chester C.
    1951 Scarlet Fever. In: *A Textbook of Medicine*, edited by Russell L. Cecil and Robert F. Loeb. Philadelphia: W. B. Saunders, pp. 145–53.

Kempe, C. Henry
    1975 Variola and Vaccinia. In: *Textbook of Medicine*, edited by Paul B. Beeson and Walsh McDermott. 14th ed. Philadelphia: W. B. Saunders, pp. 206–11.

Kent, Susan, and David Dunn
    1996 Anemia and the Transition of Nomadic Hunter-Gatherers to a Sedentary Life Style: Follow-up Study of a Kalahari Community. *American Journal of Physical Anthropology* 99 (3): 455–72.

Kilbourne, Edwin D.
    1975 Influenza. In: *Textbook of Medicine*, edited by Paul B. Beeson and Walsh McDermott. 14th ed. Philadelphia: W. B. Saunders, pp. 193–99.

Kilbourne, Edwin D.
    1987 *Influenza*. New York: Plenum Medical Books.

Kinney, Thomas R., and Russel E. Ware
    1994 Compound Heterozygous States. In: *Sickle Cell Disease: Basic Principles and Clinical Practice*, edited by Stephen H. Embury, Robert P. Hebbel, Narla Mohandas, and Martin H. Steinberg. New York: Raven Press, pp. 437–51.

Kirschmann, John D.
    1975 *Nutritional Almanac*. New York: McGraw-Hill.

Klos, Heinz-Georg, and Ernest M. Lang
    1976 *Handbook of Zoo Medicine*. New York: Van Nostrand Reinholdt.

Knight, Vernon
    1975 Brucellosis (Undulant Fever, Malta Fever). In: *Textbook of Medicine*, edited by Paul B. Beeson and Walsh McDermott. 14th ed. Philadelphia: W. B. Saunders, pp. 388–91.

Koenig, Robert
  1996 Koch Keeps New Watch on Infections. *Science* 272: 1412–14.
Kolker, Steven E., Herbert J. Manz, and David A. Schwartz
  1997 Syphilis. In: *Pathology of Infectious Diseases*, Vol. 1, edited by Daniel
        H. Conner, Francis W. Chandler, David A. Schwartz, Herbert J. Manz,
        and Ernest E. Lack. Stamford: Appleton & Lange, pp. 833–46.
Krause, Richard M.
  1992 The Origin of Plagues: Old and New. *Science* 257: 1073–78.
Kreiswirth, Barry N., and Andrew Moss
  1996 Genotyping Multidrug-Resistent M. Tuberculosis in New York City.
        In: *Tuberculosis*, edited by William N. Rom and Stuart M. Garay.
        Boston: Little, Brown, pp. 199–209.
Kuhn, Raymond E.
  1974 Immunology of Trypanosoma Cruzi Infections. In: *Parasitic Diseases,*
        Volume 1: *The Immunology*, edited by John M. Mansfield. New York:
        Marcel Dekker, pp. 137–66.
Lack, Ernest E., and Daniel H. Conner
  1997 Tuberculosis. In: *Pathology of Infectious Diseases*, Vol. 1, edited
        by Daniel H. Conner, Francis W. Chandler, David A. Schwartz,
        Herbert J. Manz, and Ernest E. Lack. Stamford, Conn.: Appleton &
        Lange, pp. 857–68.
LaForce, F. Marc
  1990 Bacillus Anthracis (Anthrax). In: *Principles and Practice of Infectious
        Diseases*, edited by Gerald Mandell, R. Gordon Duoglas, Jr., and John
        E. Bennett. 3rd ed. New York: Churchill Livingstone, pp. 1593–95.
Lambrecht, Frank L.
  1967 Trypanosomiasis in Prehistoric and Later Human Populations,
        a Tentative Reconstruction. In: *Diseases in Antiquity*, edited
        by Don Brothwell and A. T. Sandison. Springfield, Ill.: Charles
        C. Thomas, pp. 132–51.
Langman, Rodney E.
  1989 *The Immune System*. San Diego: Academic Press.
Lederberg, Joshua
  1993 Viruses and Humankind: Intracellular Symbiosis and Evolutionary
        Competition. In: *Emerging Viruses*, edited by Stephen S. Morse.
        Oxford: Oxford University Press, pp. 3–9.
Lederberg, Joshua, Robert E. Shope, and Stanley Oaks, Jr.
  1992 *Emerging Infections: Microbial Threats to Health in the United States*.
        Washington, D.C.: Institute of Medicine, National Academy Press.
Levine, Arnold J.
  1992 *Viruses*. New York: Scientific American Library.
Lewis, Stuart, and Steven Field
  1996 Intestinal and Peritoneal Tuberculosis. In: *Tuberculosis*, edited by
        William N. Rom and Stuart M. Garay. Boston: Little, Brown, pp. 585–97.
Ley, Herbert L., Jr.
  1975 Scrub Typhus and Trench Fever. In: *Textbook of Medicine*, edited
        by Paul B. Beeson and Walsh McDermott. 14th ed. Philadelphia:
        W. B. Saunders, pp. 259–62.

Lichtenstein, Lawrence M.
    1993 Allergy and the Immune System. *Scientific American* 269 (3): 117–24.

Little, M. D.
    1985a Cestodes (Tapeworms). In: *Animal Agents and Vectors of Human Disease*, edited by Paul Chester Beaver and Rodney Clifton Jung. 5th ed. Philadelphia: Lea & Febiger, pp. 110–26.

Little, M. D.
    1985b Nematodes of the Digestive Tract and Related Species. In: *Animal Agents and Vectors of Human Disease*, edited by Paul Chester Beaver and Rodney Clifton Jung. 5th ed. Philadelphia: Lea & Febiger, pp. 127–70.

Liu, Jianguo
    2003 SARS, Wildlife, and Human Health. *Science* 302: 53.

Livingstone, Frank B.
    1984 The Duffy Blood Groups, Vivax Malaria, and Malaria Selection in Human Populations: A Review. *Human Biology* 56 (3): 413–25.

Livingstone, Frank B.
    1986 Anthropological Aspects of the Distribution of the Human Hemoglobin Variants. In: *Hemoglobin Variants in Human Populations*, Vol. 1, edited by William P. Winter. Boca Raton, Fla.: CRC Press, pp. 17–28.

Longmate, Norman
    1966 *King Cholera: The Biography of a Disease.* London: Hamish Hamilton.

Low, Donald E., Benjamin Schwartz, and Allison McGeer
    1998 The Reemergence of Severe Group A Streptococcus Disease: An Evolutionary Perspective. In: *Emerging Infections*, edited by W. M. Scheld, D. Armstrong, and J. M. Huges. Washington, D.C.: ASM Press, pp. 93–123.

Maat, G. J. R.
    1982 Scurvy in Dutch Whalers Buried at Spitsbergen. In: *Proceedings of the IV European Meeting of the Paleopathology Association at Middleburg-Antwerp*, p. 8 (abstract). Published by the Paleopathology Association.

Mahalanabis, Dilip, A. M. Molla, and David A. Sack
    1992 Clinical Management of Cholera. In: *Cholera*, edited by Dhiram Barua and William B. Greenough III. New York: Plenum Medical Books, pp. 253–83.

Manz, Herbert J., and Alfred A. Buck
    1997 Yaws, Bejel, and Pinta. In: *Pathology of Infectious Diseases*, Vol. 1, edited by Daniel H. Conner, Francis W. Chandler, David A. Schwartz, Herbert J. Manz, and Ernest E. Lack. Stamford, Conn.: Appleton & Lange, pp. 911–16.

Markowitz, Milton, and Edward L. Kaplan
    2000 Rheumatic Fever. In: *Streptococcal Infections*, edited by Dennis L. Stevens and Edward L. Kaplan. New York: Oxford University Press, pp. 133–43.

Marlink, Richard
    2001 The Biology and Epidemiology of HIV-2. In: *AIDS Clinical Review 2000/2001*, edited by Paul A. Volberding and Mark A. Jacobson. New York: Marcel Dekker, pp. 47–65.

Marra, C. M.
    2000 Encephalitis in the 21st Century. *Seminars in Neurology* 20 (3): 323–27.

Martin, Maureen P., and Mary Carrington
    2002 The Role of Human Genetics in HIV-1 Infection. In: *Chemokine Receptors and AIDS*, edited by Thomas O'Brien. New York: Marcel Dekker, pp. 1133–62.

Matrosovich, Mikhail, Nannan Zhou, Yoshihiro Kawaoka, and Robert Webster
    1999 The Surface Glycoproteins of H5 Influenza Viruses Isolated from Humans, Chickens, and Wild Aquatic Birds Have Distinguishable Properties. *Journal of Virology* 73 (2): 1146–55.

Mattman, Lida H.
    1993 *Cell Wall Deficient Forms: Stealth Pathogens*. 2nd ed. Boca Raton, Fla.: CRC Press.

Matsuoka, Masao
    2000 Adult T-Cell Leukemia/Lymphoma. In: *Infectious Causes of Cancer*, edited by James J. Goedert. Totowa, N.J.: Humana Press, pp. 211–29.

Mayer, Leonard W., et al.
    2002 Outbreak of W135 Meningococcal Disease in 2000: Not Emergence of a New W135 Strain But Clonal Expansion within the Electrophoretic Type-37 Complex. *Journal of Infectious Diseases* 185: 1596–1605.

McConnaughey, Janet
    2002 West Nile Found in Four Ailing Louisiana Dogs. Associated Press, printed in *Arizona Daily Star*, 20 October, p. A3.

McCullers, Jonathan A., Sergio Facchini, P. Joan Chesney, and Robert G. Webster
    1999 Influenza B Virus Encephalitis. *Clinical Infectious Diseases* 28: 898–900.

McDade, Joseph E., and Verne F. Newhouse
    1986 Natural History of Rickettsia Rickettsii. In: *Annual Review of Microbiology*, Vol. 40, edited by L. Nicholas Ornston, Albert Balows, and Paul Bauman. Palo Alto, Calif.: Annual Reviews, pp. 287–309.

McElroy, Ann, and Patricia K. Townsend
    1989 *Medical Anthropology*. 2nd ed. Boulder, Colo.: Westview Press.

McKenzie, William, and Don Brothwell
    1967 Disease in the Ear Region. In: *Diseases in Antiquity*, edited by Don Brothwell and A. T. Sandison. Springfield, Ill.: Charles C. Thomas, pp. 464–73.

McNeill, William H.
    1976 *Plagues and Peoples*. New York: Doubleday.

McNeill, William H.
    1980 Migration Patterns and Infection in Traditional Societies. In: *Changing Disease Patterns and Human Behavior*, edited by N. F. Stanley and R. A. Joske. New York: Academic Press, pp. 27–36.

McNicol, L. A., and R. N. Doetsch
    1983 A Hypothesis Accounting for the Origin of Pandemic Cholera:
        A Retrograde Analysis. *Perspectives in Biology and Medicine*
        26 (4): 542–52.

Medina, Eva, Oliver Goldmann, Manfred Rohde, Andreas Lengeling, and
    Gursharan S. Chhatwals
    2001 Genetic Control of Susceptibility yo Group A Streptococcal Infection.
        Journal of Infectious Diseases 184: 846–52.

Mertz, Gregory J.
    2002 Bunyaviridae: Bunyaviruses, Phleboviruses, Nairoviruses and
        Hantaviruses. In: *Clinical Virology*, edited by Douglas D. Richman,
        Richard J. Whitely, and Frederick G. Hayen. Washington, D.C.:
        ASM Press, pp. 921–47.

Michael, Nelson L.
    2002 Chemokine Receptors as HIV-1 Coreceptors. In: *Chemokine Receptors
        and AIDS*, edited by Thomas R. O'Brien. New York: Marcel Dekker,
        pp. 75–89.

Mignogna, Frank V., Kenneth F. Garay, and Ruth Spiegel
    1996 Tuberculosis of the Head and Neck and Oral Cavity. In: *Tuberculosis*,
        edited by William N. Rom and Stuart M. Garay. Boston: Little, Brown,
        pp. 567–75.

Miles, James S.
    1975 *Orthopedic Problems of the Wetherill Mesa Populations*. Washington,
        D.C.: National Park Service, U.S. Department of Interior.

Miller, Naomi F.
    1992 The Origins of Plant Cultivation in the Near East. In: *The Origins of
        Agriculture*, edited by C. Wesley Cowant and Patty Jo Watson.
        Washington, D.C.: Smithsonian Institution Press, pp. 39–58.

Miller, R. L., et al.
    1994 Diagnosis of Plasmodium Falciparum in Mummies Using the
        Rapid Manual ParaSight TM F Test. *Transactions of Royal Society of
        Tropical Medicine and Hygiene* 88: 31–32.

Millet, Nicholas B., Gerald D. Hart, Theodore A. Reyman, Michael R. Zimmerman,
    and Peter K. Lewin
    1980 ROM I: Mummification for the Common People. In: *Mummies, Disease
        and Ancient Cultures*, edited by Aidan Cockburn and Eve Cockburn.
        Cambridge: Cambridge University Press, pp. 71–84.

Mims, Cedric
    1980 The Emergence of New Infectious Diseases. In: *Changing Disease
        Patterns and Human Behavior*, edited by N. F. Stanley and R. A. Joske.
        New York: Academic Press, pp. 231–50.

Mitchison, Avrion
    1993 Will We Survive? *Scientific American* 269 (3): 136–44.

Mlot, Christine
    1996 Chlamydia Linked to Atherosclerosis. *Science* 272: 1422.

Moller-Christensen, Vilhelm
    1967 Evidence of Leprosy in Earlier Peoples. In: *Diseases and Antiquity*,
        edited by Don Brothwell and A. T. Sandison. Springfield, Ill.:
        Charles C. Thomas, pp. 295–306.

Molner, Stephen
  1972 Tooth Wear and Culture: A Survey of Tooth Functions among Some
        Prehistoric Populations. *Current Anthropology* 13 (5): 511–25.

Molto, J. E.
  1997 Leprosy: A Perspective from the Dakhleh Oasis, Egypt. In: *Papers on
        Paleopathology, 24th Annual Meeting of Paleopathology Association,
        St. Louis*, p. 10. Published by the Paleopathology Association.

Monath, Thomas P.
  1991 Yellow Fever: Victor, Victoria? Conquerer, Conquest? Epidemics and
        Research in the Last Forty Years and Prospects for the Future. *American
        Journal of Tropical Medicine and Hygiene* 45: 1–43.

Monath, Thomas P.
  1995 Flaviviradae. In: *Mandell, Douglas, and Bennett's Principles and
        Practice of Infectious Diseases*, edited by Gerald L. Mandell,
        John E. Bennett, and Raphael Dolin. 4th ed. New York: Churchill
        Livingstone, pp. 1465–74.

Monath, Thomas P., and Theodore F. Tsai
  2002 Flaviviruses. In: *Clinical Virology*, edited by Douglas D. Richman,
        Richard J. Whitely, and Frederick G. Hayden. Washington, D.C.:
        ASM Press, pp. 1097–1151.

Moore, Kristine A., Craig Hedberg, and Michael T. Osterholm
  1998 Lyme Disease. In: *Bacterial Infections in Humans*, edited by
        Alfred S. Evans and Philip S. Brachman. New York: Plenum Medical
        Books, pp. 437–58.

Moore, Patrick S., and Claire V. Broome
  1994 Cerebrospinal Meningitis Epidemics. *Scientific American*
        271 (5): 38–45.

Morely, David
  1980 Severe Measles. In: *Changing Disease Patterns and Human Behavior*,
        edited by N. F. Stanley and R. A. Joske. New York: Academic Press,
        pp. 115–28.

Morgan, Herbert E.
  1952 The Salmonella. In: *Bacterial and Mycotic Infections in Man*, edited
        by René J. Dubos. Philadelphia: J. B. Lippincott, pp. 420–36.

Morris, R. J.
  1976 *Cholera 1832*. New York: Holmes & Meier.

Morse, Dan
  1967 Tuberculosis. In: *Diseases and Antiquity*, edited by Don Brothwell
        and A. T. Sandison. Springfield, Ill.: Charles C. Thomas, pp. 249–71.

Morse, Stephen S.
  1993 Examining the Origins of Emerging Viruses. In: *Emerging Viruses*, edited
        by Stephen S. Morse. New York: Oxford University Press, pp. 10–28.

Moseley, Michael E.
  1992 *The Incas and Their Ancestors*. London: Thames & Hudson.

Mott, Kenneth E.
  1987 Schistosomiasis Control. In: *The Biology of Schistosomes: From Genes
        to Latrines*, edited by David Rollinson and Andrew J. G. Simpson.
        London: Academic Press, pp. 429–50.

Muirhead-Thomson, R. C.
1951 *Mosquito Behavior in Relation to Malaria Transmission and Control in the Tropics*. London: Edward Arnold.

Murdock, George Peter
1980 *Theories of Illness: A World Survey*. Pittsburgh: University of Pittsburgh Press.

Murray, Edward S.
1975 The Typhus Group. In: *Textbook of Medicine*, edited by Paul S. Beeson and Walsh McDermott. 14th ed. Philadelphia: W. B. Saunders, pp. 249–55.

Nagel, Ronald L.
1994 Origins and Dispersion of the Sickle Gene. In: *Sickle Cell Disease: Basic Principles and Clinical Practice*, edited by Stephen H. Embury, Robert P. Hebbel, Narla Mohandas, and Martin H. Steinberg. New York: Raven Press, pp. 294–353.

Nasci, Roger S., and Barry R. Miller
1996 Culicine Mosquitoes and the Agents They Transmit. In: *The Biology of Disease Vectors*, edited by Barry J. Beaty and William C. Marquardt. Boulder: University Press of Colorado, pp. 85–97.

Neustadt, Richard E., and Harvey V. Fineberg
1978 *The Swine Flu Affair*. Washington, D.C.: U.S. Department of Health, Education, and Welfare.

Nizet, Victor, Patricia Ferrieri, and Craig E. Rubens
2000 Molecular Pathogenesis of Group B Streptococcal Disease in Newborns. In: *Streptococcal Infections*, edited by Dennis L. Stevens and Edward L. Kaplan. New York: Oxford University Press, pp. 180–221.

Nomile, Dennis
2004 Viral DNA Match Spurs China's Civet Roundup. *Science* 303: 292.

Nossal, Sir Gustav J. V.
1993 Life, Death and the Immune System. *Scientific American* 269 (3): 53–60, 62.

Novgorodskaya, E. M., and Yu. E. Polotsky
1977 Escherichia Coli. In: *Pathogenesis of Intestinal Infections: Microbiological and Pathological Principles*, edited by M. V. Voino-Yasenetsky and T. Bakacs. Budapest: Akademiaikiado, pp. 257–76.

O'Brien, A. D., et al.
1992 Shiga Toxin: Biochemistry, Genetics, Mode of Action, and Role in Pathogen. In: *Pathogenesis of Shigellosis*, edited by P. J. Sansonetti. Berlin: Springer Verlag, pp. 65–94.

Ogilvie, Bridget M., and Charles D. McKenzie
1981 Immunology and Immunopathology of Infections Caused by Filarial Nematodes. In: *Parasitic Diseases*, Volume 1: *The Immunology*, edited by John M. Mansfield. New York: Marcel Dekker, pp. 227–89.

Ohene-Frempong and Francis K. Nkrumah
1994 Sickle Cell Disease in Africa. In: *Sickle Cell Disease: Basic Principles and Clinical Practice*, edited by Stephen H. Embury, Robert P. Hebbel, Narla Mohandas, and Martin H. Steinberg. New York: Raven Press, pp. 423–35.

Olitsky, Peter K., and Delphine H. Clarke
    1959 Arthropod-Borne Group B Virus Infections in Man. In: *Viral and Rickettsial Infections in Man,* edited by Thomas M. Rivers and Frank L. Horsfall. Philadelphia: J. B. Lippincott, pp. 305–42.

Orihel, T. C.
    1985 Filariae. In: *Animal Agents and Vectors of Human Disease,* edited by Paul Chester Beaver and Rodney Clifton Jung. 5th ed. Philadelphia: Lea & Febiger, pp. 171–91.

Oshanin, L. V.
    1964 *Anthropological Composition of the Population of Central Asia, and the Ethnogenesis of Its Peoples, Parts I–III.* Cambridge, Mass.: Peabody Museum of Harvard University.

Palfi, G., O. Dutour, M. Borreani, J.-P. Brun, and J. Berato
    1992 Pre-Columbian Syphilis from the Late Antiquity in France. *International Journal of Osteoarchaeology* 2 (3): 245–61.

Patterson, David K.
    1987 *Pandemic Influenza 1700–1900: A Study in Historical Epidemiology.* Totowa, N.J.: Rowman & Littlefield.

Patterson, Thomas C.
    1973 *America's Past: A New World Archaeology.* Glenview, Ill.: Scott, Foresman.

Paul, William E.
    1993 Infectious Diseases and the Immune System. *Scientific American* 269 (3): 91–97.

Pauling, Linus
    1994 Foreword. In: *Sickle Cell Disease: Basic Principles and Clinical Practice,* edited by Stephen H. Embry, Robert P. Hebbel, Narla Mohandas, and Martin H. Steinberg. New York: Raven Press, pp. xii–xix.

Pearson, Helen
    2004 Antibodies to SARS-like Virus Hint at Repeated Infections. *Nature* 427 (15): 185.

Pedley, J. C., and John G. Geater
    1976 Does Droplet Infection Play a Role in the Transmission of Leprosy? *Leprosy Review* 47: 97–102.

Pennington, Renee L.
    1996 Causes of Early Human Population Growth. *American Journal of Physical Anthropology* 99: 259–74.

Peters, C. J.
    2002 Arenaviruses. In: *Clinical Virology,* edited by Douglas D. Richman, Richard J. Whitely, and Frederick G. Hayden. Washington, D.C.: ASM Press, pp. 949–69.

Peterson, Richard A.
    1973 *The Industrial Order and Social Policy.* Englewood Cliffs, N.J.: Prentice-Hall.

Pfeiffer, Carl C.
    1975 *Mental and Elemental Nutrients.* New Canaan, Conn.: Keats Publishing.

Pietrusewsky, M.
1969 An Osteological Study of Cranial and Infracranial Remains from Tonga. *Records of the Auckland Institute Museum* 6 (4–6): 287–402.

Pietrusewsky, M., M. T. Douglas, and R. M. Ikehara-Quetral
1997 An Assessment of Health and Disease in the Prehistoric Inhabitants of the Mariana Islands. *American Journal of Physical Anthropology* 104: 315–42.

Pietrusewsky, M. T., M. Pietrusewsky, and R.M. Ikehara-Quetral
1997 Skeletal Biology of Apurguani, a Precontact Chamorro Site on Guam. *American Journal of Physical Anthropology* 104: 291–313.

Piggott, Stuart
1965 *Ancient Europe: From the Beginnings of Agriculture to Classical Antiquity.* Chicago: Aldine Press.

Plum, Fred
1975 Acute Anterior Poliomyelitis. In: *Textbook of Medicine,* edited by Paul B. Beeson and Walsh McDermott. 14th ed. Philadelphia: W. B. Saunders, pp. 696–701.

Polunin, Ivan V.
1967 Health and Disease in Contemporary Primitive Societies. In: *Diseases and Antiquity,* edited by Don Brothwell and A. T. Sandison. Springfield, Ill.: Charles C. Thomas, pp. 69–97.

Pomeranz, Miriam K., Philip Orbuch, Jerome Shupack, and Rena Brand
1996 Mycobacteria and the Skin. In: *Tuberculosis,* edited by William N. Rom and Stuart M. Garay. Boston: Little, Brown, pp. 657–68.

Postgate, John F. R. S.
1994 *The Outer Reaches of Life.* Cambridge: Cambridge University Press.

Potter, Christopher W.
1998 Chronicle of Influenza Pandemics. In: *Textbook of Influenza,* edited by K. G. Nicholson, R. G. Webster, and A. J. Hay. Oxford: Blackwell Science, pp. 3–18.

Powers, Darleen R.
1994 Natural History of Disease: The First Two Decades. In: *Sickle Cell Disease: Basic Principles and Clinical Practice,* edited by Stephen H. Embury, Robert P. Hebbel, Narla Mohandas, and Martin H. Steinberg. New York: Raven Press, pp. 395–412.

Prusiner, Stanley B.
1995 The Prion Diseases. *Scientific American* 272 (1): 48–57.

Quillin, Patrick
1989 *Healing Nutrients.* New York: Vintage.

Rabbani, G. H., and William B. Greenough III
1992 Pathology and Clinical Aspects of Cholera. In: *Cholera,* edited by Dhiram Baura and William B. Greenough III. Plenum Medical Books, pp. 209–28.

Rafi, A., M. Spigelman, J. Stanford, E. Lemma, H. Donoghue, and J. Zias
1994 DNA of Mycobacterium Leprae Detected by PCR in Ancient Bone. *International Journal of Osteoarchaeology* 4: 287–90.

Rao, V. V., T. S. Vasulu, and A. D. W. Rector Baba
    1996 Possible Paleopathological Evidence of Treponematosis from a
        Megalithic Site at Agripalle, India. *American Journal of Physical
        Anthropology* 100: 49–55.

Raupach, B., J. Mecsas, U. Heczko, S. Falkow, and B. B. Finlay
    1999 Bacterial Epithelial Cells Cross Talk. In: *Defense of Mucosal Surfaces:
        Pathogenesis, Immunity, and Vaccines*, edited by J. P. Kraehenbuhl and
        M. R. Neutra. Berlin: Springer Verlag, pp. 137–61.

Ray, George C.
    1984 Arthropod-Borne and Other Zoonotic Viruses. In: *Medical Microbiology:
        An Introduction to Infectious Diseases*, edited by John C. Sherris.
        New York: Elsevier, pp. 434–45.

Reader, Rachel
    1974 New Evidence for the Antiquity of Leprosy in Early Britain.
        Journal of Archaeological Science 1: 205–7.

Regush, Nicholas
    1992 Last Gasp. *Equinox* 63 (May–June): 85–97.

Reid, Ann H., and Jeffery Taubenerger
    1999 The 1918 Flu and Other Influenza Pandemics: "Over There and Back
        Again." *U.S. and Canadian Academy of Pathology* 79 (2): 95–101.

Reingold, Arthur L.
    1998 Toxic Shock Syndrome. In: *Bacterial Infections of Humans*,
        edited by Alfred S. Evans and Philip S. Brachman. New York:
        Plenum Medical Books, pp. 759–75.

Ribeiro, Jose M. C.
    1996 Common Problems of Arthropod Vectors of Disease. In: *The Biology
        of Disease Vectors*, edited by Barry J. Beaty and William C. Marquardt.
        Boulder: University of Colorado Press, pp. 25–33.

Richardson, Malcolm D., and David W. Warnick
    1997 *Fungal Infection: Diagnosis and Management*. Oxford:
        Blackwell Science.

Rizzardi, G. Paolo, and Giuseppe Pantaleo
    2002 Pathogenesis of HIV-1 Infection. In: *Chemokine Receptors and AIDS*,
        edited by Thomas R. O'Brien. New York: Marcel Dekker, pp. 51–74.

Roab-Traub, Nancy
    2000 Epstein-Barr Virus and Nasopharyngeal Carcinoma. In: *Infectious
        Causes of Cancer*, edited by James J. Goedert. Totowa, N.J.: Humana
        Press, pp. 93–111.

Rocha, Heonir
    1975 Chagas' Disease. In: *Textbook of Medicine*, edited by Paul B.
        Beeson and Walsh McDermott. 14th ed. Philadelphia: W. B. Saunders,
        pp. 484–88.

Roe, Daphne A.
    1973 *A Plague of Corn: The Social History of Pellagra*. Ithaca, N.Y.: Cornell
        University Press.

Rokhlin, D. G.
    1965 *Diseases of Ancient Men (Bones of the Men of Various Epochs—
        Normal and Pathological Change)*. Moscow: Leningrad Publishing
        House "Nauka."

Rollinson, David, and Vaughn R. Southgate
    1987 The Genus Schistosoma: A Taxonomic Appraisal. In: *The Biology of Schistosomes: From Genes to Latrines*, edited by David Rollinson and Andrew J. G. Simpson. London: Academic Press, pp. 1–49.

Rosenthal, Elisabeth
    2001 AIDS and Corruption in a Poor Province. *International Herald Tribune*, 31 May, p. 2.

Rothhammer, Francisco, Marvin J. Allison, Lautaro Numez, Vivien Standen, and Bernardo Arriaza
    1985 Chagas' Disease in Pre-Columbian South America. *American Journal of Physical Anthropology* 68: 495–98.

Rothman, Alan L., and Francis A. Ennis
    2000 Toga/Flaviviruses: Immunopathology. In: *Effects of Microbes on the Immune System*, edited by Madeleine W. Cunningham and Robert S. Fujinami. Philadelphia: Lippincott Williams & Wilkins, pp. 473–90.

Rotterdam, Heidrun
    1997 Mycobacterium Avium Complex (MAC) Infection. In: *Pathology of Infectious Diseases*, Volume 1, edited by Daniel H. Conner, Francis W. Chandler, David A. Scwartz, Herbert J. Manz, and Ernest F. Lack. Stamford, Conn.: Appleton & Lange, pp. 657–69.

Rowe, B., and R. J. Gross
    1984 Salmonellosis, Camplobacter Enertitis and Shigella Dysentery. In: *Microbes and Infections of the Gut*, edited by C. S. Goodwin. Melbourne: Blackwell Scientific, pp. 47–77.

Roy, Peter, and S. E. Lentz
    1994 Molecular Genetic Evidence Suggesting Treponematosis in Pre-Columbian, Chilean Mummies. *American Journal of Physical Anthropology* Supplement 18: 171–72.

Rubin, Frederick L., and Robert R. Muder
    1998 Staphylococcal Infections. In: *Bacterial Infections of Humans*, edited by Alfred S. Evans and Philip S. Brachman. New York: Plenum Medical Books, pp. 657–72.

Rubin, Robert H., and Louis Weinstein
    1977 *Salmonellosis: Microbiologic, Pathologic and Clinical Features.* New York: Statton International Medical Book.

Rudolph, Andrew H.
    1981 Syphilis. In: *Communicable and Infectious Diseases*, edited by Paul F. Wehrle and Frank H. Top. St Louis: C. V. Mosby, pp. 621–34.

Ruffer, Marc A.
    1910 Note on the Presence of "Bilharzia Haematobia" in Egyptian Mummies of the Twentieth Dynasty (1250–1000 B.C.). *British Medical Journal* 1: 16.

Ruffer, Marc A.
    1914 Pathological Notes on the Royal Mummies of the Cairo Museum. *Mitteilungen zur Geschichite der Medizin und der Naturwissenschaften* 13: 239.

Ruigrok, Rob W. H.
    1998 Structure of Influenza A, B and C Viruses. In: *Textbook of Influenza*, edited by K. G. Nicholson, R. G. Webster, and A. J. Hay. Oxford: Blackwell Science, pp. 29–42.

Russell, Paul F., Lloyd Rozeboom, and Alan Stone
    1943 *Keys to the Anopheline Mosquitoes of the World.* Philadelphia: American Entomological Society/Academy of Natural Sciences.

Ryan, Frank
    1997 *Virus X: Tracking the New Killer Plagues.* Boston: Little, Brown.

Sabin, Albert B.
    1959 Dengue. In: *Viral and Rickettsial Infections of Man*, edited by Thomas M. Rivers and Frank L. Horsfall. Philadelphia: J. B. Lippincott, pp. 361–73.

Sack, Bradley R.
    1992 Colonization and Pathology. In: *Cholera*, edited by Dhiram Barua and William B. Greenough III. New York: Plenum Medical Books, pp. 189–97.

Sager, P. M. Schalimtzek, and V. Moller-Christensen
    1972 A Case of Spondylitis Tuberculosa in the Danish Neolithic Age. *Danish Medical Bulletin* 19: 176–80.

Sakazaki, Riichi
    1992 Bacteriology of Vibrio and Related Organisms. In: *Cholera*, edited by Dhiram Barua and William B. Greenough III. New York: Plenum Medical Books, pp. 37–56.

Sandison, A. T.
    1967 Parasitic Diseases. In: *Diseases in Antiquity*, edited by Don Brothwell and A. T. Sandison. Springfield, Ill.: Charles C. Thomas, pp. 178–83.

Sandison, A. T., and Edmund Tapp
    1998 Diseases in Ancient Egypt. In: *Mummies, Disease and Ancient Cultures*, edited by Aidan Cockburn, Eve Cockburn, and Theodore A. Reyman. 2nd ed. Cambridge: Cambridge University Press, pp. 38–58.

Sansonetti, P. J.
    1992 Molecular and Cellular Biology of Shigella Flexneri Invasiveness: From Cell Assay Systems of Shigellosis. In: *Pathogenesis of Shigellosis*, edited by P. J. Sansonetti. Berlin: Springer Verlag, pp. 1–19.

Sasakawa, C., J. M. Buysse, and H. Watanabe
    1992 The Large Virulence Plasmid of Shigella. In: *Pathogenesis of Shigellosis*, edited by P. J. Sansonetti. Berlin: Springer Verlag, pp. 21–44

Sauer, Jonathan D.
    1993 *Historical Geography of Crop Plants: A Selected Roster.* Boca Raton, Fla.: CRC Press.

Saul, F.
    1972 *The Human Skeletal Remains from Altar de Sacrificos.* Papers of the Peabody Museum of Archaeology and Ethnology, Vol. 63, No. 2. Cambridge, Mass.: Peabody Museum of Harvard University.

Saul, F.
    1973 Disease in the Maya Area: The Pre-Columbian Evidence. In:
        The Classic Maya Collapse, edited by T. P. Culbert. Albuquerque:
        University of New Mexico Press.

Sawyer, Wilbur A.
    1951 Yellow Fever. In: *Textbook of Medicine,* edited by Russell L. Cecil
        and Robert F. Loeb. Philadelphia: W. B. Saunders, pp. 15–19.

Schlievert, Patrick M., Kathryn N. Shands, Bruce B. Dan, George P. Schmid, and
    Russell D. Nishimura
    1981 Identification and Characterization of an Exotoxin from Staphylococcus
        Aureus Associated with Toxic Shock Syndrome. *Journal of Infectious
        Diseases* 143 (4): 509–16.

Schoch-Spana, Monica
    2000 Implications of Pandemic Influenza for Bioterrorism Response. *Clinical
        Infectious Diseases* 31: 1409–13.

Schoenbach, Emanuel B.
    1952 The Meningococci. In: *Bacterial and Mycotic Infections in Man,* edited
        by René J. Dubos. Philadelphia: J. B. Lippincott, pp. 547–63.

Scholtissek, Christoph
    1992 Cultivating a Killer Virus. *Natural History,* January, pp. 2–6.

Scholtissek, Christoph
    1998 Genetic Reassortment of Human Influenza Viruses in Nature. In:
        Textbook of Influenza, edited by K. G. Nicholson, R. G. Webster,
        and A. J. Hay. Oxford: Blackwell Science, pp. 120–25.

Scholtissek, Christoph, Virgina S. Hinshaw, and Christopher W. Olsen
    1998 Influenza in Pigs and Their Role as the Intermediate Host. In:
        Textbook of Influenza, edited by K. G. Nicholson, R. G. Webster,
        and A. J. Hay. Oxford: Blackwell Science, pp. 137–45.

Schurr, Erwin, and Emil Skamene
    1996 The Role of Bcg Gene in Mycobacterial Infections. In: *Tuberculosis,*
        edited by William N. Rom and Stuart M. Garay. Boston: Little,
        Brown, pp. 247–58.

Scrimschaw, Nevin S.
    1975 Deficiencies of Individual Nutrients: Vitamin Diseases. In: *Textbook
        of Medicine,* edited by Paul B. Beeson and Walsh McDermott. 14th ed.
        Philadelphia: W. B. Saunders, pp. 1368–75.

Seemayer, Thomas A., Timothy G. Grienek, Thomas G. Gross, Jack R. Davis,
    Arpad Lanyi, and Janos Sumegi
    2000 X-Linked Lymphoproliferative Disease. In: *Infectious Causes of Cancer,*
        edited by James J. Goedert. Totowa, N.J.: Humana Press, pp. 51–61.

Sell, S., and S. J. Norris
    1983 The Biology, Pathology, and Immunology of Syphilis. *International
        Review of Experimental Pathology* 24: 203–77.

Sereny, B.
    1977 Biological Features of Enteric Bacteria Capable of Intracellular
        Parasitism. In: *Pathogenesis of Intestinal Infections: Microbiological
        and Pathological Principles,* edited by M. V. Voino-Yasenetsky and
        T. Bakacs. Budapest: Akademiaikiado, pp. 32–40.

Sharpe, Virginia A., and Alan I. Faden

    1998 *Medical Harm: Historical, Conceptual, and Ethical Dimensions of Iatrogenic Illness.* Cambridge: Cambridge University Press.

Sherlock, S.

    1998 Clinical Features of Hepatitis. In: *Viral Hepatitis,* edited by Arie J. Zuckeran and Howard C. Thomas. London: Churchill & Livingstone, pp. 1–13.

Shinar, Eilat

    1990 Differences in Pathophysiology of Hemolysis of Alpha and Beta Thalassemia Red Blood Cells. In: *6th Cooley's Anemia Symposium,* edited by Arthur Bank. Annals of the New York Academy of Sciences, Volume 612. New York: New York Academy of Sciences, pp. 118–26.

Siddique, A. K., A. H. Baqui, Abu Eusof, K. Haider, M. A. Hossain, I. Bashir, and K. Zaman

    1991 Survival of Classic Cholera in Bangladesh. *Lancet* 337: 1125–27.

Sigerist, Henry E.

    1945 *Civilization and Disease.* Ithaca, N.Y.: Cornell University Press.

Slack, John M., and Irvin S. Snyder

    1978 *Bacteria and Human Disease.* Chicago: Yearbook Medical Publishing.

Sloane, Mark F.

    1996 Mycobacteria Lymphadenitis. In: *Tuberculosis,* edited by William N. Rom and Stuart M. Garay. Boston: Little, Brown, pp. 577–83.

Small, Kenneth J.

    2002 Remembering Malthus: A Preliminary Argument for a Significant Reduction in Global Human Numbers. *American Journal of Physical Anthropology* 118: 292–97.

Smith, Frances I., and Peter Palse

    1989 Variation in Influenza Virus Genes: Epidemiological, Pathogenic and Evolutionary Consequences. In: *The Influenza Viruses,* edited by Robert M. Krug. New York: Plenum Press, pp. 319–59.

Smith, Holly B.

    1984 Patterns of Molar Wear in Hunter-Gatherers and Agriculturalists. *American Journal of Physical Anthropology* 63: 39–56.

Smith, Jerome H., and Barbara S. Reisner

    1997 Plague. In: *Pathology of Infectious Diseases,* Volume 1, edited by Daniel H. Connor, Francis Chandler, David A. Schwartz, Herbert J. Manz, and Ernst E. Lack. Stamford, Conn.: Appleton & Lange, pp. 729–38.

Smith, Karen L., and Julie Parsonnet

    1998 Helicobacter Pylori. In: *Bacterial Infections in Humans,* edited by Alfred S. Evans and Philip S. Brachman. New York: Plenum Medical Books, pp. 337–53.

Smith, Philip E. L.

    1972 The Solutrean Culture. In: *Old World Archaeology: Foundations of Civilization: Readings from Scientific American.* San Francisco: W. H. Freeman, pp. 24–32.

Snyder, John C.

    1959 The Typhus Fevers. In: *Viral and Rickettsial Infections of Man,* edited by Thomas M. Rivers and Frank L. Horsfall. Philadelphia: J. B. Lippincott, pp. 799–827.

Sodeman, William A.
  1956 Nutritional Factors: Protein and Fat Metabolism. In: *Pathologic Physiology: Mechanisms of Disease*, edited by William A. Sodeman. Philadelphia: W. B. Saunders, pp. 25–55.

Sonenshine, Daniel E.
  1993 *Biology of Ticks*, Volume 2. Oxford: Oxford University Press.

Southgate, Vaughan R., and David Rollinson
  1987 Natural History of Transmission and Schistosome Interactions. In: *The Biology of Schistosomes: From Genes to Latrines*, edited by David Rollinson and Andrew J. G. Simpson. London: Academic Press, pp. 347–78.

Spies, Tom D.
  1951 Pellagra. In: *A Textbook of Medicine*, edited by Russell L. Cecil and Robert F. Loeb. Philadelphia: W. B. Saunders, pp. 575–81.

Spink, Wesley W.
  1956 *The Nature of Brucellosis*. Minneapolis: University of Minnesota Press.

Stanley, N. F.
  1980 Man's Role in Changing Patterns of Arbovirus Infections. In: *Changing Disease Patterns and Human Behavior*, edited by N. F. Stanley and R. A. Joske. London: Academic Press, pp. 152–73.

Stearn, E. Wagner, and Allen E. Stearn
  1945 *The Effect of Smallpox on the Destiny of the Amerindian*. Boston: Bruce Humphries.

Stein, Philip L., and Bruce M. Rowe
  1989 *Physical Anthropology*. 4th ed. New York: McGraw-Hill.

Steinberg, Martin H., and Stephen H. Embury
  1994 Sickle Hemoglobin: Overview. In: *Sickle Cell Disease: Basic Principles and Clinical Practice*, edited by Stephen H. Embry, Robert P. Hebbel, Narla Mohandas, and Martin H. Steinberg. New York: Raven Press, pp. 9–11.

Steinbock, R. Ted
  1976 *Paleopathological Diagnosis and Interpretation*. Springfield, Ill.: Charles C. Thomas.

Stevens, Dennis L.
  2000a Group A Beta-Hemolytic Streptococci: Virulence Factors, Pathogenesis, and Spectrum of Clinical Infections. In: *Streptococcal Infections*, edited by Dennis L. Stevens and Edward L. Kaplan. New York: Oxford University Press, pp. 19–36.

Stevens, Dennis L.
  2000b Life-Threatening Streptococcal Infections: Scarlet Fever, Necrotizing Fasciitis, Myositis, Bacteremia and Streptococcal Toxic Shock Syndrome. In: *Streptococcal Infections*, edited by Dennis L, Stevens and Edward L. Kaplan. New York: Oxford University Press, pp. 163–79.

Stewart, T. Dale, and Alexander Spoehr
  1952 Evidence on the Paleopathology of Yaws. *Bulletin of the History of Medicine* 26: 538–53.

Stirland, Ann
    1993 Evidence for Pre-Columbian Syphilis in Medieval Europe. In *Papers of the 20th Paleopathology Association Meeting, Toronto*, pp. 13–14. Published by the Paleopathology Association.

Stollerman, Gene H.
    1975 Streptococcal Diseases. In: *Textbook of Medicine*, edited by Paul Beeson and Walsh McDermott. 14th ed. Philadelphia: W. B. Saunders, pp. 290–91.

Strauss, James H., and Ellen G. Strauss
    2002 *Viruses and Human Disease*. San Diego: Academic Press.

Stringer, Christopher B.
    1992 Evolution of Early Humans. In: *The Cambridge Encyclopedia of Human Evolution*, edited by Steven Jones, Robert Martin, and David Pilbeam. Cambridge: Cambridge University Press, pp. 241–51.

Strouhal, Eugen
    1993 Malignant Tumours in the Old World in Antiquity. *Paleopathology Newsletter* 82: 5.

Stuart-Harris, C. H.
    1965 *Influenza and Other Virus Infections of the Upper Respiratory Tract*. Baltimore: Williams & Wilkins.

Stuart-Harris, C. H., Geoffrey C. Schild, and John S. Oxford
    1985 *Influenza: The Viruses and the Disease*. Baltimore: Edward Arnold.

Stuart-Macadam, Patricia
    1992 Anemia in Past Human Populations. In: *Diet, Demography, and Disease: Changing Perspectives on Anemia*, edited by Patrica Stuart-Macadam and Susan Kent. New York: Aldine De Gruyter, pp. 151–70.

Su, Xin-zhuan, Jianbing Mu, and Deirdre A. Joy
    2003 The "Malaria's Eve" Hypothesis and the Debate Concerning the Origin of the Human Malaria Parasite Plasmodium Falciparum. *Microbes and Infection* 5 (10): 891–96.

Sugaya, Norio, Tetsushi Yoshikawa, Masaru Miura, Takehiro Ishizuka, Ckharu Kawakami, and Yoshizo Asano
    2002 Influenza Encephalopathy Associated with Infection with Human Herpesvirus 6 and/or Human Herpesvirus 7. *Clinical Infectious Diseases* 34: 461–66.

Sumner, D. R.
    1985 A Probable Case of Prehistoric Tuberculosis from Northeastern Arizona. In: *Health and Disease in the Prehistoric Southwest*, edited by Charles F. Merbs and Robert J. Miller. Anthropological Research Papers, No. 34. Tempe: Arizona State University, pp. 340–346.

Suzuki, Takao
    1984 *Paleopathological and Paleoepidemiological Study of Osseous Syphilis in Skulls of the Edo Period*. Tokyo: University of Tokyo Press.

Suzuki, Takao
    1985 Paleopathological Diagnosis of Bone Tuberculosis in the Lumbosacral Region. *Journal of Anthropological Society of Nippon* 93 (3): 381–90.

Swango, Larry J.
  1989 Canine Viral Diseases. In: *Textbook of Veterinary Internal Medicine*, edited by Stephen J. Ettinger. Philadelphia: W. B. Saunders, pp. 298–311.

Swift, Homer F.
  1951 Rheumatic Fever. In: *Textbook of Medicine*, edited by Russell L. Cecil and Robert F. Loeb. Philadelphia: W. B. Saunders, pp. 153–65.

Swift, Homer F.
  1952 The Streptococci. In: *Bacterial and Mycotic Infections of Man*, edited by René J. Dubos. Philadelphia: J. B. Lippincott, pp. 265–323.

Sydenstricker, V. P.
  1951 Dengue. In: *Textbook of Medicine*, edited by Russell L. Cecil and Robert F. Loeb. Philadelphia: W. B. Saunders, pp. 12–15.

Syrjanen, Ritva K., Terhi M. Kilpi, Tarja H. Kaijalainen, Elja E. Herva, and Aino K. Takala
  2001 Nasopharyngeal Carriage of Streptococcus Pneumoniae in Finnish Children Younger than Two Years Old. *Journal of Infectious Diseases* 184: 451–59.

Tayles, Nancy
  1996 Anemia, Genetic Diseases, and Malaria in Prehistoric Mainland Southeast Asia. *American Journal of Physical Anthropology* 101: 11–27.

Tentori, Leonardo, and Marino Marinocci
  1986 Hemoglobin Variants and Thalassemias in Italy. In: *Hemoglobin Variants in Human Populations*, Volume 1, edited by William P. Winter. Boca Raton, Fla.: CRC Press, pp. 155–64.

Thangaraj, R. H., and S. J. Yawalkar
  1986 *Leprosy for Medical Practitioners and Paramedical Workers*. Basle: Ciba-Geigy.

Tishkoff, Sarah A., et al.
  2001 Haplotype Diversity and Linkage Disequilibrium at Human G6PD: Recent Origin of Alleles That Confer Malaria Resistance. *Science* 293: 455–62.

Tomatis, L.
  1990 *Cancer: Causes, Occurrence and Control*. WHO International Agency for Research on Cancer, Scientific Publications No. 100. Lyon: WHO.

Top, Franklin H.
  1955 *Communicable Diseases*. 3rd ed. St. Louis: C. V. Mosby.

Trembly, D. L.
  1995 On the Antiquity of Leprosy in Western Micronesia. *International Journal of Osteoarchaeology* 5: 377–84.

Trembly, D. L.
  1996a Whence Came Tuberculosis to Hawaii? In: *Papers on Paleopathology, 11th Annual European Paleopathology Association Meeting, Maastricht*, p. 21. Published by the Paleopathology Association.

Trembly, D. L.
  1996b Treponematosis in Pre-Spanish Western Micronesia. *International Journal of Osteoarchaeology* 6: 397–402.

Turner, Thomas B.
    1970 Syphilis and the Treponematoses. In: *Infectious Agents and Host Reactions*, edited by Stuart Mudd. Philadelphia: W. B. Saunders, pp. 346–90.

T-W-Fiennes, Richard N.
    1967 *Zoonoses of Primates: The Epidemiology and Ecology of Simian Diseases in Relation to Man*. Ithica, N.Y.: Cornell University Press.

T-W-Fiennes, Richard N.
    1978a *The Environment of Man*. New York: St. Martin's Press.

T-W-Fiennes, Richard N.
    1978b *Zoonoses and the Origins and Ecology of Human Disease*. London: Academic Press.

Uppal, P. K.
    2000 Emergence of Nipah Virus in Malaysia. *Annals of the New York Academy of Sciences* 916: 354–57.

Van der Hoeden, J.
    1964 *Zoonoses*. Amsterdam: Elsevier.

Vanhamme, L., and E. Pays
    1995 Control of Gene Expression in Trypanosomes. *Microbiology Review* 59 (2): 223–40.

Vaughan, W. T.
    1921 *Influenza: An Epidemiologic Study. American Journal of Hygiene* Monographic Series, No. 1.

Voino-Yasenetsky, M. V.
    1977 Human Dysentery and Hypothesis on Its Pathogenesis. In: *Pathogenesis of Intestinal Infections: Microbiological and Pathological Principles*, edited by M. V. Voino-Yasenetsky and T. Bakacs. Budapest: Akademiaikiado, pp. 53–64.

Von Lichtenberg, Franz
    1987 Consequences of Infections with Schistosomes. In: *The Biology of Schistosomes: From Genes to Latrines*, edited by David Rollinson and Andrew J. G. Simpson. London: Academic Press, pp. 185–232.

Walker, Bruce D.
    2001 Can Immune Responses and Human Immunodeficiency Virus Be Preserved, Enhanced or Restored? In: *AIDS Clinical Review 2000/2001*, edited by Paul A. Volberding and Mark A. Jacobson. New York: Marcel Dekker, pp. 101–14.

Walker, David H.
    1988 *Biology of Rickettsial Diseases*, Volume 1. Boca Raton, Fla.: CRC Press.

Walker, David H., and J. Stephen Dumler
    1997 Rickettsial Infections. In: *Pathology of Infectious Diseases*, Volume 1, edited by Daniel H. Conner, Francis W. Chandler, David A. Schwartz, Herbert J. Manz, and Ernest L. Lack. Stamford, Conn.: Appleton & Lange, pp. 789–99.

Wallace, Richard J., Jr.
    1997 Nontuberculosis Mycobacterial Infections in the HIV-Negative Host.
          In: *Pathology of Infectious Diseases*, Volume 1, edited by Daniel H.
          Conner, Francis W. Chandler, David A. Schwartz, Herbert J. Manz, and
          Ernest F. Lack. Stamford, Conn.: Appleton & Lange, pp. 699–709.

Warren, Kenneth S.
    1975 Schistosomiasis (Bilharziasis). In: *Textbook of Medicine*, edited
          by Paul B. Beeson and Walsh McDermott. 14th ed. Philadelphia:
          W. B. Saunders, pp. 512–18.

Waters, M. F. R.
    1975 Leprosy (Hansen's Disease). In: *Textbook of Medicine*, edited by
          Paul B. Beeson and Walsh McDermott. 14th ed. Philadelphia:
          W. B. Saunders, pp. 412–16.

Webb, Stephen
    1995 *Paleopathology of Aboriginal Australians*. Cambridge: Cambridge
          University Press.

Webster, Robert G.
    1993 Influenza. In: *Emerging Viruses*, edited by Stephen S. Morse.
          New York: Oxford University Press, pp. 7–45.

Webster, Robert G., and William J. Bean
    1998 Evolution and Ecology of Influenza Viruses: Interspecies Transmission.
          In: *Textbook of Influenza*, edited by K. G. Nicholson, R. G. Webster,
          and A. J. Hay. Oxford: Blackwell Science, pp. 109–19.

Weech, Ashley A.
    1951 Vitamin D Deficiency. In: *Textbook of Medicine*, edited by
          Russell L. Cecil and Robert F. Loeb. Philadelphia: W. B. Saunders,
          pp. 588–92.

Weekly Epidemiological Record
    2002 Influenza Activity October 2001 to First Week in February 2002.
          77 (8): 62.

Weetman, Anthony P.
    1996 Infection and Endocrine Autoimmunity. In: *Microorganisms and
          Autoimmune Diseases*, edited by Herman Friedman, Noel R. Rose,
          and Mauro Bendinelli. New York: Plenum Press, pp. 257–75.

Weinberg, Eugene D.
    1992 Iron Withholding in Prevention of Disease. In: *Diet, Demography,
          and Disease: Changing Perspectives on Anemia* edited by
          Patricia Stuart-Macadam and Susan Kent. New York: Aldine De
          Gruyter, pp. 105–50.

Weiss, Emilio
    1988 History of Rickettsiology. In: *Biology of Rickettsial Diseases*,
          Volume 1, edited by David H. Walker. Boca Raton, Fla.: CRC
          Press, pp. 15–32.

Weiss, Rick
    1992 On the Track of "Killer" TB. *Science* 255: 148–50.

Whitby, Noela, and Michael Whitby
    2003 SARS: A New Infectious Disease for a New Century. *Australian
          Family Physician* 32 (10): 779–83.

Whitehouse, Ruth, and John Wilkins
    1986   *The Making of Civilization.* New York: Alfred A. Knopf.
Wilkins, H. A.
    1987   The Epidemiology of Schistosome Infections in Man. In: *The Biology of Schistosomes: From Genes to Latrines,* edited by David Rollinson and Andrew J. G. Simpson. London: Academic Press, pp. 279–397.
Wilkinson, P. B.
    1959   *Variations on a Theme by Sydenham: Smallpox.* Bristol: John Wright & Sons.
Willcox, R. R.
    1960   Evolutionary Cycle of the Treponematoses. *British Journal of Venereal Diseases* 36: 78–90.
Williams, Herbert U.
    1932   The Origin and Antiquity of Syphilis: The Evidence from Diseased Bones. *Archives of Pathology* 13: 779–814, 931–83.
Williams, Peter L., Roger Warwick, Mary Dyson, and L. Bannister
    1989   *Gray's Anatomy.* 37th ed. Edinburgh: Churchill Livingstone.
Wilson, J. V. Kinnier
    1967   Organic Diseases of Ancient Mesopotamia, In: *Diseases in Antiquity,* edited by Don Brothwell and A. T. Sandison. Springfield, Ill.: Charles C. Thomas, pp. 191–208.
Wilson, R. Alan
    1987   Cercariae to Liver Worms: Development and Migration in the Mammalian Host. In: *The Biology of Schistosomes: From Genes to Latrines,* edited by David Rollinson and Andrew J. G. Simpson. London: Academic Press, pp. 115–46.
Winichagoon, Pranee, Suthat Fucharoen, Varaporin Thonglairoam, Veerawar Tana Potiwirut, and Prawese Wasi
    1990   B-Thalassemia in Thailand. In: *6th Cooley's Anemia Symposium,* edited by Arthur Bank. Annals of the New York Academy of Sciences, Volume 612. New York: New York Academy of Sciences, pp. 31–42.
Wood, Corinne Shear
    1979   *Human Sickness and Health: A Biocultural View.* Palo Alto, Calif.: Mayfield Publishing.
Woodard, Theodore E.
    1988   Murine Typhus Fever: Its Clinical and Biological Similarity to Epidemic Typhus. In: *Biology of Rickettsial Diseases,* Volume 1, edited by David H. Walker. Boca Raton, Fla.: CRC Press, pp. 79–92.
Woolf, Neville
    1977   *Cell, Tissue and Disease: The Basis of Pathology.* London: Bailliere Tindall.
Wuethrich, Benice
    1995   Bacterial Virulence Genes Lead Double Life. *Science* 268: 1850.
Wukovits, John F.
    1990   Destroying Angel (Typhoid Mary). *American History Illustrated* 25: 68–72.

Yaeger, R. G.

1985 Coccidia, Malarial Parasites, Babesia, and Pneumocystis. In: *Animal Agents and Vectors of Human Disease*, edited by Paul C. Beaver and Rodney C. Jung. Philadelphia: Lea & Febiger, pp. 50–77.

Young, Lawrence E.

1975 Intracorpuscular Abnormalities. In: *Textbook of Medicine*, edited by Paul B. Beeson and Walsh McDermott. 14th ed. Philadelphia: W. B. Saunders, pp. 1436–41.

Zias, Joseph

1985 Leprosy in the Byzantine Monasteries of the Judean Desert. *Koroth* 9 (1–2): 242–47.

Zeledon, Rodrigo

1974 Epidemiology, Modes of Transmission and Reservoir Hosts of Chaga's Disease. In: *Trypanosomiasis and Leishmaniasis*. Ciba Foundation Symposium 20 (New Series). Amsterdam: Associated Scientific Publishers, pp. 51–77.

Zeuner, Frederick E.

1963 *A History of Domesticated Animals*. New York: Harper & Row.

Zinsser, Hans

1935 *Rats, Lice and History*. New York: Black Dog & Leventhal.

Zivanovic, Srboljub

1982 *Ancient Diseases: The Elements of Paleopathology*. New York: Pica Press.

Zohary, Daniel, and Maria Hopf

1993 Domestication of Plants in the Old World. 2nd ed. Oxford: Clarendon Press.

INDEX

acquired immune deficiency syndrome (AIDS). *See* AIDS

adaptability: of *E. coli*, 295; of house mouse, 53; of influenza viruses, 341–43; of microbes, 202–3, 367, 391; of mosquitoes, 67–69; of mycobacteria, 159, 161–62, 174; of rats, 238–39, 249; of staphyloccal and streptococcal bacteria, 367–68, 370; of treponemes, 202, 204; of trypanosomes, 118; of viruses, 33. *See also* stealth forms

adaptability, human, 43, 46–47, 314–16

adolescents, 24, 31; and goiter, 330; and sickle cell, 90

adults, 24; and chickenpox, 198; and malaria, 85; and pinta, 205; and tuberculosis infection, 164–65

Aedes (mosquito), 132, 399

Aedes aegypti (mosquito), 300–303, 305, 307–11

Aedes africanus (mosquito), 301

Aedes albopictus (tiger mosquito), 306–7, 310–11

Aedes niveus (mosquito), 306

Africa, 117–21, 134. *See also* slave trade

Africa, diseases originating in: Chikungunya, 311; ebola virus, 399–401; filaria infections, 131, 133; HIV/AIDS, 388–90; lassa virus, 405; malaria, 70, 75, 97; marburg virus, 402; schistosome infection, 105–10; sickle cell, 90; sleeping sickness, 117–21; smallpox, 226; treponemal infection, 216, 218; yellow fever, 300, 310

aging process, and immune system, 24

agricultural revolution, 48–52, 63–65, 67–70, 116–17, 143–44, 160, 185–86, 316

AIDS (acquired immune deficiency syndrome), 388–98. *See also* HIV (human immunodeficiency virus)

air pollution, 163, 416–18. *See also* environmental pollution

air travel, 356, 385

Akari rickettsiae, 266

alcoholism, 275

allergic reactions, 315, 417–18

alpaca, domestication of, 153–54

alphaviruses, 407–8

amastigotes, 123, 127

Amazon basin, and Chagas' disease, 135

amino acids, 314; isoleucine, 68; tryptophan, 320

ancient evidence of disease: anthrax, 151–52; bilharziosis, 107; brucellosis, 148; Chagas' disease, 124–25; diphtheria, 198; endemic goiter, 331; leprosy, 180–81; malaria, 97; measles, 193; night blindness, 329; poliomyelitis, 360; rabies, 139–40; rickets, 327–28; schistosomes, 110–11; scurvy, 325; smallpox, 227–28; syphilis, 216; thalassemia, 97; tuberculosis, 167–71

Ancycostoma duodenal (hookworm), 61

anemia, 57, 62, 80–81, 84, 95, 129, 290–91, 323. *See also* sickle cell; thalassemia

animal feed, and risk of infection, 292, 422

animal hosts, 54, 56, 68–69; for blood-sucking insects, 54–55, 118, 120; for influenza viruses, 341–43; for mycobacteria, 159; and plague, 248; for sandflies, 125; for schistosomes, 99–100, 102–3, 107, 110; for yellow fever virus, 301–2. *See also names*

diabetes, 333–34; type I, 333; type II, 333, 335

diagnosis: of leprosy, 178; of smallpox, 224, 226, 230, 235

diarrhea: from cholera, 283; from contaminated drinking water, 280; from salmonella infection, 289; from shigella infection, 293–94; "traveler's diarrhea," 294, 296

diphtheria, 196–98, 200

disease: approaches to study of, 5–6; biological interpretation of, 2–5. *See also* epidemics; pandemics

disease patterns, 51–52, 57, 65, 357, 359, 385

disease prevention, 355, 357–59

diseases: chronic, 380–85; emerging, 398; endemic, 115–17, 270; insect-borne, 54–57; noninfectious, 41–42, 62–63; rodent-borne, 52–54; water-borne, 280; work-related, 275

"diseases of affluence," 356

disfigurement: associated with leprosy, 179–80; from smallpox scars, 225, 234

distemper, canine, 139, 191

dog flea *(Ctenocephalides canis)*, 241

dogs, 60, 138–40, 150, 191

domestication of animals, 137–38, 154–55, 188; camels, 146; cats, 140–41; cattle, 144–45, 150, 159–60, 167–68, 170; dogs, 138; elephants, 146; fowl, 146–47; goats, 143–44; horses, 146, 199; llama and alpaca, 153–54; pigs, 145–46; reindeer, 146; sheep, 143–44; water buffalo, 145

drinking water, 58, 415–16; contaminated, 106, 275, 279–81, 287, 289–90, 294, 297; and ingestion of parasites, 37–39; and iodine deficiency, 331

drug treatment, for HIV/AIDS, 397

drug-resistant microbes, 98, 157, 171, 183, 249, 292, 297–98, 357, 364, 374, 386

drugs, antimalarial, 93, 98

ebola virus, 235, 399–401

ecology, 5

ecosystems, self-contained, 33

ectoparasites, 28, 35–37

education, and control of HIV/AIDS, 397

elderly, the: and pellagra, 321; and tuberculosis infection, 164; and West Nile virus, 409

elephants, domestication of, 146

Embury, Stephen, 90

emphysema, 196, 417

encephalitis, 56, 339; equine, 407–8; viral, 406–11

Entamoeba coli (protozoa), 28–29, 155

enterobacteriacene family of bacteria, 243

Enterobius vermicularis (pinworm), 61

environmental change, 28, 51, 268

environmental factors, and spread of tuberculosis, 163

environmental pollution, 358, 382, 415–18

epidemics, 200, 251–53, 270–71, 427; anthrax, 151–52; dengue fever, 307–8; human typhus infection, 252; measles, 193; meningococcal meningitis, 363–64; plague, 237–38, 248; syphilis, 213; typhus, 255–56, 268; water-borne diseases, 280; yellow fever, 302–3, 305. *See also* pandemics

epidemiology, 5

epilepsy, focal, 112

Epstein-Barr virus (herpes virus), 31–32, 383–84, 395

equine encephalitis: eastern (EEE), 407–8; western (WEE), 407–8

eradication programs, 357–59; mosquitoes, 303, 308; nonvenereal syphilis, 218; poliomyelitis, 362; smallpox, 221, 234–35, 421; tuberculosis, 157; yaws, 218

erysipelas, 190, 371

erythema nodusum leprosum, 180

Escherichia coli (E. coli) (bacteria), 30, 38, 282, 295–97; *Diffuse Adherence* strains *(DAEC)*, 296; *Enteroaggregative* strains *(EAggEC)*, 296; *Enterohemorrhagic* strains *(EHEC)*, 296; *Enteroinvasive* strains *(EIEC)*, 296; *Enteropathogenic Escherichia coli (EPEC)*, 295–96; *Enterotoxigenic* strains *(ETEC)*, 296

espundia, 128–29

syphilis, 201–4, 213–17, 275; congenital, 207, 211–12, 214; nonvenereal, 206–13, 215; treponarid or endemic, 206–7; venereal (lues), 207–8, 210–13, 215. *See also* pinta; yaws

T cells, 307–8; CD4, 21, 126–27, 162–63, 178, 391–92, 394; CD8, 21–23, 391–92

tabardillo, 259

Taenia saginata (beef tapeworm), 40, 145

Taenia solium (pork tapeworm), 40–41

tapeworm, 40–41; beef tapeworm *(Taenia saginata),* 40, 145; pork tapeworm *(Taenia solium),* 40–41

technological advances, 51, 274, 356; air conditioning, 376; firearms, 271; food processing, 317–18

teeth, diseases of, 41, 63

termites, 15

Terra Amata (Nice, France), 42

thalassemia, 94–95, 97; alpha, 94–95; beta, 95–96

Thangaraj, R. H., 182

thiamine deficiency, 318–19

thrush, 419

thyroid gland, human, 329–31

ticks, 202, 262–65, 377–79, 399; *Ixodes scapularis,* 377–79

tiger mosquito *(Aedes albopictus),* 306–7, 310–11

Togaviridae viruses, 194

tolerance, development of, 33, 51, 57

tourism, risks of, 134

toxic shock syndrome, 369

toxoplasmosis, 141–43

trachoma, 381

trade networks, 50–51, 65, 187–89, 200; and common cold, 199; and filariae, 131–32; and house mouse, 53; and leishmaniasis, 129; and leprosy, 180–81; and malaria, 91; and measles, 193; and plague, 245–47; and rats, 240–41; and schistosomes, 109; and smallpox, 226–27; and typhus, 252, 258

transmissible spongiform encephalopathy (mad cow disease), 422–25

transmission of disease: aerosol route, 158, 161, 175–76, 189, 191, 193–94, 197, 244, 338; animal-human, 137–38; blood-borne, 365, 392, 396; insect-human, 34–35; oral-fecal contamination, 58–59, 158, 189, 288–89, 291, 294–95, 365; rodent-human, 54; sexual, 204, 207, 212, 391–92, 396; water-borne, 280–81, 285–86

trauma, 41, 62

"traveler's diarrhea," 294, 296

trematodes, 38. *See also* schistosomes

Treponema (spirochete), 202–3

Treponema carateum, 205

Treponema cuniculi, 202

Treponema pallidum, 202–3

Treponema pertenue, 204

treponemal infections, 207–11, 217–19

Trichinella spiralis (parasitic worm), 39, 145

trichinosis, 39, 145–46

Trichuris trichiura (whipworm), 60

Tricula, 111

tropical eosinophilic lung (Weingarten's syndrome), 132

tropical forest, vector-borne parasites in, 34

tropical regions, and vector-borne diseases, 55

Trypanosoma brucei complex, 119

Trypanosoma gambiense brucei, 119–21

Trypanosoma rhodesiense brucei, 119–21

trypanosomes, 117–21; in New World, 122–25; in Old World, 117–21

trypomastigotes, 121, 123

tsetse flies *(Glossinae),* 117–21

Tsutsugamushi rickettsia, 266–67

tubercles, 162, 164

tuberculosis, 158–66, 171–72, 174, 182, 275, 355, 358; chronic pulmonary, 164–65

Turks, 270

typhoid fever, 289–91

"Typhoid Mary" (Mary Mallon), 290

typhus, 251–52, 257–61, 267–68; flea-borne, 253–55; louse-borne, 255–57

"typhus islands," 266–67